An Atlas of **Surgery of the Spine**

An Atlas of **Surgery of the Spine**

Edited by **Howard S An**, MD

The Morton International Professor of Orthopaedic Surgery
Department of Orthopaedic Surgery
Rush–Presbyterian St Luke's Medical Center
Chicago
Illinois, USA

and **Lee H Riley III**, MD

Assistant Professor
Department of Orthopaedic Surgery
Johns Hopkins University School of Medicine
Baltimore
Maryland, USA

With artwork by **Carole Russell Hilmer**, CMI

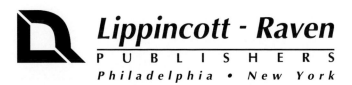

Lippincott · Raven
PUBLISHERS
Philadelphia · New York

Martin Dunitz

First published in the United Kingdom in 1998
by Martin Dunitz Ltd, The Livery House, 7–9 Pratt Street,
London NW1 0AE

First published in the United States of America in 1998 by
Lippincott-Raven Publishers

Library of Congress Cataloguing-in-Publication Data
applied for

ISBN 0-7817-1219-X

Composition by Scribe Design, Gillingham, Kent, UK

Printed and bound in Singapore by Imago

Contents

List of contributors

Howard S An, MD
The Morton International Professor of Orthopaedic Surgery
Department of Orthopaedic Surgery
Rush–Presbyterian St Luke's Medical Center
Chicago
Illinois, USA

Michael J Botte, MD
Assistant Professor
Department of Orthopaedics
University of California at San Diego
San Diego
California, USA

Thomas Byrne, OTC
Department of Orthopaedics
University of California at San Diego
San Diego
California, USA

H Alan Crockard, FRCS
Department of Surgical Neurology
The National Hospital for Neurology and Neurosurgery
London, UK

Steven R Garfin, MD
Professor and Chairman
Department of Orthopaedics
University of California at San Diego
San Diego
California, USA

Alexander J Ghanayem, MD
Assistant Professor of Orthopaedic Surgery
Loyola University
Chicago
Illinois, USA

Kiyoshi Kaneda MD
Professor and Chairman
Department of Orthopaedic Surgery
Director, University of Wisconsin Spine Center
Madison
Wisconsin, USA

John Kostuik, MD
Professor and Director
Division of Spine Surgery
Department of Orthopaedic Surgery
Johns Hopkins University School of Medicine
Baltimore
Maryland, USA

Alan M Levine, MD
Professor
Department of Orthopaedic Surgery
University of Maryland Hospital
Baltimore
Maryland, USA

Don M Long, MD, PhD
Professor and Director
Department of Neurosurgery
Johns Hopkins University School of Medicine
Baltimore
Maryland, USA

Paul C McAfee, MD
Associate Professor of Orthopaedic Surgery
Assistant Professor of Neurosurgery
Johns Hopkins University School of Medicine
Baltimore
Maryland, USA

John A McCulloch, MD, FRCS(C)
Professor of Orthopaedics
Northeastern Ohio Universities College of Medicine
Akron
Ohio, USA

Patrick S McNulty, MD
Scoliosis and Spine Center
Baltimore
Maryland, USA

Nigel Mendoza, FRCS
Department of Neurosurgery
Charing Cross Hospital
London, UK

Lee H Riley III, MD
Assistant Professor
Department of Orthopaedic Surgery
Johns Hopkins University School of Medicine
Baltimore
Maryland, USA

Harry L Shufflebarger, MD
Clinical Professor of Orthopaedic Surgery
Department of Orthopaedic Surgery
University of Miami School of Medicine
Miami
Florida, USA

Frederick A Simeone, MD
Professor of Neurological Surgery
Chairman, Department of Neurosurgery
Thomas Jefferson University
Jefferson Medical College
Chief, Department of Neurological Surgery
The Pennsylvania Hospital
Philadelphia
Pennsylvania, USA

J Michael Simpson, MD
Assistant Clinical Professor
Department of Orthopaedic Surgery
Medical College of Virginia
Richmond
Virginia, USA

Alexander R Vaccaro, MD
Associate Professor
Department of Orthopaedic Surgery
Thomas Jefferson University
Philadelphia
Pennsylvania, USA

Rongming Xu, MD
Visiting Research Associate
Department of Orthopaedic Surgery
Medical College of Ohio
Toledo
Ohio, USA

Thomas A Zdeblick, MD
Professor
Division of Orthopaedic Surgery
Director, University of Wisconsin Spine Center
Madison
Wisconsin, USA

Preface

This atlas is designed to cover the technical aspects of contemporary spinal operations. Over the past decade, there has been significant progress in the techniques of spine surgery such as fusion procedures, spinal instrumentation, cervical spine procedures, and minimally invasive techniques.

The editors were fortunate to recruit a superb medical illustrator, Carole Hilmer, who spent countless hours to provide brilliant artwork. The illustrations depict beautifully the basic surgical approaches and newer techniques of today. The editors would like to thank the contributors, international authorities in the field of spine surgery, for their insight and expertise.

This book is organized to cover pertinent anatomy, indications, step-by-step surgical techniques with illustrations, and complications. The most important factors for successful spine surgery is proper patient selection and appropriate indications for surgery. Meticulous surgical techniques are also important in successful outcome and preventing complications. The authors and editors have stressed these points throughout the book. We believe that this book is a valuable asset to orthopaedic surgeons, neurosurgeons, and any trainee that would like to study the field of spine surgery in more detail.

We are grateful to the publisher, Martin Dunitz Ltd, and particularly Robert Peden and Yasmin Khan-Chowdhury for their contribution to this work.

HSA
LHR III

1

Patient positioning and application of tongs and halo

Howard S An
Michael J Botte
Thomas Byrne
Steven R Garfin

Introduction

Patient positioning is an important initial consideration for any spine surgery. The optimal position for
spinal surgery can facilitate exposure, minimize bleeding, and avoid potential complications associated with
positioning. For the posterior thoracolumbar spinal
surgery, the intra-abdominal pressure must be
minimized to avoid venous congestion and excess
intraoperative bleeding, while allowing adequate
ventilation of the anesthetized patient. There are
numerous frames that can be used for the prone
position, including the chest rolls, the Wilson frame,
the Relton-Hall frame, Hastings frame, the Heffington
frame, the Andrews frame, etc. In our institution,
operations for degenerative disc disease are performed in a modified knee-chest position utilizing the
Heffington or Andrews frame, and surgical procedures
for thoracolumbar trauma or deformities are
performed on the Relton-Hall or Jackson's table. A
lateral decubitus position is required for the anterior
exposure of the thoracolumbar spine, and a supine
position can be utilized for the direct anterior
exposure of the lower lumbar spine and for the
lumbosacral junction. For the posterior cervical spine
surgery, the head is secured with the Mayfield pin
holder or horseshoe types of head holder, and the
patient is placed prone in a reverse Trendelenburg
position. The sitting position can also be utilized for
posterior cervical laminectomy or foraminotomy
cases. The anterior approach to the cervical spine
may require a Gardner-Wells tong for traction during
surgery. The application of tongs and halo will be
described in detail in this chapter.

Modified knee-chest positioning (Fig. 1.1)

This position is mostly for lumbar procedures, and its
greatest advantage is decompression of the abdominal
contents to minimize bleeding. Potential disadvantages include difficulty with obtaining an AP
radiograph, excessive stresses on the hips and knees,
and difficulty with maintenance of lumbosacral lordosis. Patients with a history of abnormal hips or knees
should avoid this position. For fusion and instrumentation down to the sacrum, the knee-chest position
may not give the optimum lumbosacral lordotic angle,
and four poster like frames are preferable.

Indications

1. Lumbar laminotomy and discectomy for
   herniated disc
2. Lumbar laminectomy for spinal stenosis
3. Microsurgical lumbar laminotomy or laminectomy for herniated disc
4. Lumbar fusion and instrumentation for
   spondylolisthesis, degenerative disc disease,
   and spinal stenosis.

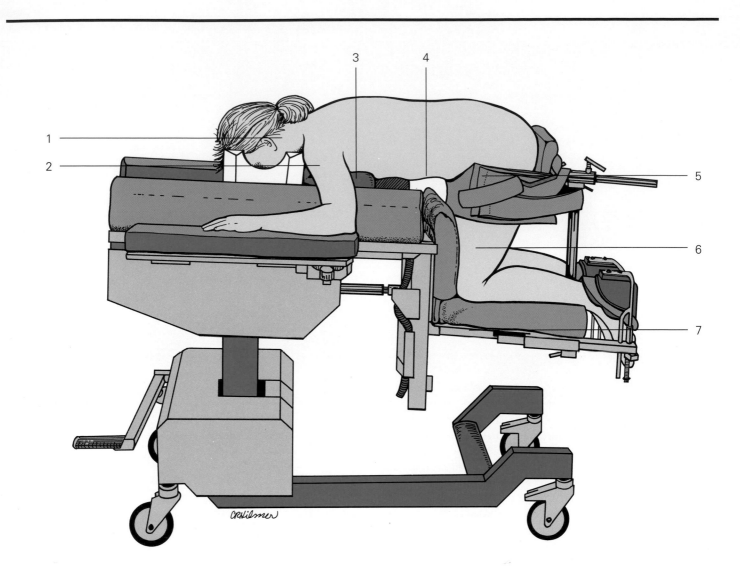

Figure 1.1

A kneeling position for lumbar surgery.

1 The neck is in a neutral position and not hyperextended.
2 The arms are positioned at 90° or less of abduction and slightly hanging down.
3 The axillae and ulnar nerves are padded.
4 This position allows the abdomen to hang free.
5 The thighs are stabilized with pads.
6 The hips and knees are flexed beyond 90°.
7 The height of the legs may be adjusted to flatten the lumbar spine region.

Technique

After anesthesia, the patient is rolled to a prone kneeling position. This kneeling position is stabilized with three-point contacts. The chest is laid against a padded table, the knees are rested on the table, and the buttocks are stabilized against a padded frame. The hips and knees are bent past 90° for increased stability. The height of the table that the knees are resting on is adjusted so that the lumbar spine is horizontalized. The entire table can also be adjusted in a Trendelenburg or reverse Trendelenburg position so that the back is as horizontal as possible. The abdomen is allowed to hang free in order to reduce venous pressure and bleeding. The shoulders and elbows are bent to 90° to relax the brachial plexus. The axillae and ulnar nerves are carefully padded. The head and neck are placed in a neutral position to prevent neck strain.

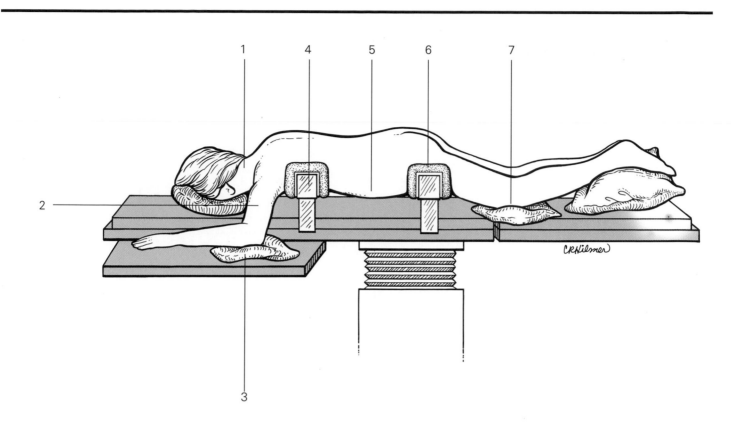

Figure 1.2

A prone position utilizing a four poster frame.

1 The neck is in a neutral position and not hyperextended.
2 The arms are positioned at 90° or less of abduction and slightly hanging down.
3 The ulnar nerves are padded.
4 The proximal pads will support the chest just distal to the axilla and slightly lateral to the nipple line.
5 This position allows the abdomen to hang free.
6 The distal pads are against the proximal thighs just distal to the iliac crests.
7 The hips and knees are flexed slightly.

Indications

1. Posterior fusion and instrumentation for scoliosis and kyphosis
2. Posterior fusion and instrumentation for thoracolumbar spine fractures
3. Costotransversectomy for biopsy, thoracic disc disease, or débridement
4. Lumbar laminotomy and discectomy for herniated disc
5. Lumbar laminectomy for spinal stenosis
6. Lumbar fusion and instrumentation for spondylolisthesis, degenerative disc disease, and spinal stenosis.

Prone positioning utilizing a four poster frame (Fig. 1.2)

This positioning device can be used for virtually any posterior thoracolumbar procedures. The four poster type of frame also decompresses the abdomen better than chest rolls or the Wilson frame. Additionally, the hips can be extended to provide a reduction maneuver in fractures or osteotomy cases. This frame preserves lumbar lordosis better than kneeling position frames. The potential disadvantages include excessive pressures on the chest and anterior thighs in long cases, and possible brachial plexus stretch if the arms are not properly positioned.

Technique

The four posts should be adjusted so that the proximal pads will support the chest just distal to the axilla and slightly lateral to the nipple line and the distal pads against the proximal thighs just distal to the iliac crests. A blanket is placed over the entire frame to distribute the pressures on the pads, but the blanket should be loose under the abdomen. For women, the breasts should be placed medial to the pads. The distal pads should not rest on the iliac crest to avoid excess pressure on the lateral femoral cutaneous nerve. The distal pads should be lateral enough to avoid occluding femoral vessels. Pads are placed under the knees and legs so that the hips and knees are slightly flexed. It is important to place enough pads under the arms that the arms are not hanging, and the shoulders are abducted no more than 90° in order to avoid brachial plexus stretch.

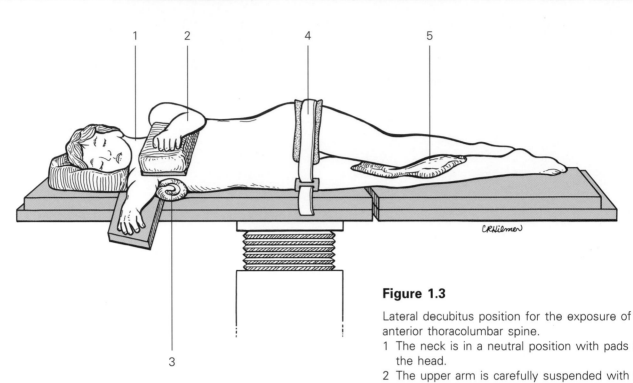

Figure 1.3

Lateral decubitus position for the exposure of the anterior thoracolumbar spine.
1 The neck is in a neutral position with pads under the head.
2 The upper arm is carefully suspended with pads under the elbows.
3 An axillary roll must be placed to protect neurovascular structures in the axilla of the lower arm.
4 The pelvis is strapped for stability.
5 The hips and knees are flexed and cushions are placed under the fibular head below the lower leg and between the legs.

Lateral decubitus positioning (Fig. 1.3)

The exposure of the anterior aspects of the thoracolumbar spine is routinely accomplished by transthoracic, thoracoabdominal, or retroperitoneal flank approaches. These surgical approaches are performed with the patient in a lateral decubitus position. The rightsided transthoracic approach is utilized for the exposure of the upper thoracic spine, and the left-sided thoracoabdominal or retroperitoneal flank approaches are utilized for the exposure of the thoracolumbar junction and the lumbar spine. For cases requiring both anterior and posterior exposures of the spine, the table may be turned into a semi-prone position, and simultaneous anterior and posterior exposures of the spine may be accomplished without repreparing and redraping the patient.

Indications

1. Right sided thoracotomy, anterior discectomy, corpectomy, fusion or instrumentation for thoracic disc herniation, burst fractures, deformities, tumors, infections of the thoracic spine
2. Left sided thoracoabdominal or retroperitoneal approach for anterior discectomy, corpectomy, fusion, and instrumentation of the thoracolumbar junction and the lumbar spine.

Technique

This position is inherently unstable, and all steps should be taken to secure the patient in a stable position, while avoiding undue pressures to the vital structures. For strut grafting cases, the bend of the table should be at the same level as the strut graft site to facilitate the insertion of the graft. By bending the table, the corpectomy defect can be widened, and unbending the table can lock the graft in compression. A bean bag is helpful to secure the patient in the lateral position. An additional strap is secured over the hips. It is important to place padding under the fibular head to avoid peroneal nerve compression. A pad is also placed between the legs. An axillary roll must be placed to protect neurovascular structures in the axilla. The upper arm is carefully suspended with pads under the elbows.

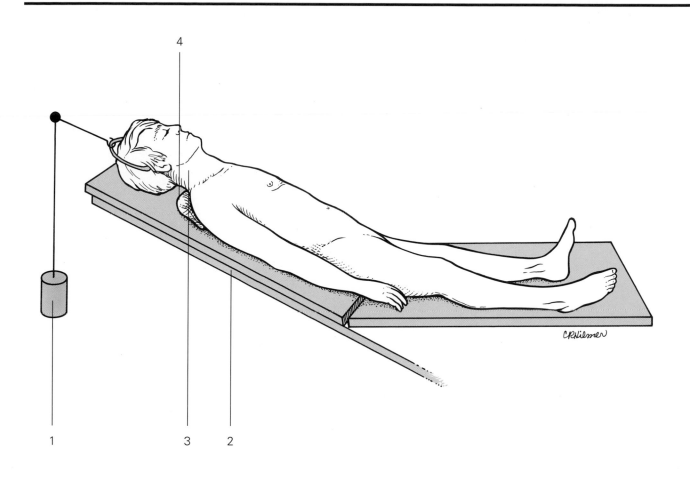

Anterior cervical spine procedures (Fig. 1.4)

The most common anterior approach is the Smith–Robinson approach for the exposure of the middle and lower cervical spine. Approaches to the upper cervical spine may require turning of the head in a more extended and rotated position.

Figure 1.4

Position for anterior cervical procedures.
1 The patient is positioned supine with Gardner–Wells traction to the head.
2 The reverse Trendelenburg position allows venous drainage and less bleeding during surgery.
3 The neck is extended and slightly rotated toward the opposite side.
4 A small pad may be placed under the upper back between the scapulae if more extension of the neck is needed.

Indications

1. Anterior discectomy and fusion for herniated disc
2. Anterior corpectomy, fusion, and instrumentation for cervical spondylotic myelopathy, burst fractures, deformities, or tumors.

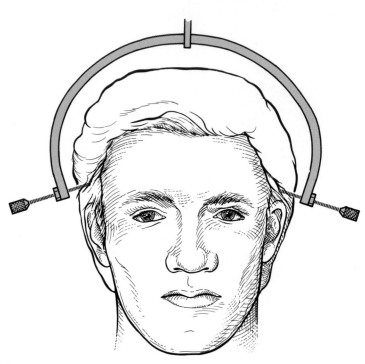

A

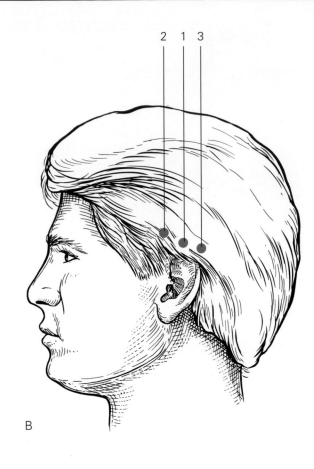

B

Figure 1.5

A
Pin sites for the Gardner–Wells tongs are about 1 cm
superior to the pinna of the ear below the maximal
circumference of the skull. The pins should be tightened until
the pressure indicator protrudes 1 mm.

B
1 For straight traction, pins are inserted 1 cm superior to the
  middle of the pinna of the ear.
2 For extension moment, pins can be inserted slightly
  anterior to and above the center of the pinna.
3 For flexion moment, pins are inserted slightly posterior to
  the pinna.

Technique

The patient is positioned supine with Gardner–Wells
traction to the head (Fig. 1.5). The Gardner–Wells tongs
are usually applied without removing the patient's hair.
The areas are thoroughly prepared. For straight
traction, pins are inserted 1 cm superior to the middle
of the pinna of the ear. The pins should
be tightened until the pressure indicator protrudes
1 mm. For extension moment, pins can be inserted
slightly anterior to and above the center of the pinna,
and for flexion moment, pins are inserted slightly
posterior to the pinna. The traction may also be
achieved with a halter type of device, but the amount
of traction is much more limited. The reverse
Trendelenburg position allows venous drainage and
less bleeding during surgery. The cervical spine is
extended and slightly rotated toward the opposite
side, and the amount of extension is greater for the
upper cervical spine approaches. The amount of
extension should not be greater than what was
allowed by the patient preoperatively. A small pad
may be placed under the upper back between the
scapulae if more extension of the neck is needed.
Caudal traction to the shoulders is gently applied using
the adhesive tape. In order to minimize injury to the
recurrent laryngeal nerve, the cervical spine is often
approached from the left, particularly in the C6-T1
region. Although the right handed surgeon prefers the
right sided approach, the recurrent laryngeal nerve is
then at a greater risk of injury, as it may leave the
carotid sheath at a higher level on the right side.

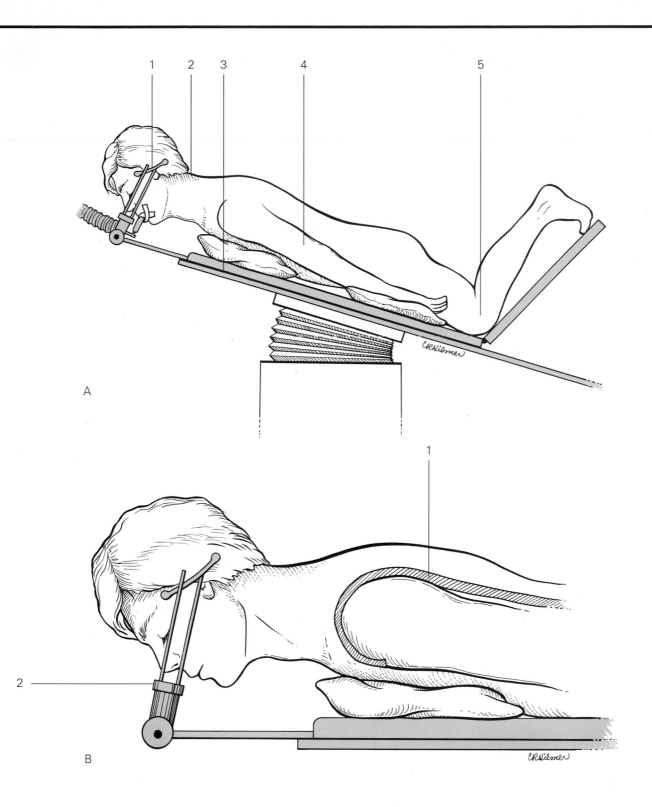

Figure 1.6

Position for posterior cervical spine procedures.

A

1 The Mayfield tongs are applied so that the head is rigidly fixed to the table.
2 The neck is slightly extended, and extreme flexion or extension of the head should be avoided.
3 The reverse Trendelenburg position allows venous drainage and less bleeding during surgery.

4 The arms and elbows must be well padded to prevent pressures on the ulnar nerves.
5 The knees are flexed to prevent distal migration of the patient.

B

1 Caudal traction to the shoulders may be gently applied using an adhesive tape.
2 The Mayfield frame is adjusted so that the forehead and the bridge of the nose are cleared by at least 2 cm. The Mayfield frame can be adjusted to provide more flexion or extension of the neck as necessary.

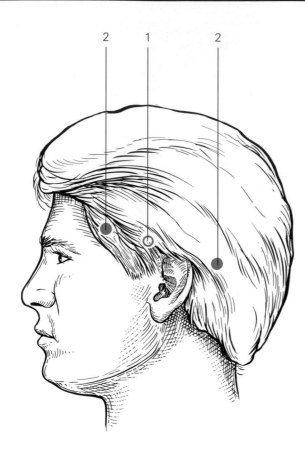

A

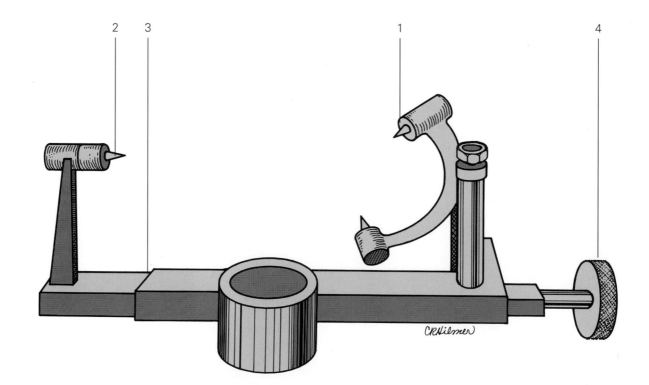

B

Figure 1.7

A
Pin sites for the Mayfield tongs.
1 The single pin is centered just above the ear.
2 The double pins are placed at the same level on the opposite side.

B
1 The two pins are fixed to a hinged yoke on one side of the frame, and
2 a third pin is fixed to the opposite side.
3 The width of the frame may be adjusted.
4 The frame is then tightened using the turning knob until the pressure indicator is at 60.

Posterior cervical spine procedures (Fig. 1.6)

The posterior cervical spine procedures are usually done in the prone position, but some surgeons prefer the sitting position. At any rate, both positions require great care to stabilize the head and neck without causing undue stresses in the pathological or injured spine.

Indications

1. Posterior foraminotomy for herniated disc or cervical spondylotic radiculopathy
2. Posterior laminectomy or laminoplasty for cervical spondylotic myelopathy
3. Posterior cervical fusion, instrumentation for fractures, dislocations, tumors, and deformities.

Technique

The posterior approach to the cervical spine requires a careful positioning to stabilize the neck and to avoid the risk of neurologic injury. The intubation must be controlled and the head should be stabilized to permit atraumatic turning to the prone position. For laminectomy or foraminotomy cases for degenerative disorders, the Mayfield tongs are applied so that the head is rigidly fixed to the table (Fig. 1.7). The application of the Mayfield three point pin headrest requires some training and practice. The frame is adjustable in width. The two pins are fixed to a hinged yoke on one side of the frame, and a third pin is fixed to the opposite side. The frame is held about one inch over the forehead with one inch space between the frame and the nose. The single pin is centered just above the ear, and the width of the frame is adjusted so that the double pins are placed at the same level on the opposite side. The frame is then tightened using the turning knob until the pressure indicator is at 60. The surgeon should apply traction and hold head and neck securely while turning. Alternatively, a horseshoe shaped headrest may be utilized but excessive pressures on the eyes must be avoided. In a patient with an unstable cervical spine, the Stryker bed or a similar turning frame may facilitate turning from the supine to the prone position. When using the Stryker bed, either a halo ring or Gardner–Wells tongs can be attached to the head to maintain traction. Extreme flexion or extension of the head should be avoided during the procedure. The elbows must be well padded to prevent pressures on the ulnar nerves. A reverse Trendelenburg position will minimize venous bleeding and lower cerebrospinal fluid pressure. Caudal traction to the shoulders may be gently applied using an adhesive tape. The knees are well padded and flexed so the legs are resting on the caudal aspect of the table. This prevents distal migration of the patient in the reverse Trendelenburg position.

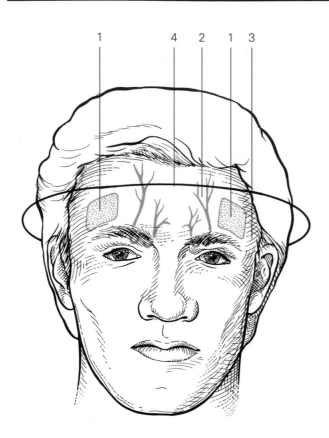

Figure 1.8

Application of the halo ring.
1 Safety zones for the anterior pin sites.
2 Medially, over the medial one-third of the orbit are the supraorbital and supratrochlear nerves and artery.
3 The temporal fossa has very thin bone which should be avoided.
4 The pins are inserted below the equator line or the largest circumference of the skull.

Halo application

The halo pins have been used for a variety of cases such as for cervical injuries and cervical deformities and as a postoperative orthosis. Even though the halo-vest is the most rigid form of external orthosis, loss of reduction may still occur in certain cases, and the specific indications and potential complications of halo-vest management must be remembered. There are different types of halo-ring and vest, and a posteriorly opened ring gives access to the occiput and the upper cervical spine and is easier to apply.

Lightweight and MR compatible rings are preferred. Pin sites are crucial, and anterior pins are placed anterolaterally approximately 1 cm above the orbital rim, below the equator of the skull and cephalad to the lateral two-thirds of the orbit (Fig. 1.8). Posterior pins should be directly opposite to anterior pins. Anterior pins should be tightened with eyes closed. Structures that are at risk anteriorly include the frontal sinus, which is located centrally cephalad to the bridge of the nose, but can extend to a variable extent above the medial aspect of the orbit. Medially, over the medial one-third of the orbit are the supraorbital and supratrochlear nerves and artery. Laterally, cephalad to the orbital ridge and eyebrow over the lateral one-half of the orbit, there are no significant structures. The temporal fossa has very thin bone which may fracture or be penetrated by a pin that is too tightly torqued. Additionally, muscles of mastication are located in the temporal fossa. Posterior to the temporal fossa, there are no significant anatomic structures in terms of alterations in pin placement. The torque of insertion should be 8 in/lb and applied at increments of 2 in/lb with opposite pins being tightened alternatively. Pins should be retightened once at 8 in/lb 24 hours later. Following halo ring application, a well fitting vest is applied. The posterior vest is applied first by log rolling or raising the patient's trunk to 30°. The connection mechanism between the halo ring and the upright posts may allow flexion–extension, anterior–posterior translation, or compression–traction controls.

Indications

1. Nonoperative management with halo-vest in C1 fractures (Jefferson's fracture), C2 hangman's fractures, odontoid fractures, compression fractures, axial loading burst fractures, and flexion–compression fractures with minimal posterior ligamentous disruption
2. Surgical stabilization with non-rigid internal fixation, as in a strut graft not supported by anterior plates and wiring procedures for the upper and lower cervical spine
3. Instabilities of the cervical spine caused by tumor or infection while medical treatment is being given.

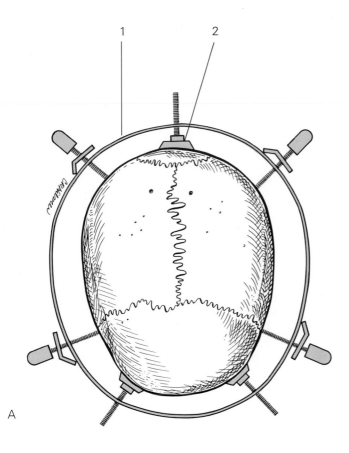

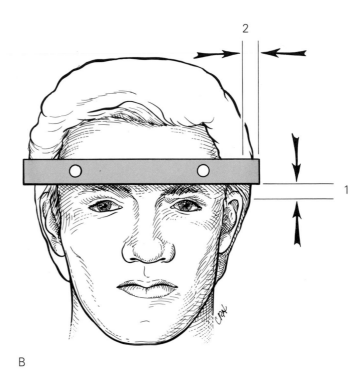

A

B

Figure 1.9

Proper positioning of the halo ring.

A
1 Top view, showing the ring with 1 cm clearance throughout the circumference of the skull.
2 Temporary positioning post.

B
1 Front view, showing the ring about 1 cm above the ear and eyebrows, and with
2 1 cm clearance from the skull.

C
The ring is placed about 1 cm above the ears, and the anterior ring is slightly more cephalad than the posterior ring so that the head is slightly extended. The ring of the halo should be inferior to the equator or widest diameter of the skull.

C

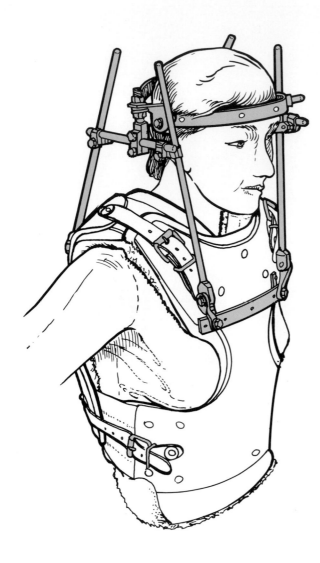

Figure 1.10

Halo-vest with the anterior and posterior vests connected to the ring with four upright posts.

Technique

1. Have the patient lie supine over the edge of the table or bed.
2. Determine the correct ring and vest sizes. The ring is placed about 1 cm above the ears, and the anterior ring is slightly more cephalad than the posterior ring, so that the head is slightly extended. The ring of the halo should be inferior to the equator or widest diameter of the skull.
3. Identify the pin site locations by holding the ring in place. A 3 cm by 3 cm hair trim, shave and preparation is carried out just superior and posterior to the ear. The halo-ring is positioned, using temporary positioning posts (Fig. 1.9).
4. Prepare pin sites with povidone–iodine solution and 1% lidocaine. Approximately 5 ml is injected down to and including the periosteum of the skull.
5. Insert the pins and tighten to 8 in/lb at 2 in/lb increments.
6. Apply the posterior vest first by by log rolling or raising the patient's trunk to 30°.
7. Apply the anterior vest and connect it to the posterior vest.
8. Apply four upright posts and tighten linkages (Fig. 1.10).
9. Obtain cervical spine radiographs to check reduction and alignment.
10. Retighten the pins to 8 in/lb and recheck all nuts and screws 24 hours later.

Bibliography

An HS (1992) Surgical exposure and fusion techniques of the spine. In: HS An, JM Cotler (eds), *Spinal Instrumentation*. Baltimore, Williams & Wilkins

An HS, Simpson JM (1994) *Surgery of the Cervical Spine*. London and Baltimore, Martin Dunitz and Williams & Wilkins

Garfin SR, Botte MJ, Waters RL et al (1986) Complications in the use of the halo fixation device. *J Bone Joint Surg* **68A**:320–5

Meyer PR Jr (1989) Emergency room assessment: Management of spinal cord and associated injuries. In: PR Meyer Jr (ed), *Surgery of Spine Trauma*. New York, Churchill Livingstone

2

Posterior cervical spine procedures

Howard S An
Rongming Xu

Introduction

Laminectomy, foraminotomy, and laminoplasty are relatively common procedures of the cervical spine. Additionally, there are numerous methods of posterior fusion and stabilization of the cervical spine. Wiring techniques have been well described in the literature in the past, but other forms of stabilization have been presented recently. There are advantages and disadvantages of each method, and the surgeon must choose a method based on the mechanism of injury, the pathoanatomy of the lesion, and the surgeon's familiarity with the technique. The purpose of this chapter is to discuss various posterior cervical procedures, and the indications, techniques, and potential complications will be presented.

Anatomy

The bony landmarks are the key to determining that the surgery will be at the appropriate levels. The bony processes are palpable posteriorly with large spinous processes at C2, C7 and T1.

Owing to the narrowed interspaces and the inferior sloping of the spinous processes, overdissection of the posterior spine may lead to unnecessary fusion of uninvolved levels. The posterior cervical spine is covered with thick muscular layers and a direct approach through the midline plane is utilized (Fig. 2.1). The superficial layer of the deep cervical fascia is found investing the trapezius posteriorly and fuses with the intermuscular septum and the spinous processes. The prevertebral fascia continues posteriorly from the intermuscular septum and inserts on the vertebral spinous processes. The ligamentum nuchae, a fibrous septum with few elastic fibers, inserts on the

spinous processes and the cervical paraspinal muscles. The supraspinous ligaments are essentially in continuity with the ligamentum nuchae and spinous processes posteriorly, and blend with the interspinous ligaments anteriorly. These ligaments are poorly defined in the upper cervical spine and become well developed in the lower cervical spine. The ligamentum nuchae acts as the primary origin or insertion point for most of the muscles in the posterior neck.

The trapezius lies most superficial just deep to the superficial fascia. The rhomboid minor and serratus attach to the seventh cervical spinous process and course distally. The intermediate muscles deep to the trapezius include the splenius capitis and splenius cervicis. The deep muscle group includes the semispinalis capitis and cervicis, and it is penetrated by the greater occipital nerve (Fig. 2.1C). The deepest group of muscles consists of the iliocostalis and longissimus muscles. A group of smaller muscles which assist in extending the head are found at the occipitocervical junction and include the rectus capitis posterior major and minor and the superior and inferior capitis obliques which all attach to the spinous process or transverse process of the axis.

The posterior approach utilizes an internervous plane in the midline which separates the muscles from the segmental innervation supplied by the right and left posterior rami of the cervical nerves. The remainder of the dissection is in this plane, and denervation is not a problem owing to the segmental pattern.

The atlantoaxial and occipitocervical region has the potential for a significant risk of complications and operative morbidity if the anatomy peculiar to that region is not understood before undertaking the exposure (Fig. 2.1F). The course of the vertebral arteries should be thoroughly understood. The course of the artery along the posterior arch of C1 makes it prone to injury if the dissection on the posterior arch is performed more than 1.5 cm from the midline of the posterior tubercle. This distance is only 1 cm in

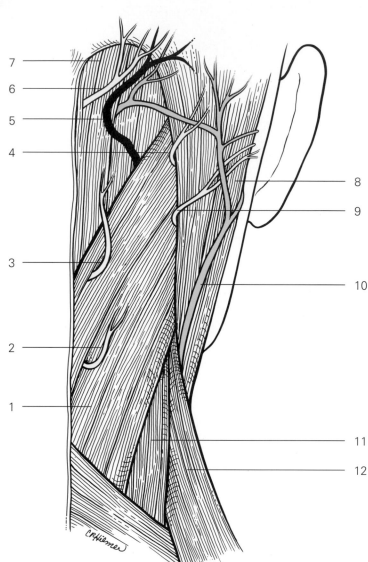

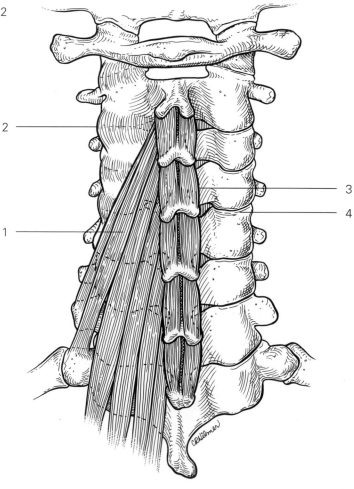

Figure 2.1

A

The anatomy of the posterior aspect of the cervical spine, showing the superficial nerves and musculature.

1   Splenius capitis m.
2   Med. br. of post. primary ramus of C5
3   Third occipital n.
4   Lesser occipital n.
5   Occipital a.
6   Greater occipital n.
7   Semispinalis capitis m.
8   Sternocleidomastoid m.
9   Greater auricular n.
10 External jugular v.
11 Splenius cervicis m.
12 Levator scapulae m.

B

Deeper structures, including the interspinous ligament, deep musculature, the articular capsule, and the facet joint.

1   Paraspinal m.
2   Articular capsule
3   Interspinous lig.
4   Facet joint

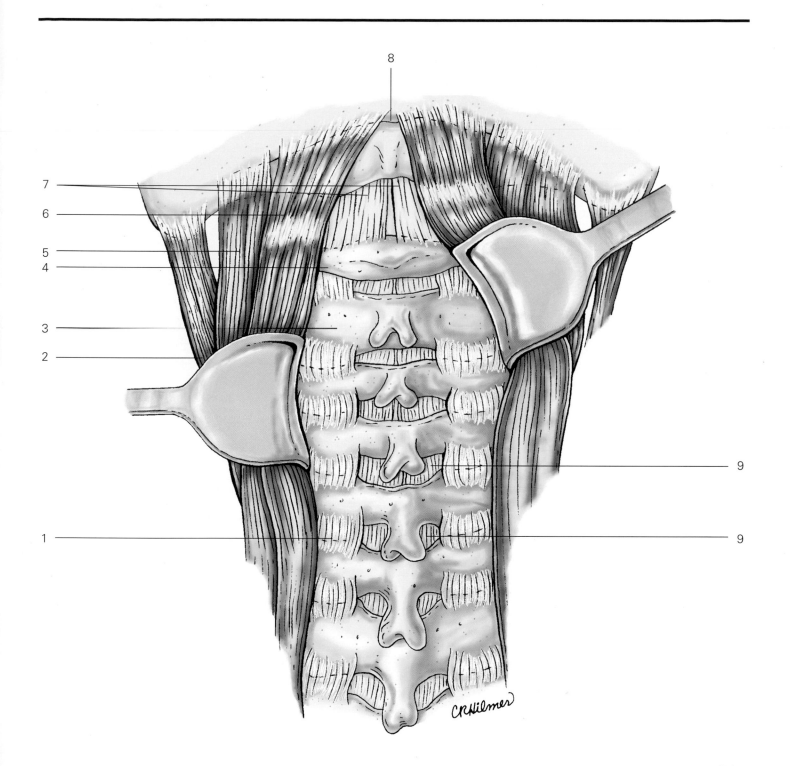

C

Muscles are arranged in layers. Deep to the superficial fascia lies the trapezius, and intermediate muscles deep to the trapezius include the splenius capitis and splenius cervicis. The deeper muscle group includes the semispinalis capitis and cervicis. The deepest group of muscles are the iliocostalis and the longissimus muscles. The capsule, ligamentum flavum and posterior atlanto-occipital membrane are illustrated.

1 Capsule of zygapophyseal lateral joint
2 Longissimus capitis m.
3 C2
4 C1
5 Splenius capitis m.
6 Semispinalis capitis m.
7 Post. atlanto-occipital memb.
8 Sup. nuchal line
9 Ligamentum flavum

Contd

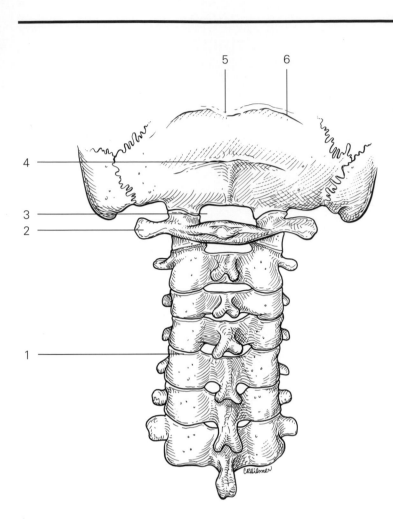

Figure 2.1 *(contd)*

D
Posterior view of the bony and articular structures.

1   Sup. articular facet
2   Transverse process of C1
3   Foramen magnum
4   Inf. nuchal line
5   Inion
6   Sup. nuchal line

E
Side view of the cervical spine, showing ligaments and bony structures.

5   Inion
7   Lateral mass
8   Post. tubercle
9   Supraspinous lig.
10 Spinous process of C2
11 Ligamentum nuchae
12 Post. atlanto-occipital lig.
13 Interspinous lig.
14 Ligamentum flavum
15 Ant. tubercle

the child. The posterior ring of C1 is also very fragile and small in size, and is therefore prone to fracture if vigorous dissecting of the ligamentum flavum is performed. Slippage of a periosteal elevator into the canal can occur on the narrow posterior arch if caution is not used. A great number of the muscles in the upper cervical spine attach to the spinous process of C2, and these should be preserved if this level is not involved in the fusion, to prevent the possibility of instability developing at C2–C3.

The posterior approach requires careful positioning to minimize the risk of neurologic injury and maxi-mize exposure of the required level. The positioning for the posterior approach has been discussed in Chapter 1. The posterior approach utilizes a longitu-dinal midline incision which extends above and below the segments required for the procedure. This extension of the skin and subcutaneous tissues is necessary as the skin of the posterior neck is less mobile and thicker for retraction. The skin is incised sharply and then electrocautery is used to dissect to the ligamentum nuchae. The ligamentum nuchae is incised in the midline and dissection is subperiosteally down the spinous processes. Care should be taken to

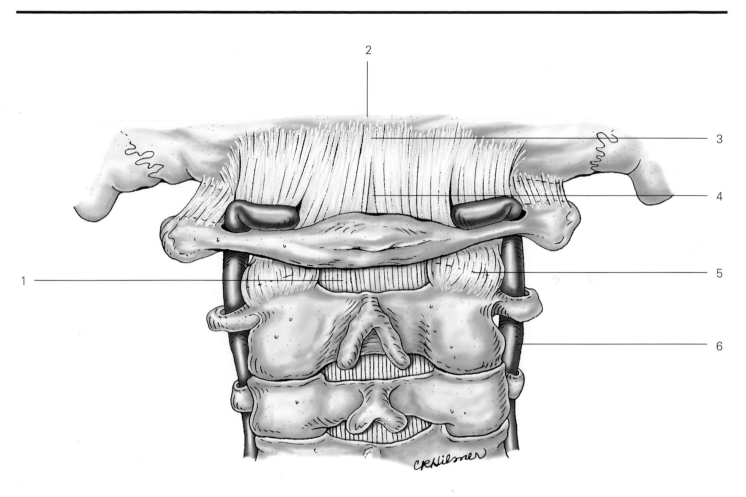

F

The anatomy of deeper structures at the craniocervical junction.

1   Ligamentum flavum
2   Inion
3   Inf. nuchal line
4   Post. atlanto-occipital memb.
5   C1–C2 articular facet
6   Vertebral a.

stay subperiosteal, as the bifid nature of the spinous processes may result in a bulbous expanse and the dissection may err into the paraspinal musculature. A superficial plexus of veins may be encountered and should be cauterized as necessary. A wide flat periosteal elevator such as a Cobb elevator should be used to carefully dissect the paraspinal muscles off the spinous processes using the electrocautery knife for the attachments to the interspinous ligament. The laminae of the cervical spine are angulated at 45° from medial to lateral and cephalad. In the cervical spine, the laminae do not override each other as much as in the thoracic spine; therefore the interlaminar space may be inadvertently penetrated if caution is not taken during the exposure of the laminae. The dissection is carried out laterally to expose the lateral edge of the facet joints and lateral masses. The facet capsule is preserved if the joint is not to be fused.

Various retractors may be used to facilitate exposure, and a small Taylor retractor may be used at the lateral edge of the articular mass to facilitate a unilateral exposure. Care must be taken not to insert the tip of the Taylor retractor too anteriorly, to safeguard the nerve roots. After the appropriate procedure has been performed, the closure includes an initial irrigation of the wound and then a tight closure in layers with the muscle and ligamentum nuchae closed separately to avoid dead space. Nonabsorbable sutures may be used to close the ligamentum nuchae. A strong suture should be used on the ligamentum nuchae, since the incision tends to spread with time from the strong broad pull of the trapezius. A bloodless field should be accomplished prior to closure by cautery to minimize the formation of a hematoma that might compromise any of the neural structures. A drain can be placed deep and removed in 24–48 hours.

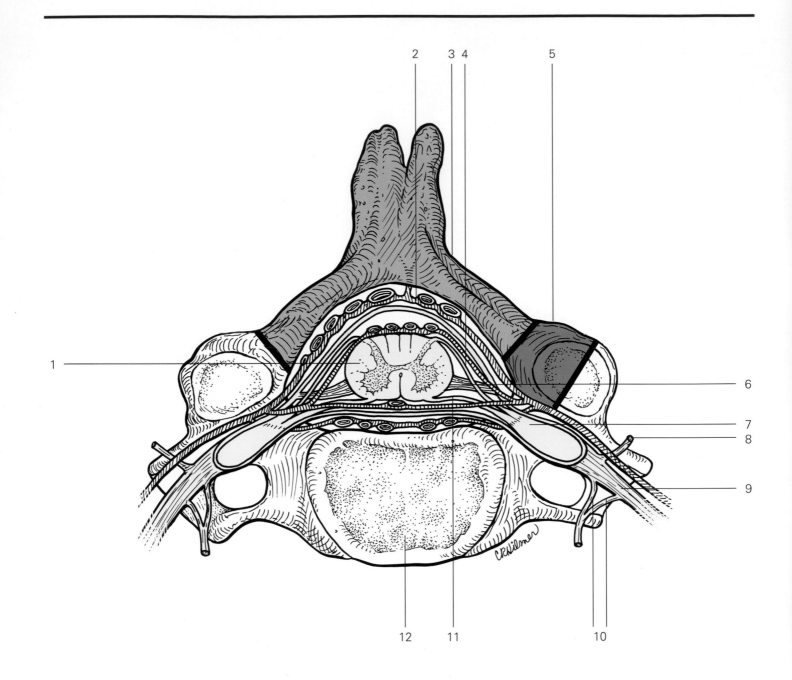

Figure 2.2

Cross-section of the cervical spine showing the lamina, facet, spinal cord and neural branches, and the vertebral body. The laminectomy procedure removes the entire lamina, and the foraminotomy procedure removes 50% of the facet joint.

1　Spinal cord
2　Epidural venous plexus
3　Laminectomy
4　Dorsal root of spinal n.
5　Foraminotomy
6　Dentate lig.
7　Spinal ganglion
8　Dorsal ramus
9　Ventral ramus of spinal n.
10　Ramus communicans
11　Ventral root of spinal n.
12　Vertebral body

Posterior foraminotomy, laminectomy, and laminoplasty (Fig. 2.2)

Posterior foraminotomy is a relatively simple procedure with a predictable good result, provided that patient selection has been strictly defined. A patient who has persistent radiculopathy due to a herniated disc or osteophyte is a good candidate for this procedure. The procedure is indicated when the patient failed an appropriate course of conservative treatment and if an imaging study confirmed the clinical radiculopathy. If the patient has a significant axial neck pain in addition to radiculopathy, the relief of neck pain is less predictable following foraminotomy, and therefore anterior discectomy and fusion is preferred in this case. Laminectomy or laminoplasty is indicated for patients with progressive myelopathy due to multi-level cervical spondylosis. If the involved levels are fewer than three, anterior corpectomy and strut fusion is recommended. If there is a kyphotic deformity, laminectomy or laminoplasty is contraindicated, and an anterior procedure is required. If there are associated problems such as degenerative spondylolisthesis or angular instability, or if facet excision has been performed in addition to laminectomy, concomitant lateral mass fusion or laminoplasty is recommended to prevent post-laminectomy deformities.

Indications

1. Foraminotomy for a herniated disc
2. Foraminotomy for cervical spondylotic radiculopathy
3. Laminectomy or laminoplasty for cervical spondylotic myelopathy.

Surgical techniques

In decompressive procedures, the dissection of the neural structures is done under 3.5× loupe magnification or a microscope.

For foraminotomy, a Kerrison rongeur may be used to remove a portion of the inferior and superior laminae (Fig. 2.3A). Partial facetectomy or foraminotomy is performed by thinning the facets with a power burr. The authors' preferred method is to use an air powered high-speed burr to thin the cortex over the foramen or laminae involved and then finish the thinning with a diamond-tip burr (Fig. 2.3B–D). Caution during the use of power instruments is vital. The surgeon should hold the instrument with both hands and rest the wrists or forearms on the patient carefully to provide proprioceptive feedback to the surgeon and avert any unexpected deviation of the instrument. The lamina and thinned bone should then be gently lifted off the cord or nerve with small angled curets. Placement of a Kerrison rongeur under the lamina may result in injury to the neural elements. Once the bone is removed, the dura and nerve root are exposed and the abundant venous plexus in the cervical canal may need to be cauterized with the bipolar cautery to minimize bleeding (Fig. 2.3E). Meticulous hemostasis is essential to avoid complications due to lack of exposure or hematoma formation, which may lead to an epidural hematoma and spinal cord compression. The nerve root is usually well decompressed by removal of the overlying facet, and removal of disc material is not routinely necessary. If the removal of disc is deemed necessary, the nerve root is gently retracted in a cephalad direction, and the disc tissue can be removed (Fig. 2.3F). Too vigorous manipulation of the nerve root may cause neurological injuries.

Laminectomy is performed by thinning of the cortices at the lamina and facet junction with a power burr (Fig. 2.4). A small Kerrison rongeur may be used to finish the cut and a small angled curet is then used to lift the lamina. Somatosensory evoked potentials should be monitored in most cases of laminectomy. The adherent underlying venous plexus should be cauterized to minimize hematoma formation.

For laminoplasty, the tips of the spinous processes should be resected to facilitate the closure later. As in laminectomy, laminoplasty is performed by thinning the cortices at the lamina and facet junction (Fig. 2.5A). The hinged side is thinned without completing the cut. The lamina is gently opened (Fig. 2.5B), and either 22 gauge wires or heavy nonabsorbable sutures may be used to secure the spinous processes to the facet joints or capsules (Fig. 2.5C). If foraminotomy is needed, it can be performed on the opening side. An additional bone block may be inserted in the opening and secured to prevent the closure of the lamina. The authors prefer using the rib or iliac crest allograft as a bone block. The graft should be fashioned to have grooves on each side to fit between the opened lamina and the medial edge of the lateral mass.

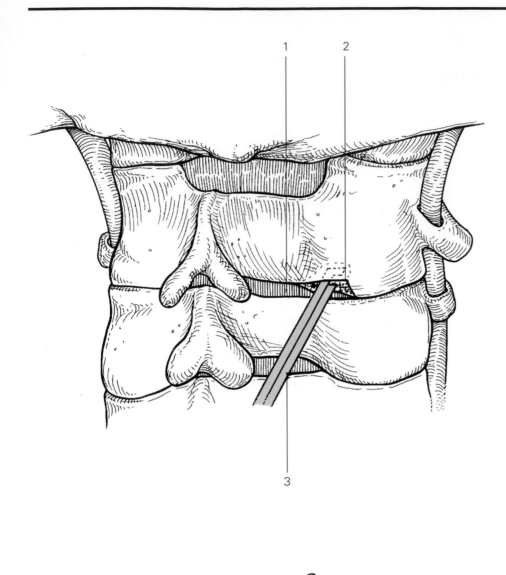

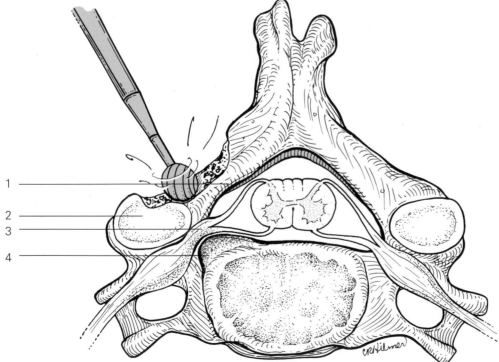

Figure 2.3

Posterior foraminotomy

A
A Kerrison rongeur may be used to remove a portion of the inferior and superior laminae.

1 Ligamentum flavum
2 Laminotomy
3 Kerrison rongeur

B
Partial facetectomy or foraminotomy is performed by thinning the facets with a power burr. Thin the cortex over the foramen; then finish the thinning with a diamond-tip burr.

1 Lamina
2 Facet
3 Nerve root
4 Osteophyte

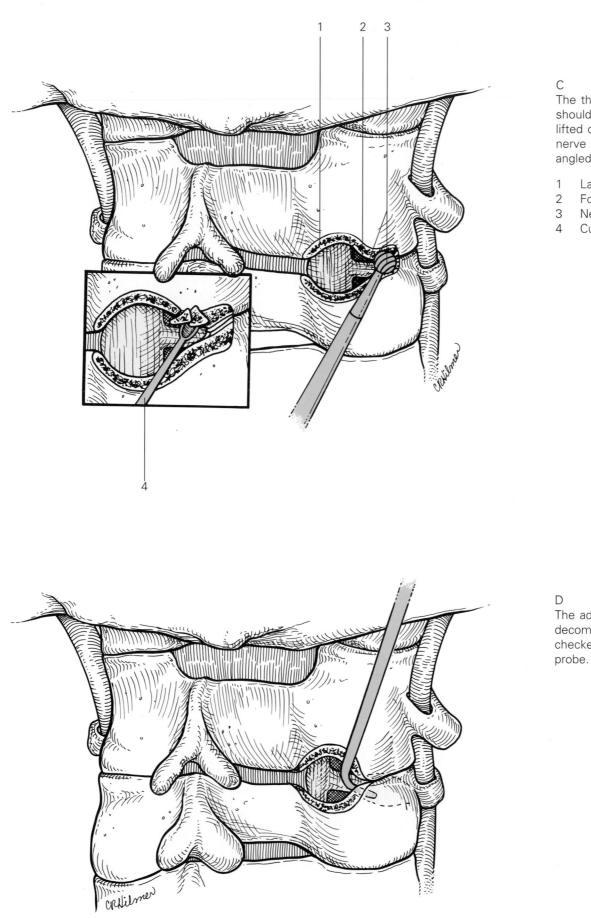

C
The thinned bone should then be gently lifted off the cord and nerve root with a small angled curet.

1   Laminotomy
2   Foraminotomy
3   Nerve root
4   Curet

D
The adequacy of decompression is checked with an angled probe.

Contd

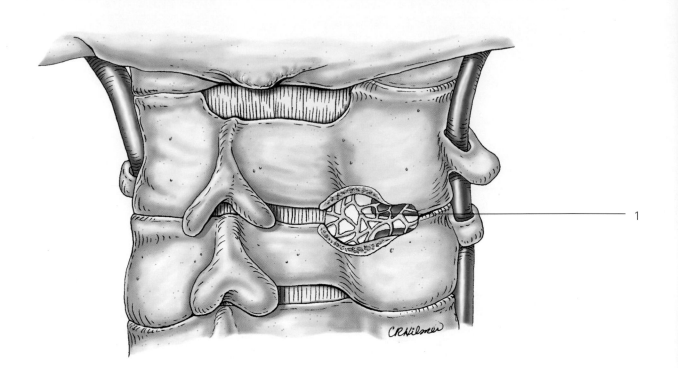

Figure 2.3 *(contd)*

E
Once the bone is removed, the dura and nerve root can be
exposed and the overlying venous plexus in the cervical canal
may need to be cauterized with the bipolar cautery.

1   Venous plexus

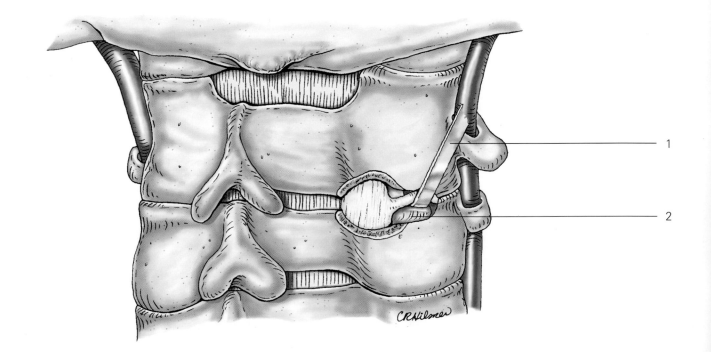

F
If the removal of disc is deemed necessary, the nerve root is
gently retracted in a cephalad direction, and the disc
fragments can be removed.

1   Penfield probe
2   Disc prolapse

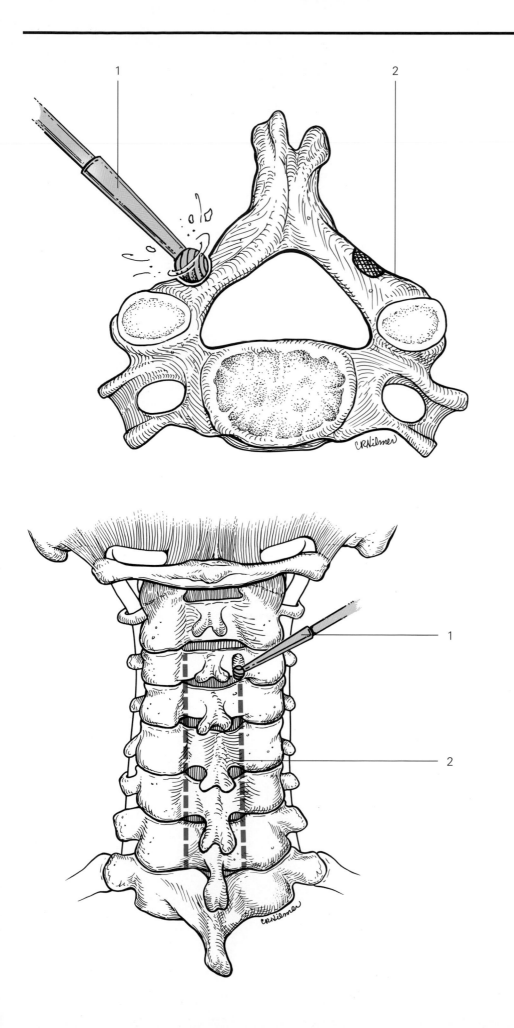

Figure 2.4

Laminectomy

A
The cortical bone at the lamina and facet junction is thinned with a power burr.

1 Power burr
2 Lamina–facet junction

B
Laminectomy is usually performed at multiple levels.

1 Power burr
2 Laminectomy line

Contd

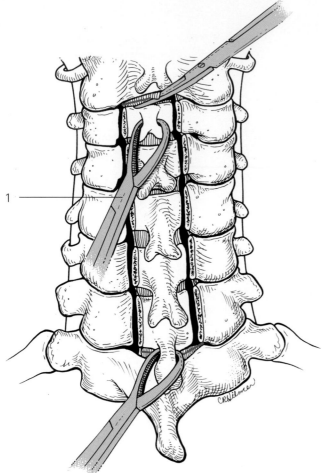

1

Figure 2.4 *(contd)*

C
A small Kerrison rongeur or a small angled curet may be used to finish the cut. Towel clips are used to lift the lamina, and the ligamentum flavum is divided at the end of laminectomy.

1   Towel clip

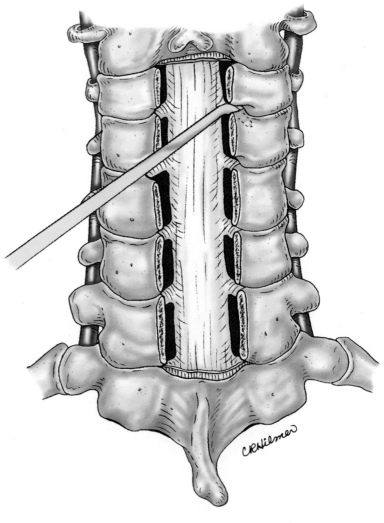

D
Following removal of the lamina, the foramen may be checked with an angled probe. Foraminotomy may be performed if necessary.

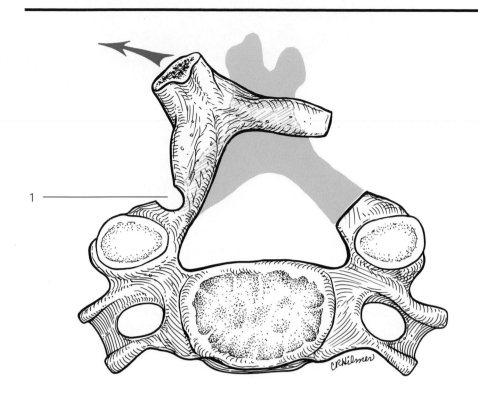

Figure 2.5

Laminoplasty.

A
The tips of the spinous processes should be resected to facilitate the closure later. Laminoplasty is performed by thinning the cortices at the lamina and facet junction and opening on one side and hinging on the other side.

1   Hinged side

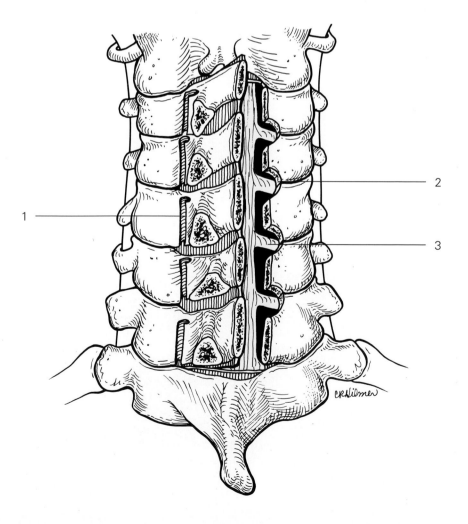

B
The lamina is gently opened, and foraminotomy may be performed on the opened side.

1   Hinged side
2   Foraminotomy
3   Nerve root

Contd

Figure 2.5 *(contd)*

C
Either 22 gauge wires or heavy nonabsorbable sutures may
be used to secure the spinous processes to the facet
joints or capsules.

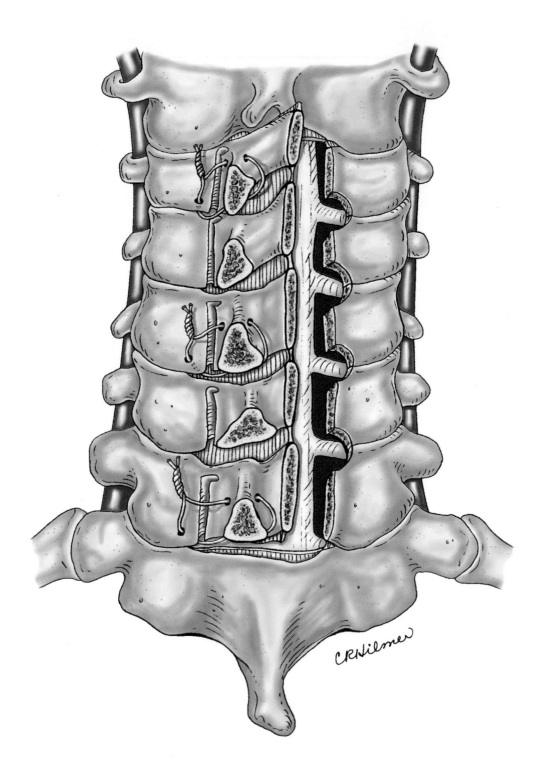

Posterior atlantoaxial arthrodesis

Most upper cervical injuries are best treated non-operatively. Cervical orthoses including the halo-vest are often utilized to provide stability until bony and soft tissue heal. The primary indication for posterior atlantoaxial fusion is acute or chronic instability due to the disruption of the transverse ligament that jeopardizes the function of the spinal cord, as in an isolated rupture of the transverse ligament or a Jefferson fracture with rupture of the transverse ligament. Another indication for posterior atlantoaxial stabilization may include acute type II odontoid fracture or nonunion of odontoid fracture with atlantoaxial instability. Atlantoaxial instabilities may also be caused by nontraumatic disorders such as rheumatoid arthritis, congenital anomalies, and metabolic disorders. The authors recommend atlantoaxial arthrodesis for an acute injury with an atlantoaxial interval greater than 5 mm, but for a chronic condition clinical findings along with other tests such as flexion–extension views and MRI should be investigated first. Basically, if the patient has neurologic symptoms or the space available for the spinal cord becomes less than 14 mm in either static or dynamic imaging studies, surgery is indicated. The indications for surgery in odontoid fractures are controversial, but the authors recommend prompt reduction and halo-vest immobilization as the first-line treatment; but surgery is recommended for the failure of reduction or the development of symptomatic nonunion.

Indications

1. Traumatic atlantoaxial instabilities with rupture of the transverse ligament
2. Type II odontoid fractures with a high risk of nonunion, as in an old patient with a significant displacement
3. Late atlantoaxial instabilities caused by Jefferson's fracture of the C1 ring or odontoid nonunion
4. Nontraumatic atlantoaxial instabilities caused by rheumatoid arthritis, congenital anomalies, or metabolic problems.

Surgical techniques

Modified Gallie fusion

A Gallie fusion provides an adequate stability, particularly against flexion. Because of its relative inferior stability against extension and rotation, a halo-vest is recommended postoperatively. Other more rigid internal fixation may be preferred if the atlantoaxial instability is severe or the instability is in the posterior direction. The modified Gallie fusion involves a doubled U-shaped 18 or 20 gauge wire that is passed under the arch of C1 from inferior to superior (Fig. 2.6A). Then, an H-type graft is taken from the posterior iliac crest and shaped to fit between C1 and C2. The loop of the wire is passed over the bone block and the spinous process of C2 (Fig. 2.6B). The end of the wire is tightened around the graft between C1 and C2 (Fig. 2.6C). Grafts of cancellous strips are added. The deep cancellous surfaces of the graft must be contoured to fit over the curved posterior surfaces of the C1 and C2 so that the graft is in firm contact with the underlying vertebrae, immobilizing the involved segment. This modified Gallie fusion may be performed using a cable or heavy nonabsorbable thread instead of wire (Fig. 2.7). The cable or thread gives more flexibility than wire for sublaminar passage. The tightening mechanism may be more cumbersome and requires a special instrument.

Brooks fusion

The Brooks fusion requires sublaminar passage of the wire at both C1 and C2, but gives a better stability against rotation and extension than the Gallie fusion. After exposing the posterior elements of C1 and C2, the surfaces of C1 and C2 which will be in contact with the bone grafts are decorticated gently. Doubled-twisted 24 gauge wires are passed under the arch of C1 and then under the lamina of C2. Two pieces of rectangular iliac crest bone grafts (1.25 cm × 3.5 cm) are harvested and beveled to fit in the interval between the arch of C1 and each lamina of C2. The wires are then tightened, securing the graft in proper position.

Segmental wire fusion technique

This technique involves segmental double wiring at both C1 and C2. The spinous process is utilized at C2 wiring instead of sublaminar passage. After exposure, a 20 or 22 gauge looped wire is passed under the arch of C1 from inferior to superior. The end of the wire is fed through the loop and tightened down to the arch of C1 (Fig. 2.8A). Another wire is then passed through the base of the spinous process of C2. Two full thickness corticocancellous bone grafts are taken

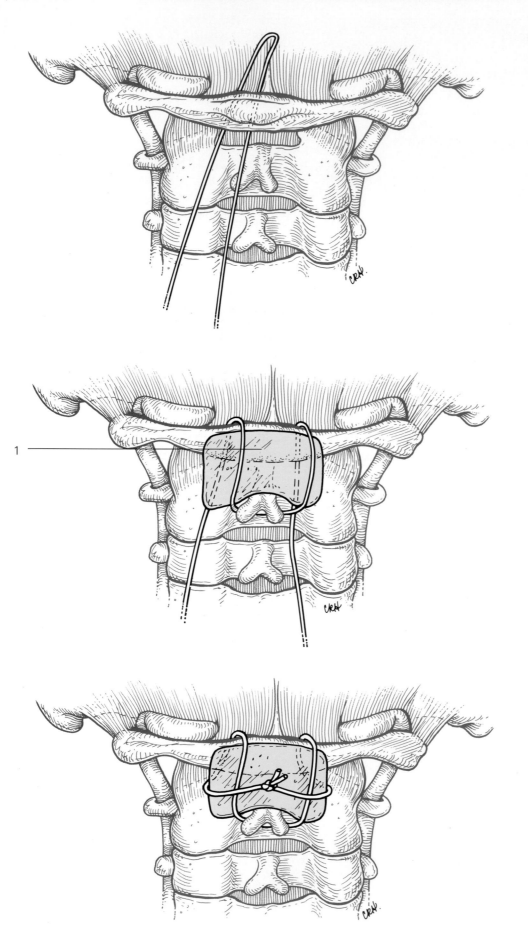

Figure 2.6

The modified Gallie fusion

A
A doubled **U**-shaped 18 or 20 gauge wire is passed under the arch of C1 from inferior to superior.

B
An **H**-type graft is taken from the posterior iliac crest and shaped to fit between C1 and C2. The loop of the wire is passed over the bone block and the spinous process of C2.

1   Bone graft

C
The end of the wire is tightened around the graft between C1 and C2.

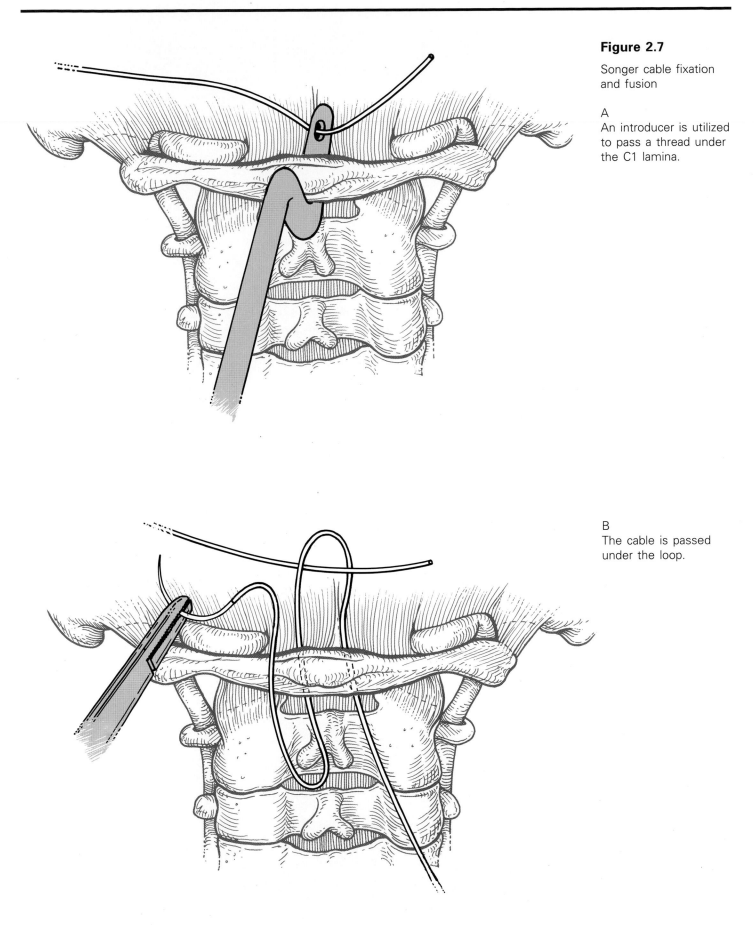

Figure 2.7

Songer cable fixation and fusion

A
An introducer is utilized to pass a thread under the C1 lamina.

B
The cable is passed under the loop.

Contd

Figure 2.7 *(contd)*

C
The cable is then passed under the C1 lamina and looped over the C2 lamina and under the C2 spinous process.

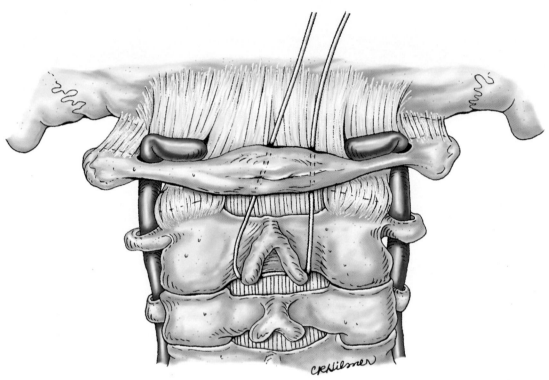

D
Bone graft is fitted between C1 and C2, and the cable is looped over the bone graft.

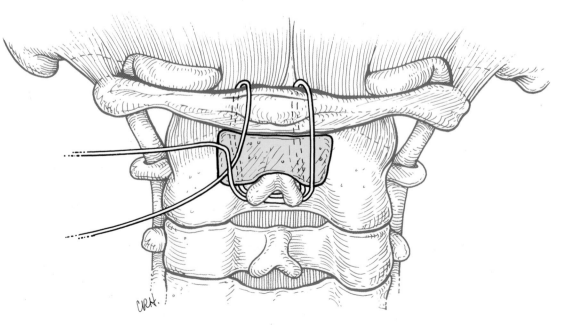

E
The cable is tightened with a special instrument.

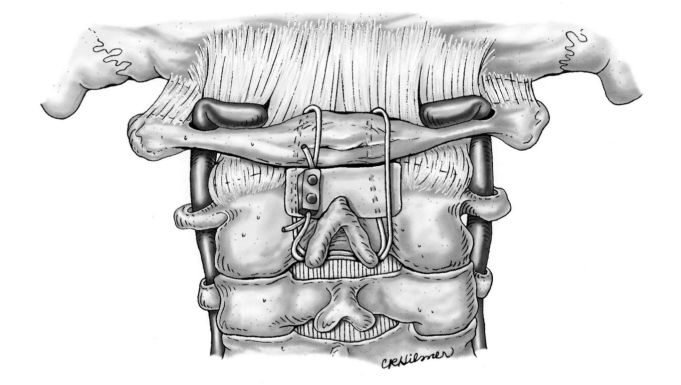

from the posterior iliac crest and are placed on the posterior laminae of C1 and C2, and then the ends of the wires are fed through the holes in the grafts (Fig. 2.8B). Finally, the C1 and C2 wires are tightened on the grafts (Fig. 2.8C).

Magerl's transarticular screw fixation

Magerl's transarticular screw technique provides the most rigid internal fixation but may be associated with a greater risk.

A midline approach is used to expose the occiput to C3. The subcutaneous exposure should extend down to C4 to facilitate the cephalad angulation of the drill. Subperiosteal dissection is done on the cranial aspect of C2 to expose the C1–C2 facet joints bilaterally. K-wires are used to retract the soft tissues containing the greater occipital nerve and its accompanying venous plexus. The screws are inserted by entering C2 at the inferior aspect and exiting at the posterior aspect of the upper articular process. The screws are placed through the facet joints into the lateral masses of C1 (Fig 2.9). Fluoroscopy is recommended during drilling. Gallie-type fusion is recommended in addition to transarticular screws in patients with an intact C1 ring.

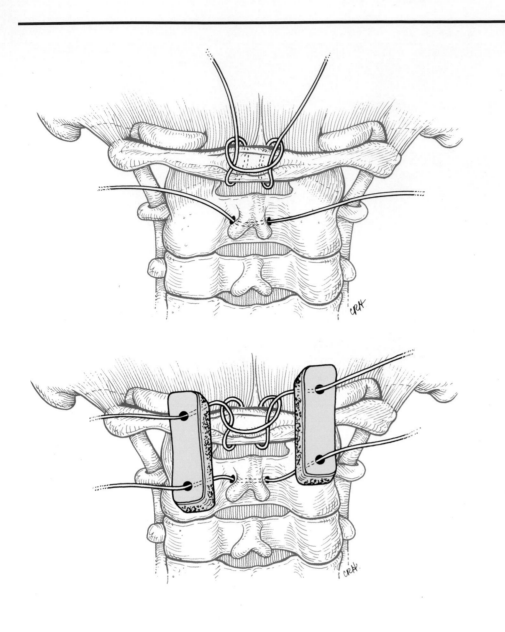

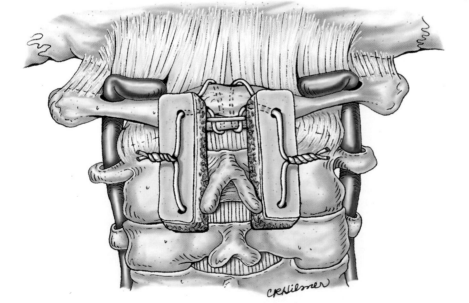

Figure 2.8

Segmental wire fusion technique

A
A 20 or 22 gauge looped wire is passed under the arch of C1 from inferior to superior. The end of the wire is fed through the loop and tightened down to the arch of C1. Another wire is then passed through the base of the spinous process of C2.

B
Two full thickness corticocancellous bone grafts are taken from the posterior iliac crest and are placed on the posterior laminae of C1 and C2, and then the ends of the wires are fed through the holes in the grafts.

C
The C1 and C2 wires are tightened on the grafts.

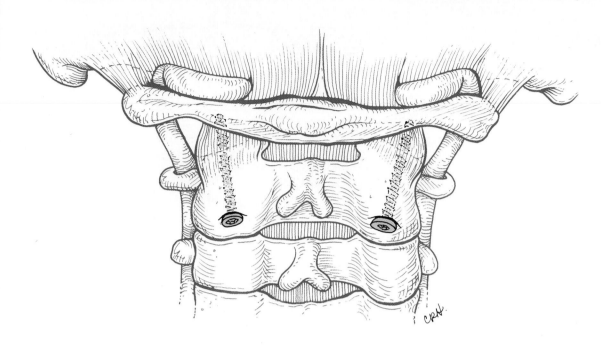

Figure 2.9

Magerl's transarticular screw fixation

A
After exposure, the screws are inserted by entering C2 at the inferior aspect and exiting at the posterior aspect of the upper articular process. The screws are placed through the facet joints into the lateral masses of C1.

B
Lateral view of the transarticular screw fixation.

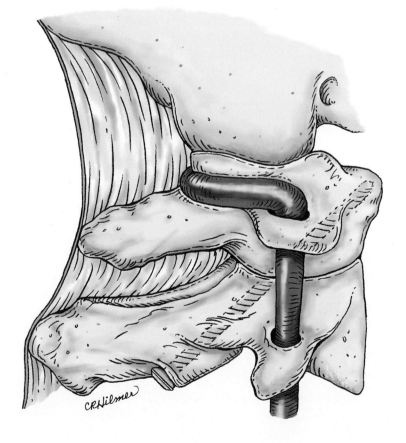

Posterior occipitocervical arthrodesis

Problems at the occipitocervical region are uncommon, and disorders that require occipitocervical arthrodesis are rare. The indications for occipitocervical fusion may include basilar impression, occipitocervical instabilities, and atlantoaxial instabilities with a deficient C1 ring. Another indication for occipitocervical fusion may be basilar impression associated with cervicomedullary cord compression. Basilar impression may develop in association with rheumatologic, post-traumatic and congenital malformations, and neoplastic disorders. Among several techniques described in the literature, the method described by Wertheim and Bohlman (1987) is the safest (Fig. 2.10). Occipitocervical fusion can also be achieved by using contoured Hartshill Luque-type rectangle instrumentation (Fig. 2.11A). Occipitocervical plate–screw fixations have been reported recently (Fig. 2.11B–D). Screw fixation into the occiput gives a better stability and may be advantageous in patients undergoing laminectomy or who require multiple level fixation from the occiput to the lower cervical spine (Fig. 2.11B–D).

Figure 2.10

Triple wiring technique for occipitocervical fusion

A

Indications

1. Occipitocervical instability caused by trauma, rheumatoid arthritis, congenital anomalies, neoplasia and infections
2. Basilar impression due to rheumatoid arthritis, congenital anomalies, or metabolic disorders
3. Atlantoaxial instability associated with a deficient arch of the atlas or failed atlantoaxial arthrodesis.

Wiring technique

The midline posterior approach is made, exposing the area from the external occipital protuberance to the fourth cervical vertebra. The base of the occiput and the cervical laminae are decorticated with a high speed burr to enhance fusion. It may be necessary to remove the posterior border of the foramen magnum or the arch of the atlas if decompression is indicated. Wiring is performed through the thick external occipital protuberance, which represents the ideal location for the passage of wires without having to go through both tables of the skull. A high-speed burr is used to create a trough on both sides of the occipital protuberance at a level 2 cm above the foramen magnum. A towel clip is used to create a hole in the ridge without penetrating the inner table. A second wire loop is passed around the arch of C1 and a third is passed through and around the base of the spinous process of C2 (Fig 2.10A). The posterior iliac crest is then exposed and a large, thick, slightly curved graft

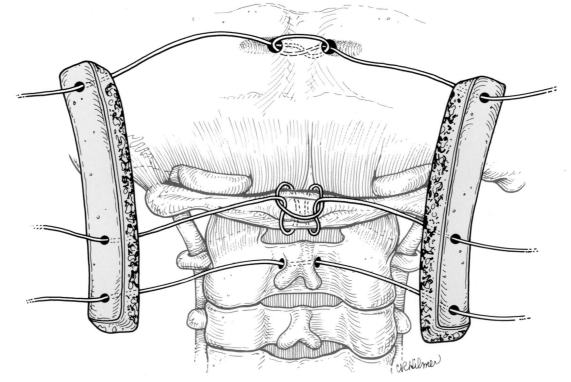

of corticocancellous bone of appropriate width and length is obtained from the outer table (Fig. 2.10B). The graft is then divided and three drill holes are placed in each graft. The occiput is decorticated and the grafts anchored in place by the wires (Fig. 2.10C). Additional cancellous bone is then packed between the two grafts. Halo-cast immobilization is required for 12 weeks.

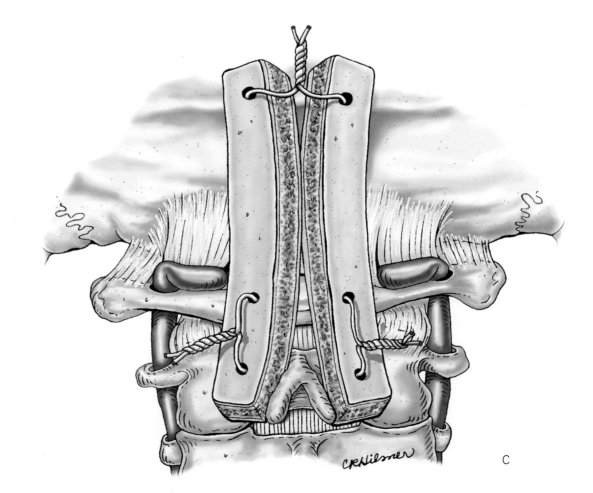

B

C

Occipitocervical plate fixation

Roy-Camille et al (1992) devised an occipitocervical plate that is contoured to fit the occipitocervical junction. The premolded plates, which are reinforced in their middle at the apex of the curve, are designed to restore the normal curvature of the occipito-cervical region, with a 105° angulation. Others have modified the Roy-Camille technique to incorporate the occipital screws in the midline, in which longer screws can be inserted (Fig. 2.11B–D). Through a midline posterior approach, the occiput and the arch of C1 and C2, as well as the lower vertebrae with their articular masses, are exposed. A 2.8 mm drill bit is used for drilling holes on the articular masses down to the desired level bilaterally, and two plates or a Y-plate are then placed on the cervical spine. The lateral mass drilling techniques in the lower cervical spine are detailed later. At the C2 level, the pedicle is used for screw fixation. The entry point is at the upper and inner quadrant, and the drill is angled at 10–15° medially and 35° superiorly to avoid injury to the vertebral artery (Fig. 2.11E). The drilling of the occiput is made through the plate hole after the plate is screwed to the cervical spine, and two or three 12–14 mm-long screws are inserted into the occiput. The second plate is secured with same technique. Corticocancellous and cancellous bone grafts are directly packed into the area between the two plates (Fig 2.11D).

Figure 2.11

Alternative occipitocervical fixations

A
Hartshill rectangle: wires are used to stabilize the contoured rod at the occiput and the lower cervical spine.

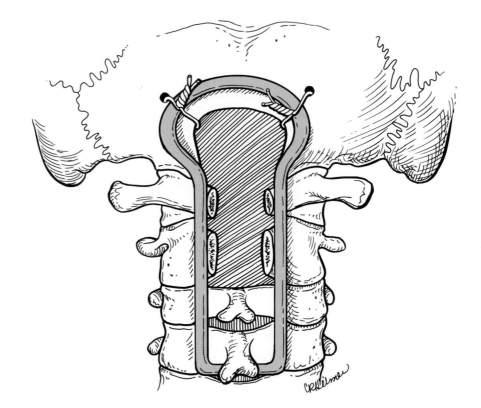

B
Occipitocervical plate–screw fixations using contoured AO reconstruction plates. The drilling of the occiput is made through the plate hole after the plate is screwed to the cervical spine.

1   AO reconstruction plate
2   Cancellous bone chips

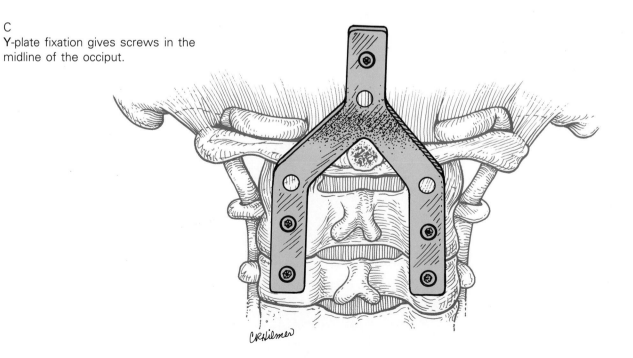

1
2

C
Y-plate fixation gives screws in the midline of the occiput.

Contd

Figure 2.11 *(contd)*

D
Additional wires may be used to
attach bone grafts over the plate.

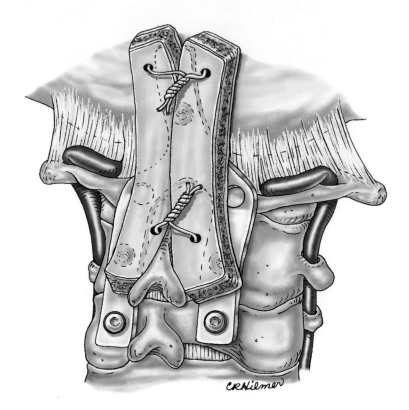

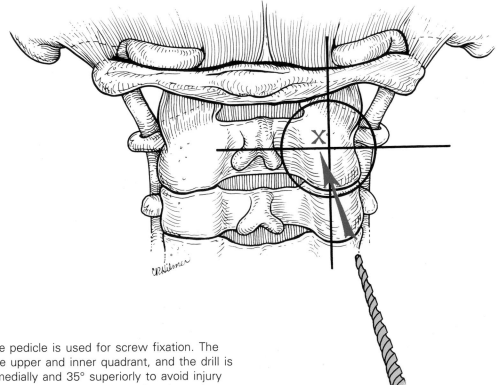

E
At the C2 level, the pedicle is used for screw fixation. The
entry point is at the upper and inner quadrant, and the drill is
angled at 10–15° medially and 35° superiorly to avoid injury
to the vertebral artery. The drilling of the occiput is made
through the plate hole after the plate is screwed to the
cervical spine, and two or three 12–14 mm-long screws are
inserted into the occiput.

Posterior lower cervical spine arthrodesis

Posterior fusion of the lower cervical spine may be indicated in patients with facet dislocations or tear drop fractures, post-laminectomy instabilities, or neoplasms. Flexion–distraction injuries such as unilateral or bilateral facet dislocations are quite unstable, and the authors recommend prompt reduction by skull tongs traction and posterior arthrodesis. In subluxation or dislocation cases with an associated herniated disc, the spinal cord should be decompressed anteriorly first. Progressive cervical kyphosis associated with trauma, laminectomy or neoplasms may require either anterior or posterior cervical fusion. If the kyphotic deformity is rigid, anterior fusion is required, but if the kyphotic deformity is flexible, then either anterior or posterior fusion may be utilized. In a severely unstable injury such as tear drop fractures, a combined anterior and posterior fusion may be indicated. With the advent of more rigid fixation techniques, the combined anterior and posterior fusion may not be necessary. Additionally, the moored rigid implants may obviate the use of the halo-vest postoperatively.

There are numerous methods of posterior stabilization of the cervical spine. Wiring techniques are quite effective in preventing flexion, but less effective in preventing extension or rotation. The authors favor a triple wire technique which secures the spinous processes and the bone grafts (Fig. 2.12). This triple wiring technique has been shown to be safe and effective, and biomechanically superior to many other constructs. Alternative fixations include Wisconsin button-wires with the Hartshill rectangle (Fig. 2.13A,B) and Halifax clamp (Fig. 2.13C). Another fixation is known as the Dewar procedure (Fig. 2.13D), in which Kirschner wires are inserted through the bases of the spinous processes and secured with wire in a loop fashion. Facet fracture or subluxation can be managed with an oblique wiring technique or a wire loop by passing the wire through the lateral mass (Fig. 2.14 A,B). In post-laminectomy conditions requiring stabilization, interfacet wiring and fusion can be performed (Figs 2.14C,D; 2.15). Although the majority of patients with an instability of the cervical spine can be treated with wiring methods, more rigid internal fixation techniques can be achieved with plate–screw techniques (Figs 2.16, 2.17). Postural cervical plating may be indicated in cases where the spinous processes are fractured or deficient, as in post-laminectomy cases. More rigid fixation may also offer early rehabilitation and decrease the need for a halo-vest postoperatively.

Indications

1. Traumatic instabilities
2. Extensive laminectomies for neural decompression
3. Destruction of bony elements by neoplasm
4. Cervical spine deformities.

Surgical techniques

Triple wire fusion technique

After exposure of the spinous processes, laminae, and facets of the involved area, a 3 to 4 mm burr is used to drill a hole at the base of the spinous process on both sides. The drill hole site should be at the proximal aspect of the cephalad spinous process and at the distal aspect of the caudad spinous process. A towel clip is gently passed through the holes to create a tunnel for wires. An 18 or 20 gauge wire is then passed from one side to the other and tightened in a simple circular or figure of 8 fashion (Figs 2.12A,B). If more than one level is to be fused, the figure of 8 wiring is used to incorporate the middle spinous process in the wiring construct. If the middle spinous process or lamina are fractured, wiring should be avoided at this level. The second and third wires are passed through the cephalad and caudad holes in the base of the processes, respectively (Fig. 2.12C). Decortication of the lamina and facets is performed carefully using a power burr. Then corticocancellous bone grafts of appropriate length are taken from the outer table of the iliac crest. The bone grafts are drilled to make two holes and laid down on the lamina bilaterally. The wires are passed through the holes in the bone grafts and tightened down (Fig. 2.12D). Additional cancellous chips are laid down on the exposed lamina or facets. The patient is usually kept in a cervicothoracic orthosis or halo-vest for 6 weeks, depending on the stability of the construct and the compliance of the patient.

Interfacet wiring fusion technique

For facet dislocation cases or if the spinous process and lamina are fractured, or laminectomy has been performed, interfacet wiring fusion can be performed (Fig. 2.14). The facet wire is passed by placing a small Penfield dissector into the facet joint, and then a 2 mm drill hole is made into the facet from superior to inferior (Fig. 2.14A). A 20 or 22 gauge wire is passed through this hole and looped around the inferior spinous process for one-level fusion as in unilateral facet dislocation (Fig. 2.14B). Facet wires may be extended to adjacent facets for interfacet facet stabilization as in postlaminectomy instability (Fig. 2.14C,D). The facet wires may be tied to bone grafts for fusion and also can be tied to rods for multi-level stabililization (Fig. 2.15).

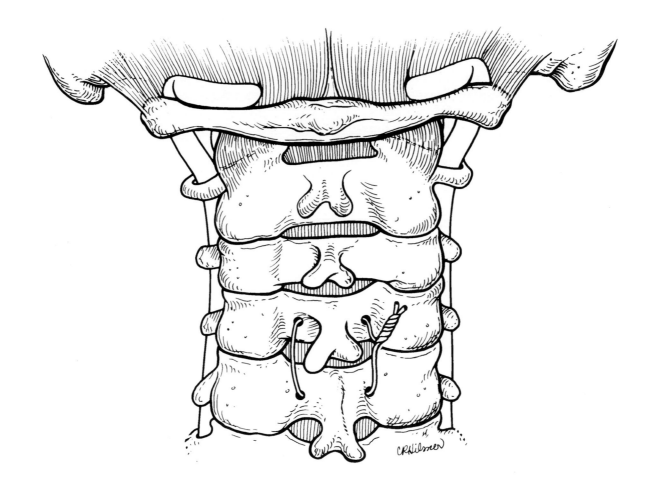

Figure 2.12

Triple wire fusion technique

A
After exposure, a 3 to 4 mm burr is used to drill a hole at the base of the spinous process on both sides. The drill hole site should be at the proximal aspect of the cephalad spinous process and at the distal aspect of the caudad spinous process. A towel clip is gently passed through the holes to create a tunnel for wires. An 18 or 20 gauge wire is then passed from one side to the other and tightened in a simple circular fashion.

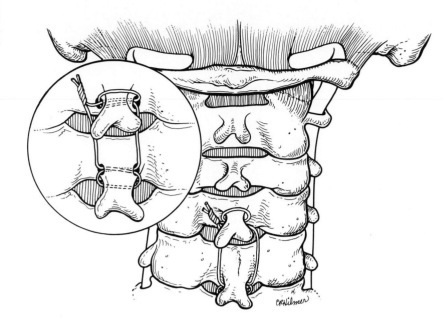

B
Alternatively, wiring may be done in a figure of 8 fashion.

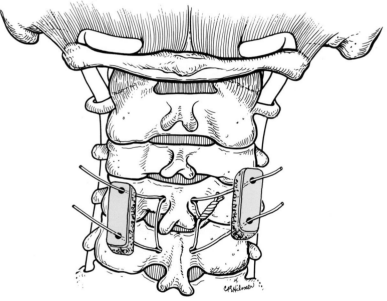

C
The second and third wires are passed through the cephalad and caudad holes in the base of the processes, respectively. The corticocancellous bone grafts from the iliac crest are drilled to make two holes and laid down on the lamina bilaterally. The wires are passed through the holes in the bone grafts.

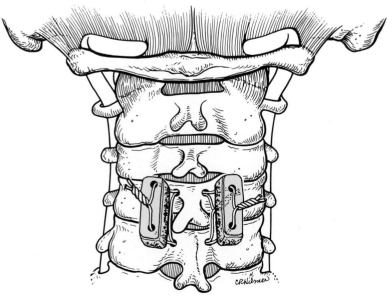

D
The grafts are tightened down with wires.

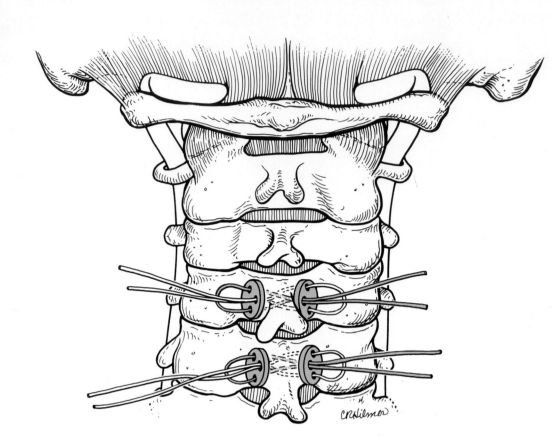

Figure 2.13

Alternative lower cervical fixations

A
Wisconsin button-wires are passed through the base of spinous processes.

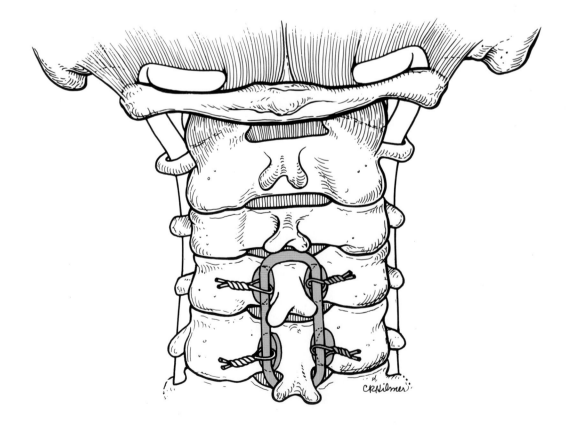

B
A Hartshill rectangle is tightened with wires.

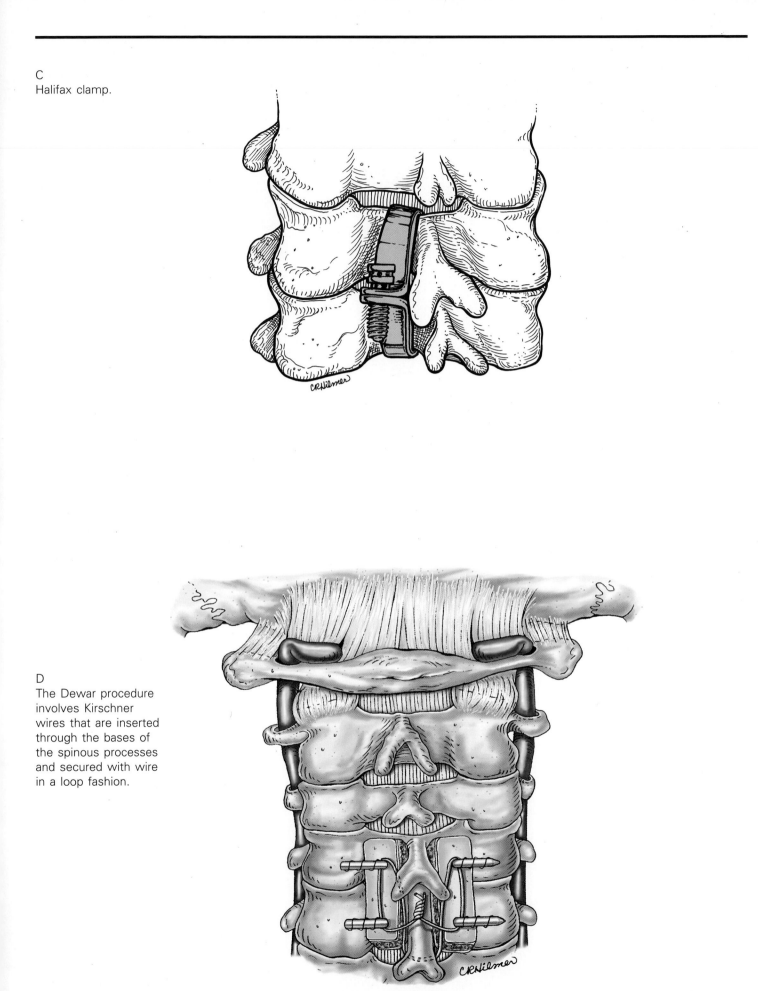

C
Halifax clamp.

D
The Dewar procedure involves Kirschner wires that are inserted through the bases of the spinous processes and secured with wire in a loop fashion.

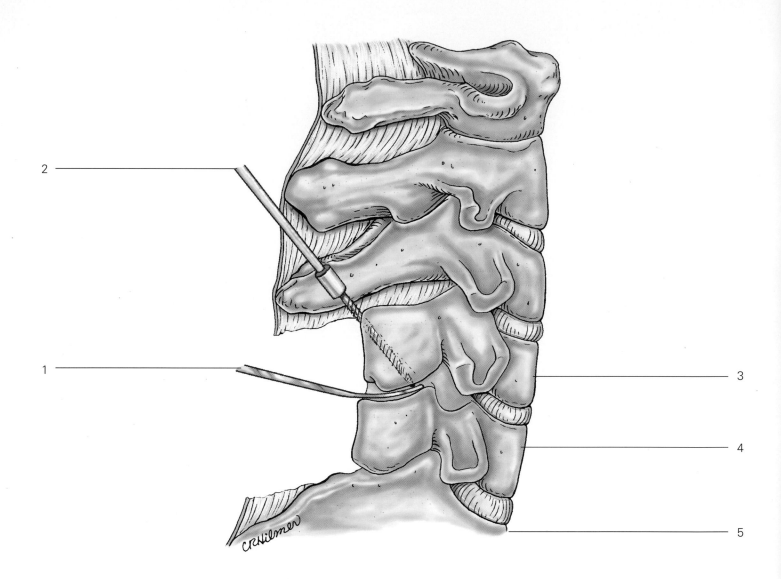

Figure 2.14

Interfacet wiring fusion technique.

A
The facet wire is passed by placing a small Penfield dissector
into the facet joint, and then a 2 mm drill hole is made into
the facet from superior to inferior.

1 Penfield dissector
2 Drill
3 C4
4 C5
5 C6

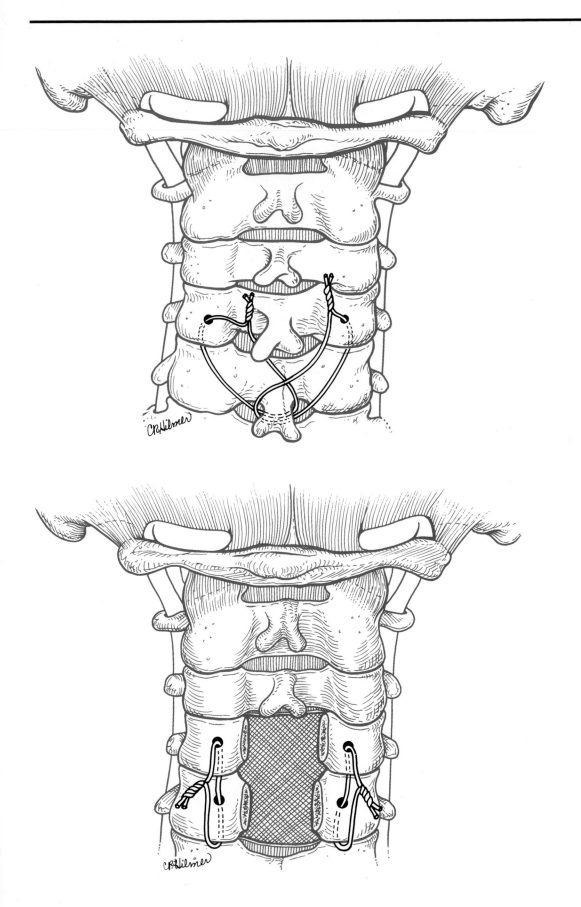

B
A 20 or 22 gauge wire is passed through this hole and looped around the inferior spinous process for one-level fusion as in unilateral facet dislocation.

C
Posterior view of interfacet wiring.

Contd

Figure 2.14 *(contd)*

D
Lateral view of interfacet wiring.

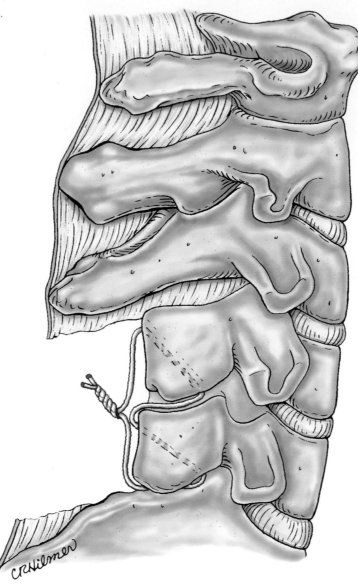

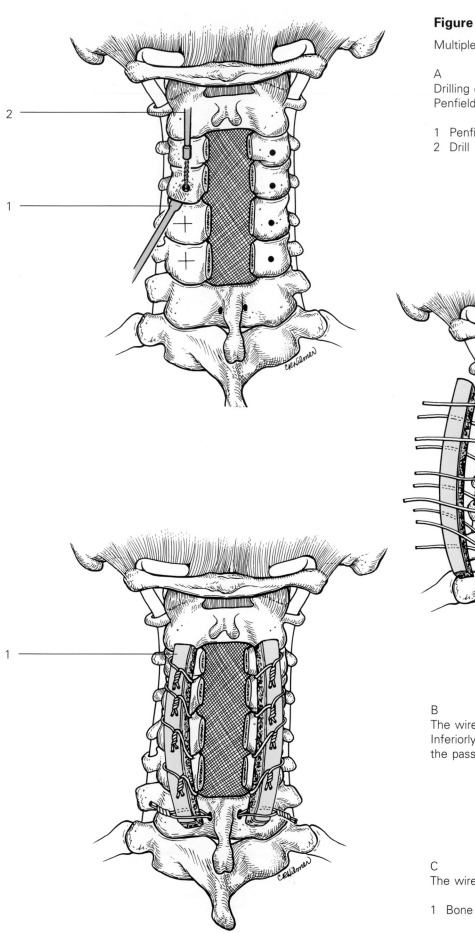

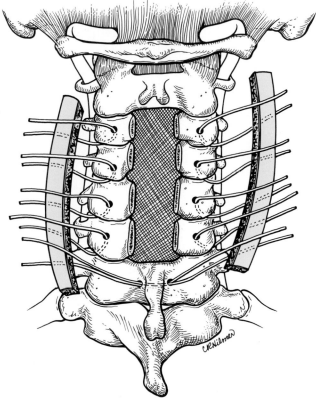

Figure 2.15

Multiple level interfacet wiring and fusion

A
Drilling of the inferior articular process with a Penfield dissector in the facet joint.

1 Penfield dissector
2 Drill

B
The wires are segmentally passed at each level. Inferiorly, the spinous process may be utilized for the passage of the wire.

C
The wire may be tied to bone grafts for fusion.

1 Bone graft

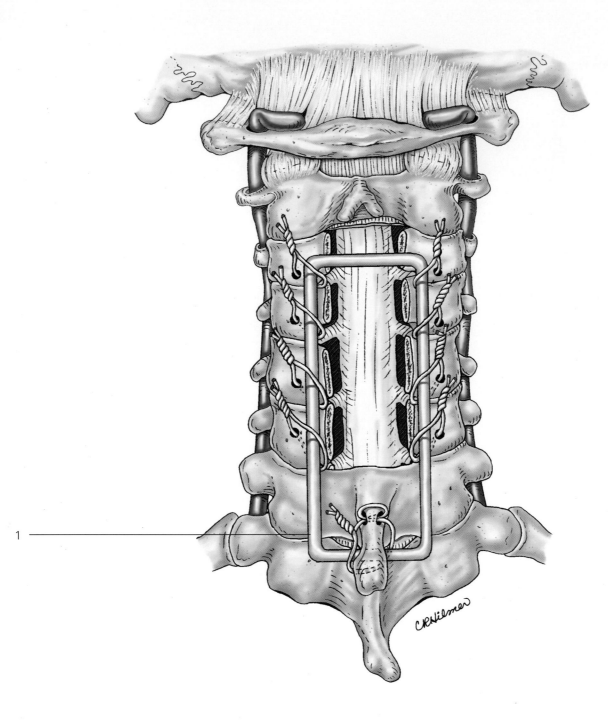

D
The wires may be tied to a rod for greater stability, and cancellous bone grafts are laid for fusion.

1 Luque rod

Posterior cervical plating

Posterior stabilization of the cervical spine using screws and plates has been pioneered by Roy-Camille in Paris (1989). Roy-Camille utilized the center of lateral mass for the entry point of drilling and angles 10° laterally (Fig. 2.16A). Magerl (1987) devised a plate–screw system for the cervical spine, in which the inferior end of the plate is a hook configuration (Fig. 2.17). Magerl recommends that drilling angles should be 25° laterally and 45° superiorly. Anderson et al (1991) presented a technique utilizing the AO reconstruction plates. Posterior plate–screw fixation of the cervical spine must be done with thorough knowledge of lateral mass anatomy. Bilateral exposure to the limits of the lateral masses is made. The center of the articular pillar is located, and the cortex pierced with an awl or small burr 1 mm medial to the center of the lateral mass (Fig. 2.16B). As mentioned before, there are many techniques of drilling favored by various authors. On the basis of anatomical dissection to avoid injury to the nerve root, the present authors use the technique of 30° laterally and 15° cephalad for C3–C6 (Fig. 2.16B,C). The opposite cortex is usually penetrated, using a drill with a stop guide. The drill hole is tapped with a 3.5 mm tap. A contoured posterior cervical plate and 3.5 mm diameter cortical screws of appropriate length are placed and secured (Fig. 2.16 D,E). In patients without lamina, cancellous chips are placed within the facet joints after using a small burr in order to achieve arthrodesis (Fig. 2.16 D,E). The posterior elements adjacent to the plates are decorticated and bone grafts are added. After surgery, a simple rigid collar is used for 6–12 weeks. For the Magerl hook-plate technique, a small notch is made in the inferior edge of the lamina for hook insertion. In the upper vertebra, the point for drilling is slightly medial and inferior to the center of the lateral mass, and the screw is then inserted 25° laterally and 45° cranially. After an H-shaped bone graft is placed between the spinous processes, the screws are tightened (Fig. 2.17).

Complications

1. Unnecessary exposure of the cervical levels resulting in fusion extension
2. Inadvertent penetration into the dura
3. Dural penetration or tearing caused by a wire or hook
4. Injuries of the spinal cord, vertebral artery, or the nerve root caused by screw–plate fixation
5. Loosening or breakage of the implant and recurrence of the deformity
6. Pseudarthosis.

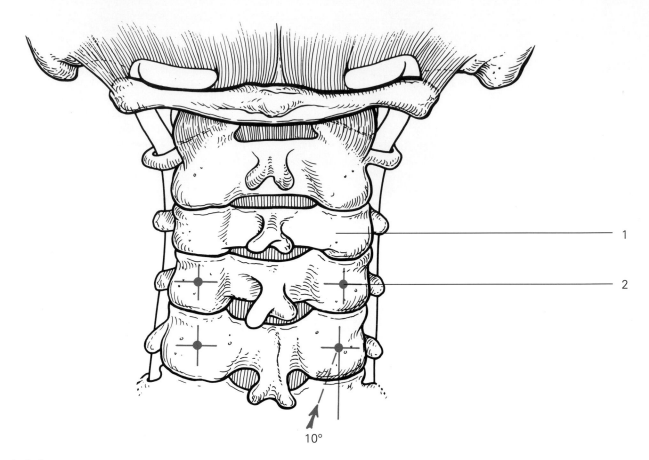

Figure 2.16

Posterior cervical plating.

A
Roy-Camille technique: bilateral exposure to the limits of the lateral masses is made. The center of the lateral mass is utilized for the entry point of drilling.

1 Lat. mass
2 Center of lat. mass

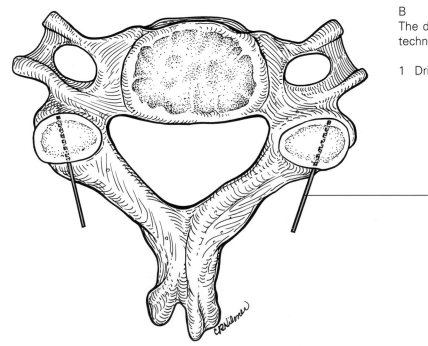

B
The drilling is directed 10° laterally for the Roy-Camille technique.

1 Drilling 10° lat.

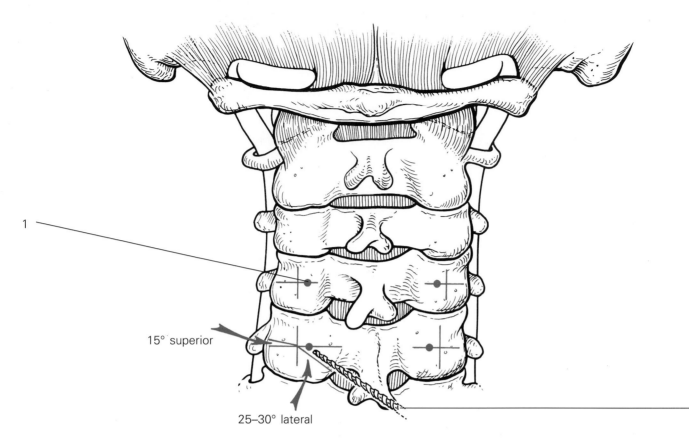

1
15° superior
25–30° lateral

C
To safeguard the nerve root and facet joint, the drilling is directed at 25-30° laterally and 15° cephalad for C3–C6, starting 1 mm medial to the center of the lateral mass.

1 1 mm med. from the center
2 Drill

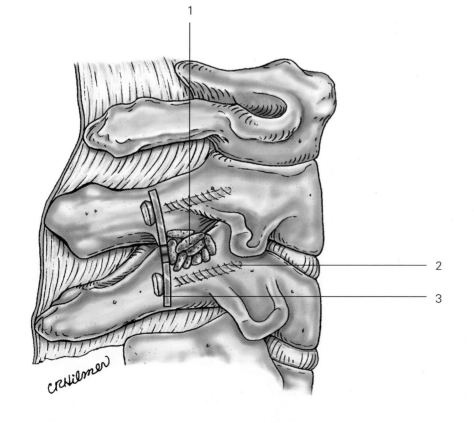

D
A contoured posterior cervical plate and 3.5 mm diameter cortical screws of appropriate length are placed and secured.

1 Bone chips
2 Screw
3 Plate

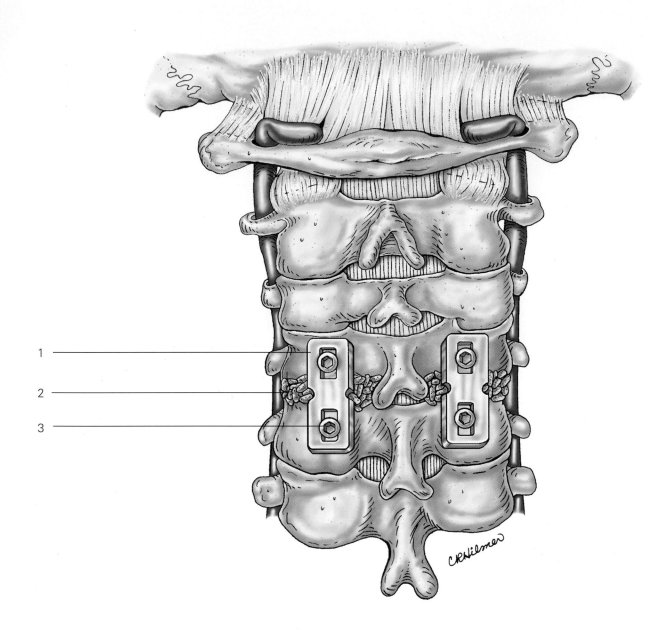

E
Cancellous bone chips are inserted between the facets and
the interlaminar space.

1 Plate
2 Bone chips
3 Screw

Figure 2.17

The Magerl hook-plate technique

A
The entry point of drilling is 1 mm medial and inferior to the center of the lateral mass, and the drilling is angled 25° laterally and 45° superiorly.

1   25° lateral and 45° superior

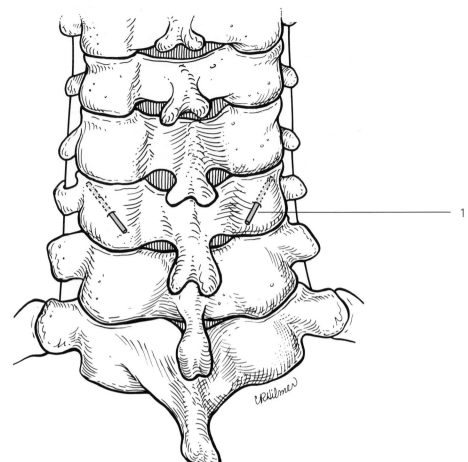

B
A small notch is made in the inferior edge of the lamina for hook insertion.

1   Bone graft
2   Hook-plate

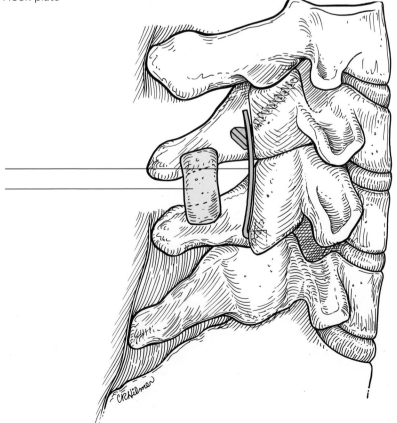

C
An H-shaped bone graft is placed between the spinous processes, and the screws are tightened.

1 Screw
2 Hook-plate
3 Bone graft

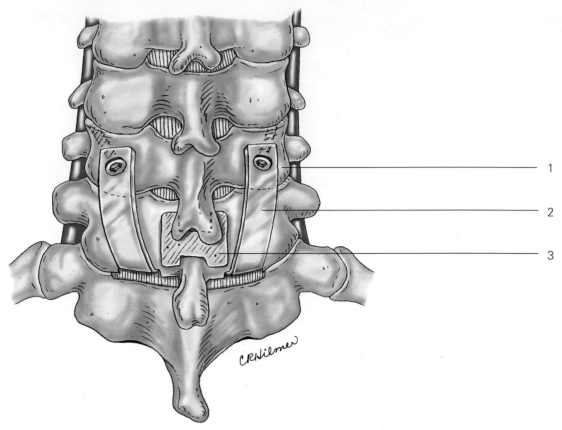

1

2

3

Bibliography

An HS (1992a) Surgical exposure and fusion techniques of the spine. In: HS An, JM Cotler (eds), *Spinal Instrumentation*. Baltimore, Williams & Wilkins

An, HS (1992b) Internal fixation of the cervical spine. *Sem Spin Surg* **4**: 142–52

An HS, Simpson JM (1994) *Surgery of the Cervical Spine*. London and Baltimore, Martin Dunitz and Williams & Wilkins

An HS, Gordin R, Renner K (1991) Anatomic consideration for plate–screw fixation of the cervical spine. *Spine* **16**:548–51

Anderson PA, Henley MB, Grady MS et al (1991) Posterior cervical arthrodesis with AO reconstruction plates and bone graft. *Spine* **16**:S72-S79

Brooks AL, Jenkins EB (1978) Atlanto-axial arthrodesis by the wedge compression method. *J Bone Joint Surg* **60A**:279–84

Gallie WE (1939) Fractures and dislocations of the cervical spine. *Am J Surg* **46**:494–9

Grob D, Dvorak J, Panjabi M et al (1994) The role of plate and screw fixation in occipitocervical fusion in rheumatoid arthritis. *Spine* **19**:2545–51

Jeanneret B, Magerl F, Halterward E et al (1991) Posterior stabilization of the cervical spine with hook plates. *Spine* **16**:S56–S63

Magerl F, Seemann P (1987) Stable posterior fusion of the atlas and axis by transarticular screw fixation. In: P Kehr, A Weidner (eds), *Cervical Spine 1*, p322. New York, Springer-Verlag

Meyer PR Jr (1989) Surgical stabilization of the cervical spine. In: PR Meyer (ed), *Surgery of Spine Trauma*, pp397–524. New York, Churchill Livingstone

Ransford AO, Crockard HA, Pozo JL et al (1986) Craniocervical instability treated by contoured loop fixation. *J Bone Joint Surg (Br)* **68**:173–7

Rogers WA (1957) Fractures and dislocations of the cervical spine: An end-result study. *J Bone Joint Surg (Am)* **39**:341–76

Roy-Camille R, Mazel C (1989) Stabilization of the cervical spine with posterior plates and screws. In: HH Sherk (ed), *The Cervical Spine* 2nd edn, pp579–80. Philadelphia, JB Lippincott

Roy-Camille R, Sailant G, Laville C et al (1992) Treatment of lower cervical spinal injuries – C3 to C7. *Spine* **17**:S442–S446

Weiland DJ, McAfee PC (1991) Posterior cervical fusion with triple-wire strut graft technique: One hundred consecutive patients. *J Spinal Disorders* **4**:15–21

Wertheim SB, Bohlman HH (1987) Occipitocervical fusion. *J Bone Joint Surg (Am)* **69**:833–6

3

Anterior transoral procedures

Nigel Mendoza
H Alan Crockard

Introduction

An anterior transoral procedure allows surgical exposure of the midline between the arch of the atlas and the C2–C3 intervertebral disc. The exposure may be increased in a cephalad direction by dividing the soft and hard palate to allow access to the foramen magnum and the lower half of the clivus and even further to the sphenoid sinus with an extended 'open door' maxillotomy. The transoral approach allows excellent midline access but is limited laterally by the vertebral arteries within the spine, and as they cross the craniocervical junction, the carotid arteries within the carotid canal and the jugular bulb surrounded by the lower cranial nerves (Fig. 3.1A).

The transoral procedure is a technically demanding operation which requires a complete understanding of the surgical anatomy and careful patient selection following appropriate preoperative assessment and investigation. While the need for such an operation is uncommon, a thorough understanding of and facility with the procedure is mandatory for any surgical unit that provides a comprehensive management program for pathology of the upper vertebral column.

Indications

1. Irreducible atlantoaxial subluxation (alone or in combination with posterior stabilization)
2. Midline anterior extradural spinal cord compression
3. As part of a 360° approach for bone tumour resection
4. Midline anterior intradural spinal cord compression
5. Mid-basilar artery aneurysms.

Anatomy

The anterior tubercle on the arch of C1 is separated from the oropharynx by the pharyngeal mucosa and muscles, which take their origin from the pharyngeal tubercle on the occipital bone and the medial pterygoid plates (Fig. 3.1B,C). In the midline the pharyngeal muscles insert into the pharyngeal raphe and, cephalad to the pharyngeal, to the back of the clivus. The prevertebral fascia lies ventral to the prevertebral muscles and is attached laterally to the tips of the transverse processes. Between the prevertebral fascia and the pharynx is the retropharyngeal space, which contains loose connective tissue through which infection may spread into the mediastinum. The anterior longitudinal ligament has a pointed attachment to the anterior tubercle of the atlas which widens as it descends to its insertion at the sacrum. Lateral to the anterior longitudinal ligament are the longus colli muscles, extending from the atlas to the third thoracic vertebra. Further laterally the longus capitis muscles arise from the anterior tubercles of the transverse processes of C3 to C6 and are inserted into the basilar part of the occipital bone ventral to the foramen magnum. The rectus capitis anterior muscle lies dorsal to the longus capitis arising from the lateral mass of the atlas inserting into the occipital bone ventral to the atlanto-occipital joint.

Dorsal to the arch of the atlas lies the median atlantoaxial joint, a synovial articulation between the odontoid peg and an oval facet on the posterior surface of the arch of the atlas, and between the posterior surface of the odontoid peg and the transverse ligament (Fig 3.1D). The transverse ligament of the atlas is attached to tubercles on the medial aspect of the lateral masses of the atlas and holds the odontoid peg firmly in place. Arising from the transverse ligaments is the superior crus, which is attached to the anterior edge of the foramen magnum, and the

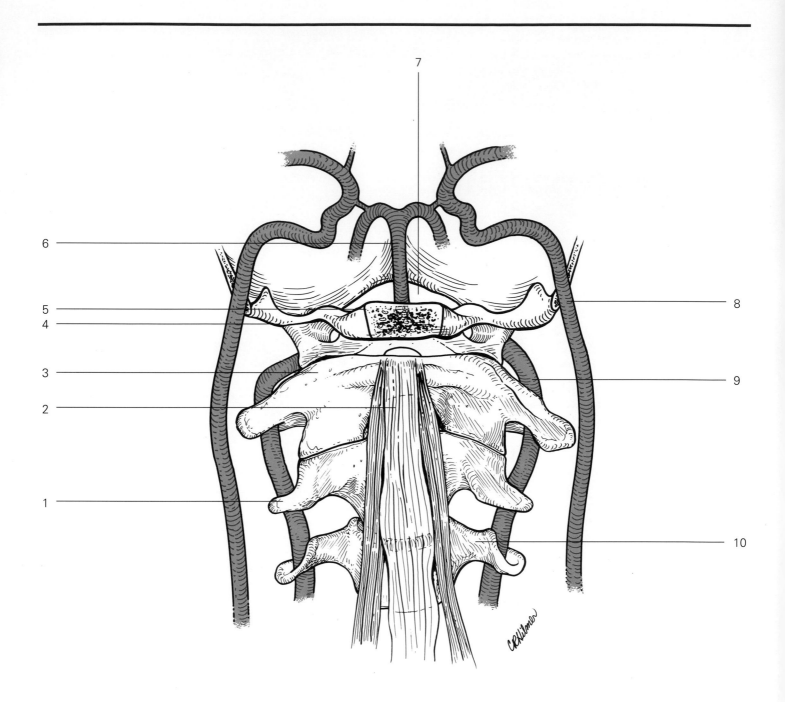

Figure 3.1

A

The key surgical landmark is the tubercle on C1 to which the longus colli muscles are attached. The vertebral artery is at a minimum of 1 cm from the midline.

1   Axis
2   Tubercle
3   Atlas
4   Lat. portion of occipital bone
5   Basilar portion of occipital bone
6   Basilar a.
7   Foramen magnum
8   Internal corotid a.
9   Vertebral a.
10 Longus colli m.

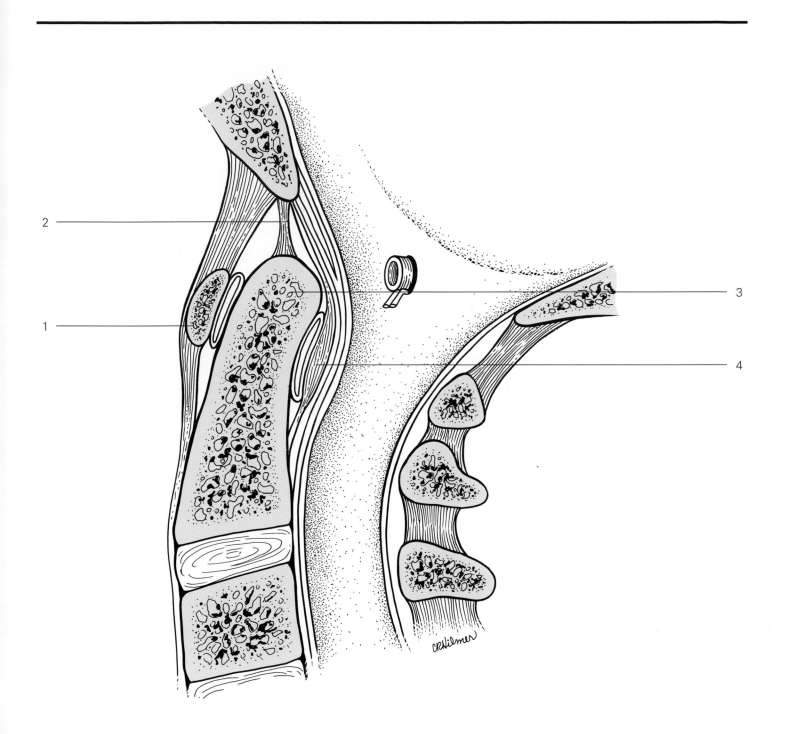

B
Sagittal section of craniocervical junction to illustrate the
articular and ligamentous relations of the dens.

1 Ant. arch of C1
2 Apical lig.
3 Odontoid
4 Transverse lig.

Contd

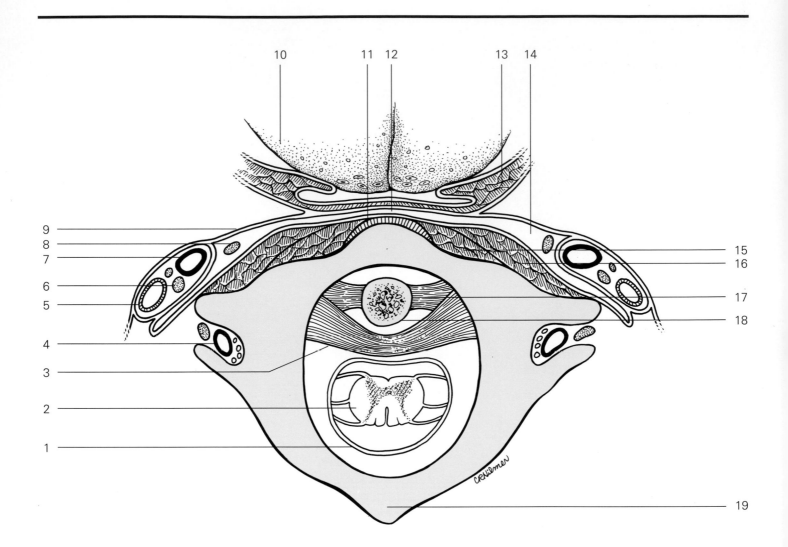

Figure 3.1 *(contd)*

C
Axial section through the atlas

1   Dura
2   Spinal cord
3   Transverse lig.
4   Vertebral a.
5   Internal jugular v.
6   Vagus n.
7   Internal carotid a.
8   Sup. cervical ganglion
9   Prevertebral fascia
10 Tongue
11 Ant. longitudinal lig.
12 Pharyngeal raphe
13 Pharyngeal m.
14 Retropharyngeal space
15 Longus capitis m.
16 Longus colli m.
17 Alar lig.
18 Odontoid peg
19 Arch of atlas

inferior crus, which is attached to the body of the axis. The tectorial membrane is the upward extension of the posterior longitudinal ligament and is attached within the anterior edge of the foramen magnum behind the superior crus.

The alar ligaments arise from either side of the apex of the odontoid peg and are inserted into the occipital condyles. The apical ligament lies between the two alar ligaments and is attached to the anterior margin of the foramen magnum between the superior crus and the anterior atlanto-occipital membrane. The three ligaments represent a 'fan-shaped' ligamentum continuum enveloping the tip of the peg.

The vertebral arteries follow a hexagonal-shaped course; they pass through the foramen transversarium of C2 and C1 ventral to the nerve roots, and lie in the vertebral groove of C1, dorsal to the atlanto-occipital joint, before entering the dura at the foramen magnum (Fig. 3.1A). In the non-rotated head the average distance from the midline of the vertebral artery is 14 mm at the axis, 22 mm at the atlas and 14 mm at the foramen magnum.

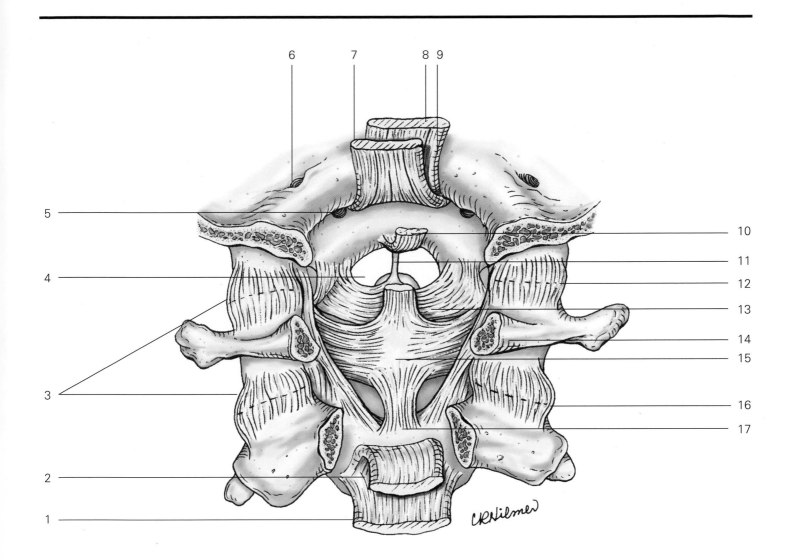

D
Upper cervical and craniocervical articulations and ligamentous structures.

1   Longitudinal lig.
2   Tectorial memb.
3   Articular capsules
4   Top of dens
5   Hypoglossal canal
6   Jugular foramen
7   Tectorial memb.
8   Longitudinal lig.
9   Post. longitudinal lig.
10   Sup. crus of cruciform lig.
11   Apical dental lig.
12   Atlanto-occipital joint
13   Alar lig.
14   Post. arch of atlas
15   Transverse lig. of atlas
16   Atlantoaxial joint
17   Inf. crus of cruciform lig.

Surgical technique

Dental sepsis must be eradicated before elective surgery, since this has been associated with both postoperative wound infection and septicemia. The interdental space should be greater than 25 mm to allow placement of the instrumentation. In the presence of severe temporomandibular disease it may be necessary to perform a midline mandibular split to allow adequate exposure. Baseline somatosensory evoked potentials are measured to compare to intra-operative monitoring values. Fiberoptic nasotracheal intubation is employed so as to reduce the risk to the unstable craniocervical junction and spinal cord that may occur with direct laryngoscopy and orotracheal intubation. A nasogastric tube is passed so as to prevent postoperative wound contamination and empty swallowed blood from the stomach.

The patient is placed in the 3/4 supine position with the head held in the Mayfield frame, making full use of the lateral tilt facility of the operating table, which allows both a transoral and a posterior

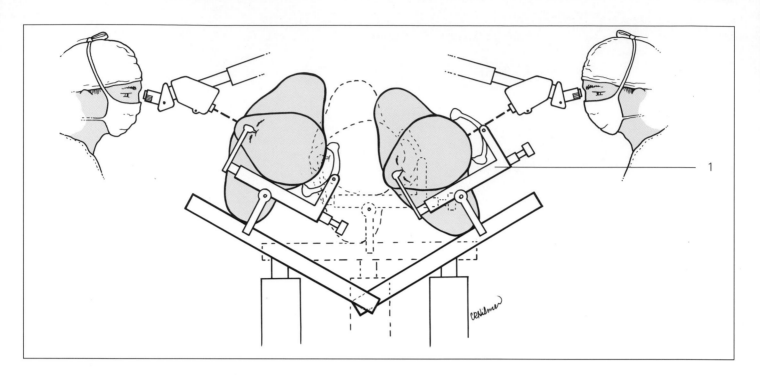

Figure 3.2

A

The patient is placed in the lateral position with the head held in the Mayfield frame. This allows both a transoral and a posterior exposure while maintaining stability and drainage of blood from the surgical field by gravity, whilst the surgeon may be seated using the operating microscope to perform the transoral procedure.

1   Mayfield frame

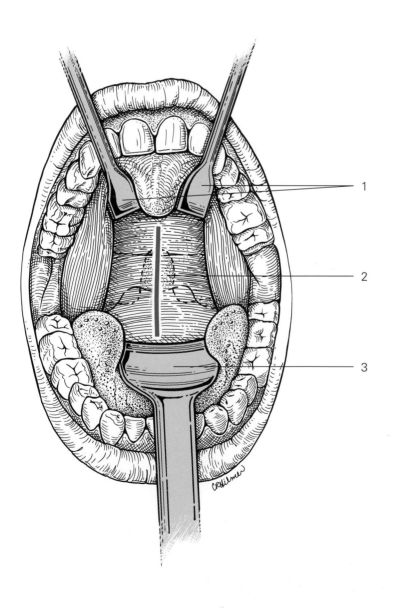

B

A 3 cm midline vertical pharyngeal incision is made centered on the anterior tubercle of the atlas.

1   Soft palate retractors
2   Incision
3   Tongue retractor

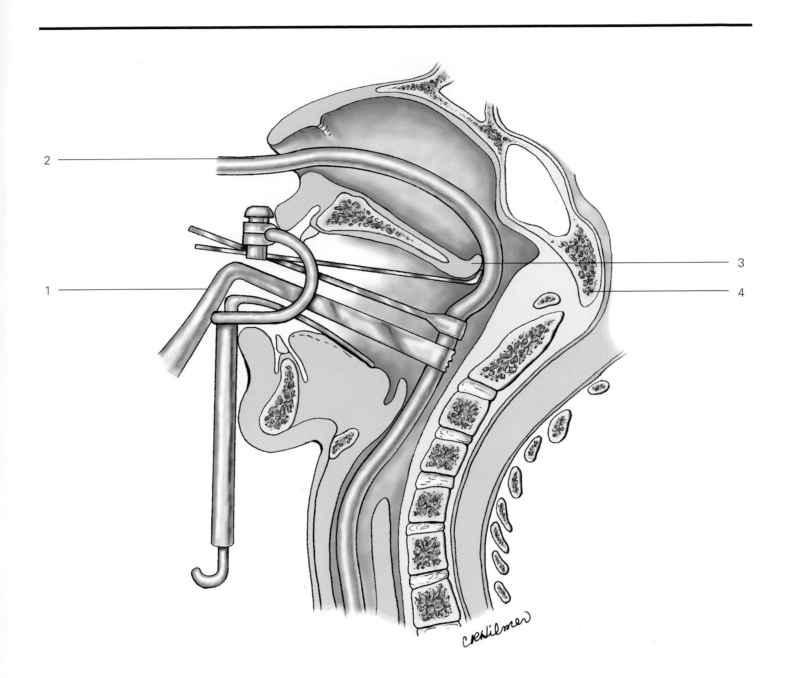

C
The sagittal view with insertion of the retractor blades. Note the retraction of the nasoendotracheal tube to a lateral position in the oropharynx to facilitate the exposure and elevation of the soft palate to expose the anterior rim of the foramen magnum.

1   Pharyngeal retractor
2   Nasoendotracheal tube
3   Soft palate
4   Ant. rim of foramen magnum

Contd

exposure (Fig. 3.2A). This position allows simultaneous anterior and posterior approaches by turning the table 45° to either side of the horizontal plane (Fig. 3.2A). This position also allows drainage of blood from the surgical field by gravity while the surgeon is seated using the operating microscope to perform the transoral procedure. Alternatively, if the transoral procedure is performed alone, the patient is positioned supine with the head slightly extended. Attention and protection must be given to the pressure areas to prevent neuropraxia and pressure sores from developing.

The oral cavity is cleansed with aqueous chlorhexidine. One per cent hydrocortisone ointment is applied to the lips and tongue to prevent postoperative edema, and is continued for 48 hours following

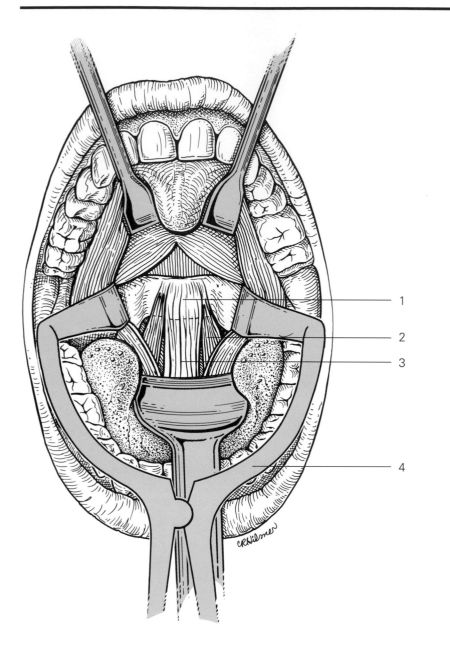

Figure 3.2 *(contd)*

D
The pharyngeal retractor converts the vertical incision into a hexagon and will expose the tubercle of the atlas, the anterior longitudinal ligament and the longus colli muscles.

1   Tubercle of atlas
2   Ant. longitudinal lig.
3   Left longus colli m.
4   Pharyngeal retractor

the operation. Perioperative antibiotics, with an intravenous cephalosporin and metronidazole, are instituted for 72 hours as prophylaxis against wound infection. They are then stopped even in the presence of a CSF leak, and only recommended when there is evidence of local or systemic infection.

The key surgical landmark is the anterior tubercle on the atlas, to which the anterior longitudinal ligament and longus colli muscles are attached. The vertebral artery is at a minimum of 20 mm from this point in the midline. The transoral tongue retractor is then inserted, exposing the posterior oropharynx. If the handle of the tongue retractor is elevated away from the chest further caudal retraction is obtained, allowing exposure of the C2 and C3 intervertebral disc. The palatal retractors are inserted to elevate the

soft palate to expose the anterior rim of the foramen magnum, the atlas and axis (Fig. 3.2B). The retractors also keep the nasotracheal and nasogastric tubes to one side so that they may be kept out of the operative field. The retractors are attached to the base ring so that they become self retaining (Fig. 3.2C). The area of the incision is infiltrated with 1:200 000 adrenalin. A midline 3 cm vertical incision centered on the anterior tubercle is made through the pharyngeal mucosa and muscle. The pharyngeal retractor is inserted, converting the vertical incision into a hexagon to expose the tubercle of the atlas, the anterior longitudinal ligament and the longus colli muscles (Fig. 3.2D). The origins of the anterior longitudinal ligament and the longus colli muscles are then divided with cutting diathermy, remaining as close as

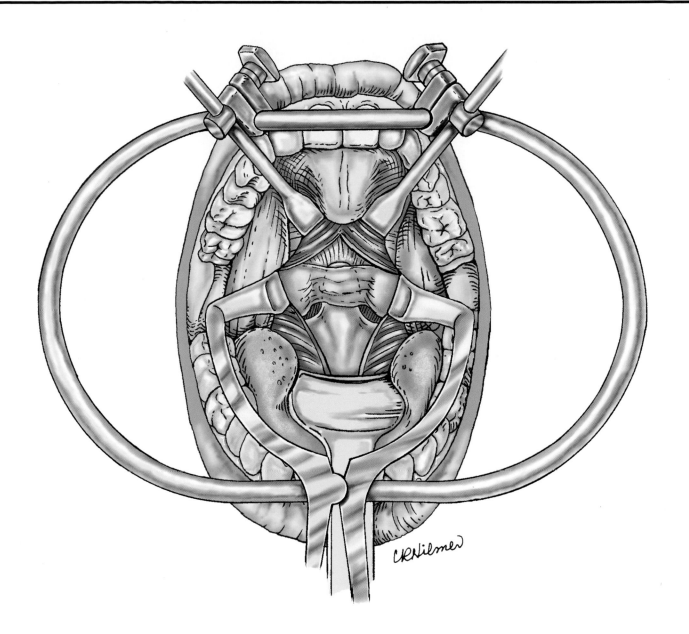

possible to bone, and reflected with a sharp dissector to complete the exposure of the arch of the atlas (Fig. 3.2E).

A high speed air drill is used to remove 10–15 mm of the anterior arch of the atlas to expose the odontoid peg or the lesion that lies in the predental space. If there is odontoid peg instability it may be held in the odontoid peg grasper as it is excised (Fig. 3.3A). Tumours found in this region such as a chordoma or chondrosarcoma are, fortunately, quite soft and well circumscribed, and may well be removed with relative ease using rongeurs or an ultrasonic aspirator or with a laser. If the odontoid peg is to be removed it is shelled out using a high speed cutting burr and then a diamond drill at the posterior cortex in order to prevent inadvertent damage to the poste-

E

The anteroposterior view following division and dissection of the anterior longitudinal ligament and longus colli muscles from the origin so as to expose the arch of the atlas.

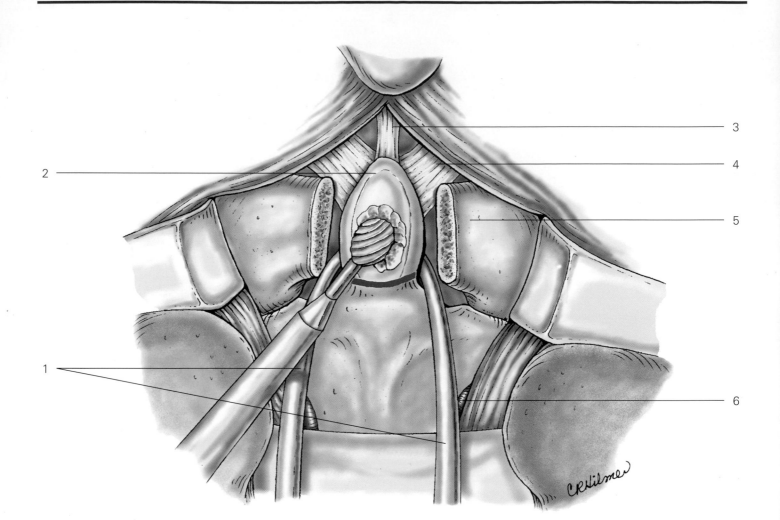

Figure 3.3

A

10–15 cm of the anterior arch of the atlas is removed by a high speed air drill to expose the odontoid peg, which itself may be stabilized in the odontoid peg grasper as it is excised.

1   Odontoid peg grasper
2   Odontoid
3   Apical lig.
4   Alar lig.
5   Arch of atlas
6   Vertebral a.

rior longitudinal ligament and dura (Fig. 3.3B). The alar and apical ligaments may then be identified at the apex of the odontoid peg and are divided using cutting diathermy, again remaining as close to the odontoid bone surface as possible. The remnants of the odontoid peg may then be removed using 1 mm and 2 mm Kerrison rongeurs (Fig 3.3C). Further decompression may then be performed by removal of the transverse ligament, posterior longitudinal ligament or tumor until it is deemed to be adequate as suggested by pulsation of the dura in phase with the cardiac cycle. If an intradural procedure is proposed the dura may then be opened with a midline vertical incision and the dura held back with stay sutures. When the odontoid peg is translocated, as it often is in patients with rheumatoid arthritis, it may be excised without removal of the anterior rim of the foramen magnum by drilling through the base of the odontoid peg, division of the alar and apical ligaments, and removal *en bloc* of the peg by traction with the grasper (Fig. 3.3D).

In order to achieve good wound healing the pharyngeal mucosa and muscle should be closed

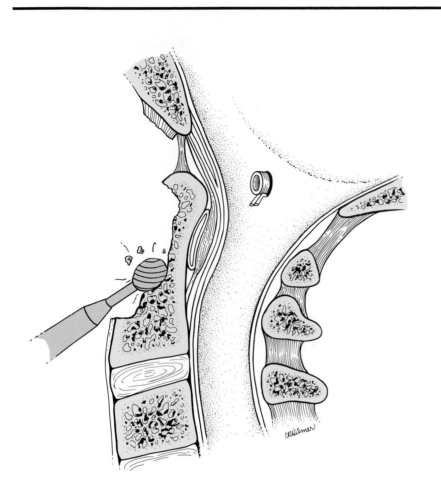

B
The odontoid peg may be removed by drilling out a shell with a high speed metal drill and then a diamond drill at the posterior cortex.

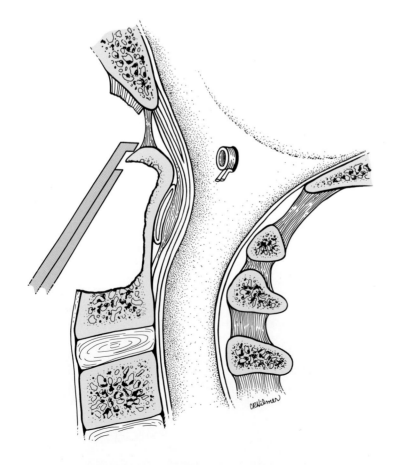

C
After division of the alar and apical ligaments the shell of the odontoid peg may be removed with a Kerrison rongeur.

Contd

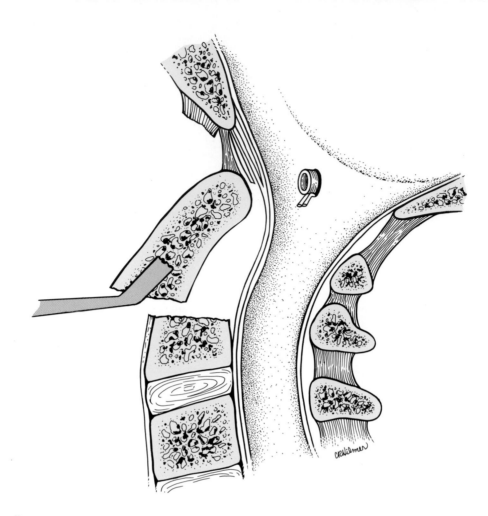

Figure 3.3 *(contd)*

D

The translocated odontoid peg may be excised by drilling through the base, division of the alar and apical ligaments, and removal *en bloc* of the peg by traction with the grasper. This technique does not require removal of the anterior rim of the foramen magnum.

carefully in two layers using interrupted 3/0 absorbable sutures, one layer for muscle and one for mucosa. It is usually only necessary to use 3 or 4 sutures in each layer (Fig 3.4A). The dura may be opened as part of a planned procedure, in which case a lumbar drain is inserted before surgery, or inadvertently, when a lumbar drain should be inserted at the end of the operation (Fig. 3.4A). It is usually not possible to achieve a watertight closure of the dura, and so prevention of a cerebrospinal fluid (CSF) fistula requires meticulous attention to detail. The dural breach is covered with an appropriately sized graft of fascia lata, which in turn is covered with hemostatic agents. A fat graft is then placed on these and a thrombin/fibrinogen glue applied to this multi-layer closure. The pharyngeal mucosa and muscle can then be closed in the usual way in two layers (Fig. 3.4B). To allow continuous drainage of CSF and a low CSF pressure a lumbar drain is inserted for at least five days, at a level to allow a flow rate of 10–20 ml/hr. On occasion it is necessary to convert this to a lumboperitoneal shunt, if the CSF leak persists.

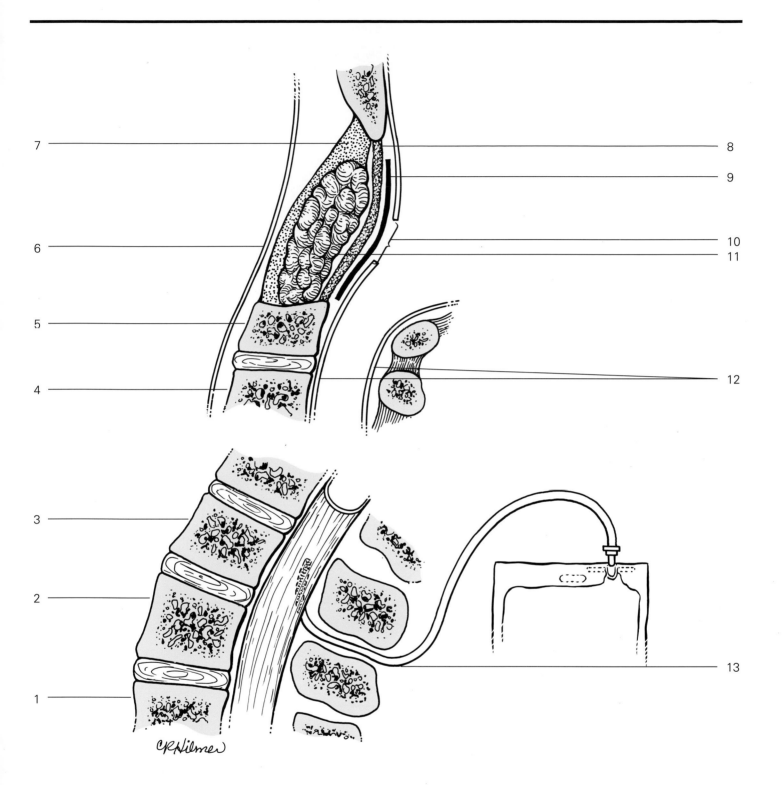

Figure 3.4

A

A dural tear and CSF leak may be repaired with multiple
layers as demonstrated. A lumbar drain is also inserted for at
least five days. The pharyngeal wall is closed in two layers,
as if there were no dural tear.

1   L5
2   L4
3   L3
4   C2
5   C3
6   Mucosa
7   Thrombin/fibrinogen glue
8   Surgicel
9   Fascia lata graft
10 Dural tear
11 Fat graft
12 Dura
13 Lumbar drain

Contd

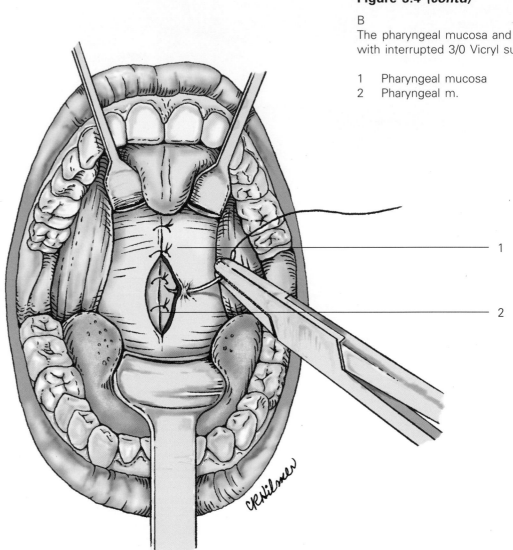

Figure 3.4 *(contd)*

B

The pharyngeal mucosa and muscle are closed in two layers with interrupted 3/0 Vicryl sutures.

1   Pharyngeal mucosa
2   Pharyngeal m.

Complications

Hemorrhage

Intraoperative venous hemorrhage usually arises from epidural veins, which may be controlled by tamponade using small pieces of oxidized cellulose and a cottonoid pattie. Once hemorrhage has been controlled, the operation should proceed at another site for at least five minutes until hemostasis is achieved. If the dura is to be opened, reflection of the dura using stay sutures will control epidural hemorrhage.

Venous hemorrhage will also improve following an adequate decompression.

Arterial hemorrhage may be due to an injury of the vertebral artery or its branches to the dura, tumor or inflammatory pannus. Although this may be controlled by tamponade using hemostatic agents and bone wax the patient may be at risk of a late reactionary hemorrhage, or development of a false aneurysm, necessitating urgent surgical intervention or balloon embolization. If hemorrhage from the vertebral artery is uncontrollable it is necessary to expose the vertebral artery in the foramen transversarium for it to be ligated, or compressed whilst preparation is made for balloon embolization.

Airway obstruction

Oropharyngeal edema may be reduced by the topical application of hydrocortisone and also by ensuring that the tongue and lip are not trapped between the tongue retractor and the teeth. The policy in our Unit is to keep the nasotracheal tube in place for at least 24 hours, during which time the patient is nursed in the intensive care unit. A lateral cervical radiograph is then obtained, and if the postoperative swelling is minimal the tube may be removed.

Infection

The risk of wound infection may be minimized with meticulous surgical technique and prophylactic antibiotics. Contamination of the wound may also be prevented by maintaining the nasogastric tube for at least five days or until there is evidence of mucosal healing. At this stage the patient may be allowed to commence oral fluids.

Spinal instability

Under normal circumstances excision of the odontoid peg does not compromise spinal stability. However, in many patients undergoing transoral surgery there is evidence of subluxation, and odontoidectomy further jeopardizes stability. Thus consideration should be given to the need for spinal fixation at the time of transoral surgery, or postoperative spinal stability should be assessed with plain flexion and extension radiographs.

Temporomandibular joint dislocation

After the transoral procedure has been performed jaw closure and dental occlusion should be assessed to ensure that a temporomandibular joint dislocation has not occurred. If present the dislocation should be reduced at that time.

Bibliography

Calder I (1987) Anaesthesia for transoral and craniocervical surgery. In: *Baillière's Clinical Anaesthesiology*, vol 2, pp441–57. Philadelphia, WB Saunders

Crockard HA (1988) Anterior approaches to lesions of the upper cervical spine. *Clinical Neurosurgery* **34**:389–416

Crockard HA, Sen C (1991) The transoral approach for the management of intradural lesions at the craniocervical junction: Review of 7 cases. *Neurosurgery* **28**:88–98

Crockard HA, Calder I, Ransford AO (1990) One stage transoral decompression and posterior fixation in rheumatoid atlanto-axial subluxation. *J Bone Joint Surg* **72(B)**:682–5

Crockard HA, Koksel Y, Warkin N (1991) Transoral transclival clipping of anterior inferior cerebellar artery aneurysm using new rotating applier. *J Neurosurg* **75**:483–5

Crockard HA, Heilman A, Stevens JM (1993) Progressive myelopathy secondary to odontoid fractures: Clinical, radiological and surgical features. *J Neurosurg* **78**: 579–86

de Oliveira E, Rhoton AL Jr, Peace DA (1985) Microsurgical anatomy of the region of the foramen magnum. *Surg Neurol* **24**:293–352

Dickman CA, Locantro J, Fessler RG (1992) The influence of transoral odontoid resection on stability of the craniovertebral junction. *J Neurosurg* **77**:525–30

DiLorenzo N (1992) Craniocervical junction malformation treated by transoral approach: A survey of 25 cases with emphasis on postoperative instability and outcome. *Acta Neurochir* **118**:112–16

Fang HSY, Ong GB (1962) Direct approach to the upper cervical spine. *J Bone Joint Surg* **44B**:1588–1604

James D, Crockard HA (1991) Surgical access to the base of skull and upper cervical spine by extended maxillotomy. *Neurosurgery* **29**:411–16

Kanaval AB (1919) Bullet located between the atlas and the base of the skull: Technique for removal through the mouth. *Surg Clin* **1**:361–6

Menezes AH, Van Gilder JC, Graf CJ et al (1980) Craniocervical abnormalities. A comprehensive surgical approach. *J Neurosurg* **53**:444–55

Pasztor E (1985) The transoral approach for epidural craniocervical pathological process. In: L Symon (ed), *Advances and Technical Standards in Neurosurgery*, vol 12, pp126–70. Vienna, Springer-Verlag

Pasztor E (1992) Transoral approach to anterior brain stem compression. *Acta Neurochir* **118**:7–19

Scoville WB, Sharman IJ (1951) Platybasia: A report of ten cases with comments on familial tendency, a special diagnostic sign and end results of operations. *Ann Surg* **133**: 469–502

4

Anterior retropharyngeal exposure of the upper cervical spine

Patrick S McNulty
Paul C McAfee

Introduction

The anterior retropharyngeal approach to the upper cervical spine allows adequate exposure for removal and stabilization of lesions extending from the clivus to C3. This approach is a superior extension of the approach described by Southwick and Robinson (1957) for exposing the middle and lower cervical spine. Because it is also entirely extramucosal, the approach can be used to effectively decompress the spinal canal anteriorly and insert an anterior stabilizing strut graft. The extramucosal aspect of the approach avoids the high infection rate (50%) associated with the transoral approach (Fang and Ong 1962), making it especially advantageous if bone grafting is to be done. The approach does not require an osteotomy of the mandible and tongue splitting, or dislocation of the temporomandibular joint, as described with other anterior approaches to the upper cervical spine (Riley 1973, Hall et al 1977). Although the lateral approach by Whitesides (1983) is extramucosal, it does not easily allow for long anterior strut grafting, nor does it allow for easy visualization and access to both vertebral arteries.

Indications

1 Decompression and stabilization of fixed atlantoaxial subluxation
2 Anterior upper cervical tumor excision
3 Débridement and stabilization of anterior upper cervical spine infections.

Anatomy and general considerations

This approach is a superior extension of the Robinson approach to the lower cervical spine and crosses the same fascial layers. These layers are: (1) the superficial fascia containing the platysma; (2) the superficial layer of the deep cervical fascia surrounding the sternocleidomastoid; (3) the middle layer of the deep cervical fascia investing the omohyoid, sternohyoid, sternothyroid, and thyrohyoid muscles; (4) the visceral fascia enclosing the trachea, esophagus, and recurrent laryngeal nerves; and (5) the deep layer of the deep cervical fascia, which is divided into the alar fascia, connecting the two carotid sheaths via midline fusion to the visceral fascia, and the prevertebral fascia, covering the longus colli and scalene muscles. In addition to being familiar with the anatomy of the neck as it applies to the classic anterior approach to the mid and lower cervical spine, the surgeon should also be familiar with the anatomy of the anterior triangle of the neck. In particular the superficial relationship of the mandibular branch of the facial nerve to the anterior facial vein and the retromandibular vein should be understood, so that denervation of the orbicularis oris muscle and ipsilateral facial droop does not occur. Overall, the approach is submandibular, anterior to the common and external carotid arteries, posterior to the pharynx, and inferior to the hypoglossal nerve.

Arteriography is often an essential part of preoperative planning. It should be considered if preoperative radiographs demonstrate involvement of the foramen transversarium at the second cervical level. Arteriography is also useful in identifying the major feeder vessels to tumors in this region, as well as clearly identifying the location of vertebral arteries displaced by tumors.

Surgical technique

The most important factor to be kept in mind when positioning the patient is preventing neurologic injury due to an unstable spine. Principles to be adhered to are minimizing movement of the patient while under anesthesia and using appropriate spinal cord monitoring. Either Gardner–Wells tongs or a halo ring are placed on the patient while awake. If postoperative stabilization is to include a halo, then a halo ring may be placed at this time so that the patient does not unnecessarily have to go through transfer to a halo ring from Gardner–Wells tongs. Once the head is secured, the patient is then transferred in the supine position to the operative wedge turning frame, where careful neurologic examination is repeated. With the patient awake, the neck is carefully extended as far as possible, but not to the point neurologic symptoms or Lhermitte's sign or changes in spinal cord monitoring potentials are provoked. This position is designated as the maximum amount of extension allowed during the procedure, and this must never be exceeded during intubation or during the operation. Typically, 10 lb of traction is used with either the Gardner–Wells tongs or the halo ring to stabilize the head and neck. Appropriate padding may be used behind the head, neck, and scapula to allow for necessary neck extension. Fiberoptic nasotracheal intubation is performed under local anesthesia. Once the airway has been secured, the patient is placed under general anesthesia and the mouth is kept free of all tubes, such as esophageal stethoscopes, oral airways and endotracheal tubes. Similarly, any dentures should be removed preoperatively. Any objects placed in the oral cavity will cause the mandible to move inferiorly, making the operative exposure more difficult.

For a righthanded surgeon, the approach is typically from the patient's right side. The head may be turned slightly to the left to aid in exposure, but this position should be cleared for neurologic compromise by checking head rotation with the patient awake before induction. The opposite is true for a lefthanded surgeon. If the surgeon does not intend to go below C5, then the rightsided approach will avoid inadvertent injury to the right recurrent laryngeal nerve. If the surgeon intends to extend the approach below C5, then a leftsided approach is safer, to avoid inadvertent injury to the recurrent laryngeal nerve. Accessory

taping should be used at this time to secure the amount of extension and rotation of the head desired. Also, countertraction is applied to the shoulders with tape to the distal end of the operating room table. Again, take care not to exceed the limit of extension and rotation determined prior to induction.

A modified transverse submandibular incision is made (Fig. 4.1A). If exposure is needed to more inferior levels of the cervical spine, the vertical limb may be used. The incision is made through the platysma muscle, and the superficial fascia and skin are mobilized in the subplatysmal plane. The mandibular branch of the facial nerve is now identified with the aid of a nerve stimulator by ligating and dissecting the retromandibular vein superiorly (Fig. 4.1B). It is important to use bipolar cautery on the retromandibular and facial veins to avoid inadvertent injury to the mandibular branch of the facial nerve. If this is injured, the patient will have noticeable droop of the ipsilateral aspect of the mouth secondary to denervation of the orbicularis oris muscle. The common facial vein is usually continuous with the retromandibular vein and the mandibular branch of the facial nerve usually crosses the retromandibular vein superficially and superiorly and is superficial to the anterior facial vein (Fig. 4.1C). By ligating the retromandibular vein as it joins the internal jugular vein, via the common facial vein, and keeping the dissection deep and inferior to the retromandibular and anterior facial veins as the exposure extends superiorly to the mandible, the superficial branches of the facial nerve are protected. The submandibular gland is now dissected and the digastric muscle is divided. The facial, lingual and superior thyroid vessels with the exception of the superior thyroid artery are then isolated, ligated and divided (see Fig. 4.1C). Note that the superior laryngeal nerve may run in close approximation to the superior thyroid artery (Fig. 4.1D).

After the superficial layer of the deep cervical fascia is incised along the anterior border of the sternocleidomastoid, the superior thyroid artery and vein should be ligated (Fig. 4.1E). The hypoglossal and superior laryngeal nerves are mobilized. Remaining branches of the carotid artery and internal jugular vein are ligated to allow retraction of the carotid sheath posteriorly and laterally as the pharynx is mobilized medially. The submandibular gland is resected, its duct being sutured to prevent salivary fistula formation. Resection of the submandibular gland can be optional, and it may be possible to do the exposure by simple retraction instead of resection of the gland. Lymph nodes can be resected as they are encountered and sent for appropriate frozen section if a neoplasm is suspected. The posterior belly of the digastric muscle and stylohyoid muscle are tagged with suture for later repair. Note that the posterior belly of the digastric muscle and the stylohyoid

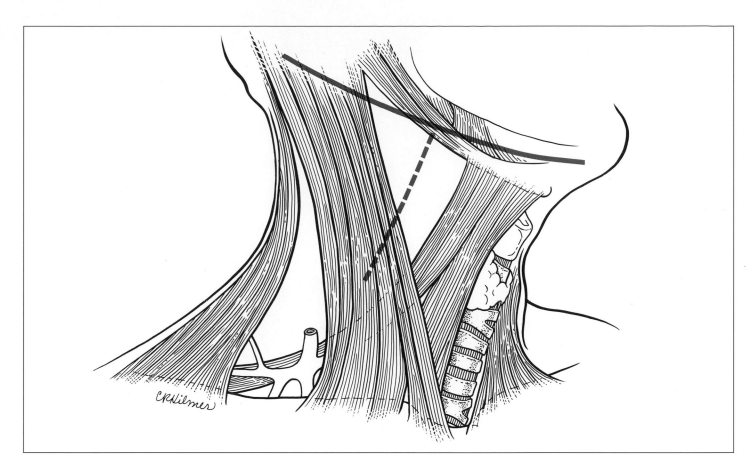

Figure 4.1

A

Submandibular incision on the right side, with optional vertical extension if exposure to mid-cervical levels is required.

Contd

muscle are confluent for all practical purposes during this approach. Care must be taken not to retract near the origin of the posterior belly of the digastric muscle and stylohyoid muscle to avoid neuropraxic injury to the facial nerve as it exits the skull. Division of the posterior belly of the digastric and stylohyoid muscles allows mobilization of the hyoid bone anteriorly and medially, thus allowing mobilization of the pharynx. This will help to avoid inadvertent injury and bacterial infection.

The hypoglossal nerve, which is identified with the aid of a nerve stimulator, is then completely mobilized from the base of the skull to the posterior border of the mylohyoid muscle. It is then retracted superiorly for the remainder of the procedure. The dissection then continues into the retropharyngeal space between the carotid sheath laterally and the pharynx, larynx and esophagus medially. There may be remain-ing smaller branches of the ascending pharyngeal artery and vein which will need to be ligated as well. The superior laryngeal nerve is mobilized with the aid of a nerve stimulator from its origin near the nodose ganglion of the vagus nerve to its entrance into the larynx.

The alar and prevertebral fascia are split longitudinally to expose the longus colli muscles that run longitudinally on the anterior lateral aspects of the spine (Fig. 4.1F). At this point, the surgeon should be oriented to the midline by noting the convergent superior attachment of the right and left longus colli muscles on the anterior tubercle of the atlas. The amount of axial rotation of the head away from the midline is gauged by palpation of the mental protuberance of the mandible. If arthrodesis involves the anterior arch of the atlas or the clivus, then any rotation of the head is undesirable and should be corrected at this time.

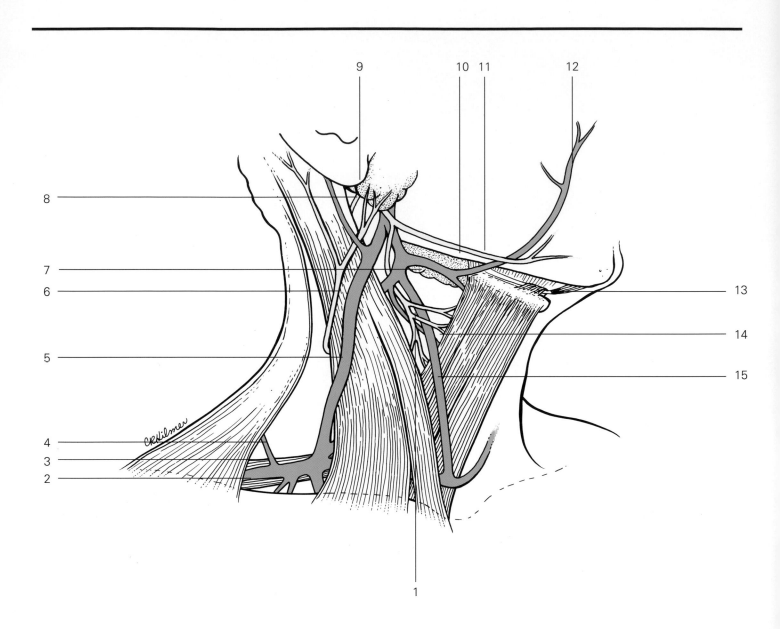

Orientation to midline of the cervical spine is maintained as the longus colli muscles are detached from the anterior surface of the atlas and axis. It is critical to maintain orientation to midline throughout the anterior decompression so that decompression is extended laterally enough to decompress the spinal cord, but not to the point of endangering the vertebral arteries. Previous radiation may make the longus colli muscles thick and fibrotic with edematous changes, making orientation to the midline difficult. The anterior atlanto-occipital membrane is not to be violated, but the anterior longitudinal ligament may be removed in order to see the cord.

Figure 4.1 *(contd)*

B

Anterolateral anatomy of the upper cervical spine, showing superficial neurovascular structures.

1   Sup. root of ansa cervicalis
2   Omohyoid m. (inf. belly)
3   Suprascapular v.
4   Transcervical v.
5   Ext. jugular v.
6   Great auricular n.
7   Submandibular gland
8   Accessory n.
9   Parotid gland
10 Mandible
11 Mandibular branch of facial n.
12 Ant. facial v.
13 Digastric ant. belly
14 Sup. thyroid v.
15 Communicating branch v.

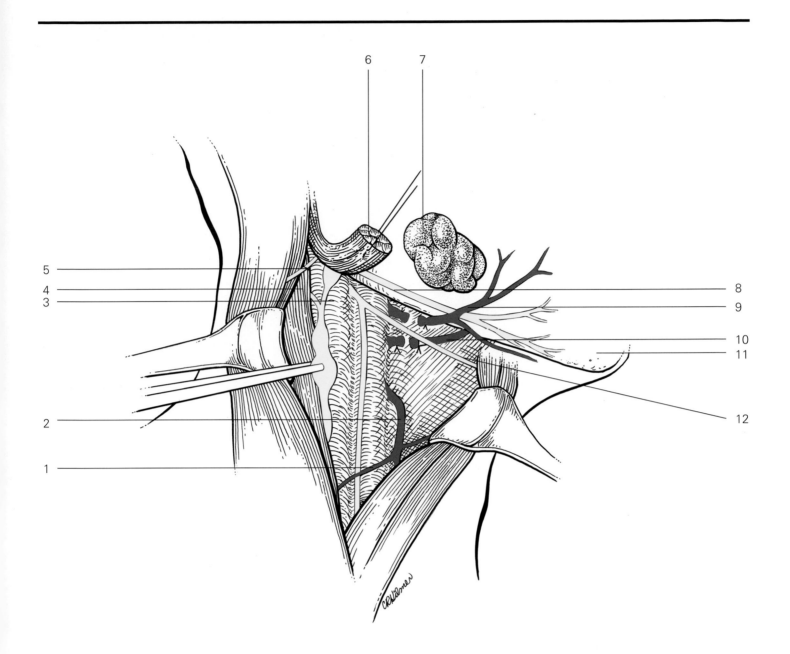

C
Initial dissection: the submandibular gland is resected
and the digastric muscle is divided. Note the
hypoglossal nerve and the marginal mandibular branch
of the facial nerve.

1   Sternomastoid branch of sup. thyroid a.
2   Sup. thyroid a.
3   Int. jugular v.
4   Sternocleidomastoid m.
5   Accessory n.
6   Divided stylohyoid and digastric m.
7   Resected submandibular gland
8   Mandibular branch of facial n.
9   Facial a.
10 Lingual a.
11 Mandible
12 Hypoglossal n.

Contd

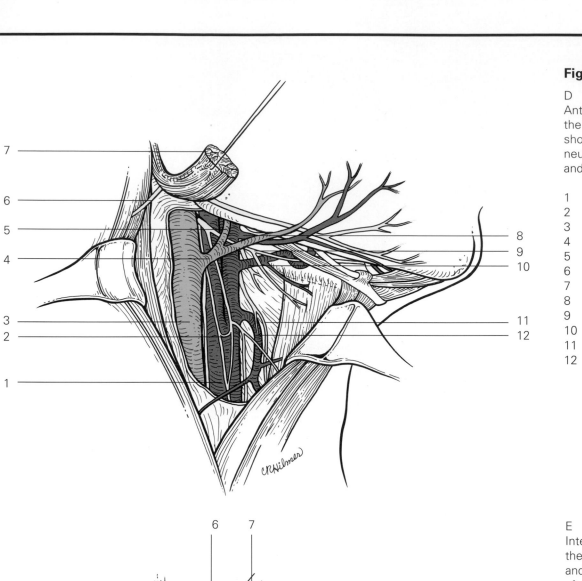

Figure 4.1 *(contd)*

D
Anterolateral anatomy of the upper cervical spine, showing deeper neurovascular structures and initial dissection.

1   Common carotid a.
2   Ansa cervicalis
3   Int. jugular v.
4   Common facial v.
5   Retromandibular v.
6   Spinal accessory n.
7   Divided digastric m.
8   Facial a.
9   Hypoglossal n.
10 Lingual a.
11 Sup. laryngeal n.
12 Sup. thyroid a.

E
Intermediate dissection: the superior thyroid vein and artery are divided after the superficial layer of the deep cervical fascia is incised along the anterior border of the sternocleidomastoid. The hypoglossal and superior laryngeal nerves are mobilized. Additional branches of the carotid artery and internal jugular vein are ligated to allow mobilization between the carotid sheath laterally and the pharynx, larynx, and esophagus medially.

1   Common carotid a.
2   Vagus n.
3   Sternocleidomastoid m.
4   Int. jugular v.
5   Spinal accessory n.
6   Sup. root of ansa cervicalis
7   Facial a.
8   Sup. laryngeal n.
9   Hypoglossal n.
10 Lingual a.
11 Sup. thyroid a.

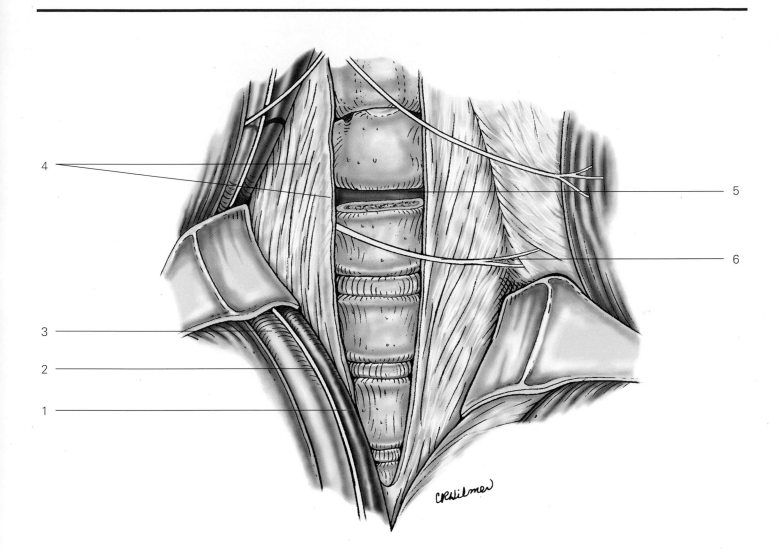

F

Initial spinal decompression: the prevertebral fascia is split longitudinally between the longus colli muscles, exposing the anterior atlas and the C2 body. Discectomy at the C2–C3 level is initially performed to obtain orientation to midline, lateral, and posterior.

1   Common carotid a.
2   Vagus n.
3   Int. jugular v.
4   Longus colli m.
5   Removal of C2–C3 disc and C1 and C2
6   Sup. laryngeal n.

The decompression is started by thoroughly removing the intervertebral disc between C2 and C3 or the first normal disc at the inferior aspect of the lesion (Fig. 4.1F). Seeing the uncovertebral joints at the initial discectomy level helps confirm midline orientation and lateral limits of decompression. The discectomy will also reveal the posterior longitudinal ligament with minimal blood loss. A C2 corpectomy is done with a high speed burr (Fig. 4.2A). Removal of odontoid is necessary for tumor cases (Fig. 4.2B,C) and for rheumatoid pannus (Fig. 4.2D).

Specimens may be sent for frozen section as the decompression progresses superiorly. Blood loss during a corpectomy can be minimized by copious use of thrombin, gelfoam, bone wax, and bipolar cauterization. If the patient does not have cranial settling secondary to basilar invagination of the odontoid, the odontoid can be partially retained to secure the superior aspect of the strut graft. A clothespin shaped strut graft is wedged superiorly into the anterior arch of the atlas and the superior remnants of the odontoid after subperiosteal dissection and decortication. A

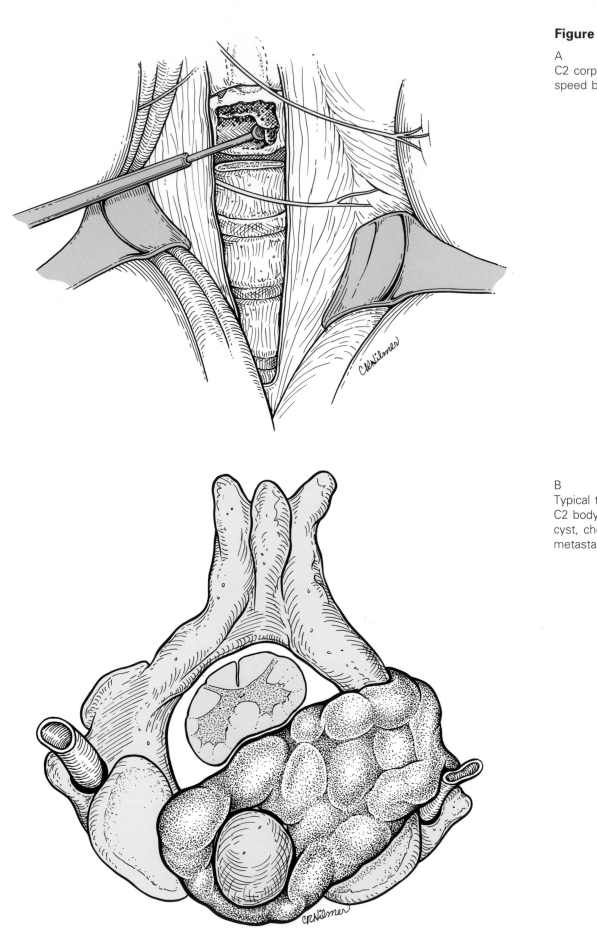

Figure 4.2

A
C2 corpectomy with high speed burr.

B
Typical tumors involving the C2 body (aneurysmal bone cyst, chordoma or metastasis).

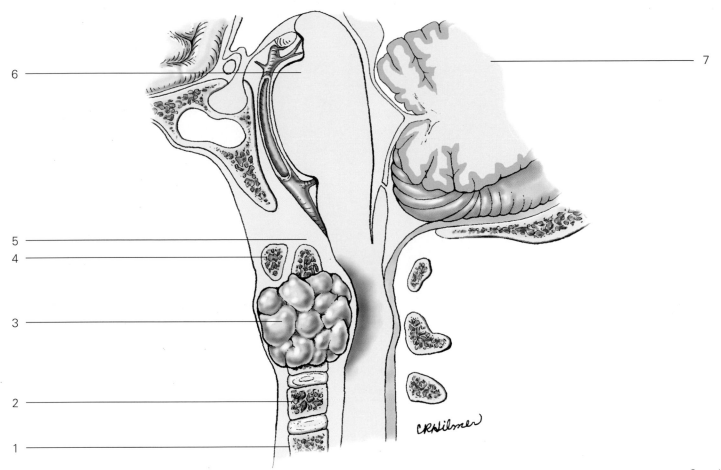

Contd

C
The anterior and middle spinal columns are affected, the spinal cord is compressed anteriorly, and the vertebral artery is occasionally involved.

1 C4
2 C3
3 Tumour in C2
4 Arch of C1
5 Top of dens
6 Pons
7 Cerebellum

clothespin type graft wedged into the clivus instead of remnants of the atlas and odontoid may be indicated in cases such as rheumatoid pannus associated with atlanto-axial subluxation and basilar invagination (Fig. 4.2E,F).

Closure is begun by reapproximation of the digastric tendon. Suction drains are placed in the retropharyngeal space and the subcutaneous space and brought out through stab incisions in the skin. The platysma and skin are sutured in a standard fashion.

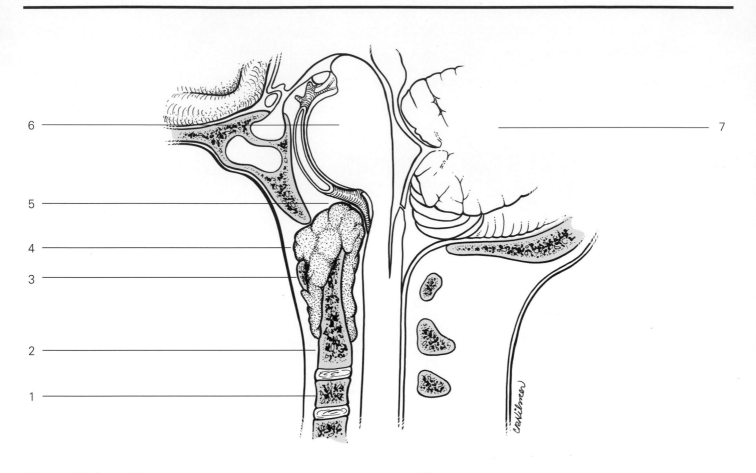

Figure 4.2 *(contd)*

D

Typical rheumatoid pannus impinging on the spinal cord: spinal cord compression secondary to rheumatoid pannus with associated atlantoaxial subluxation and basilar invagination.

1   C3
2   C2
3   Ant. arch of C1
4   Rheumatoid pannus
5   Compression of vertebral-basilar a.
6   Pons
7   Cerebellum

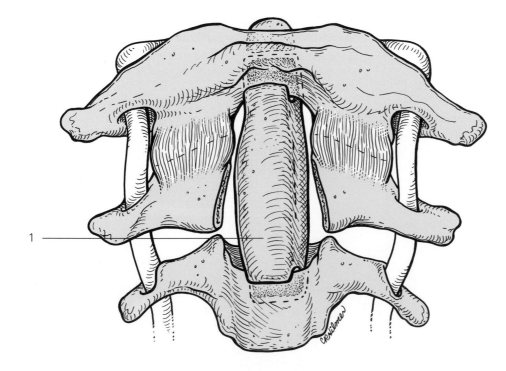

E

The front view shows a clothespin-shaped strut graft inserted into the remnants of the anterior arch of the atlas and odontoid superiorly and the C3 body inferiorly.

1   Graft

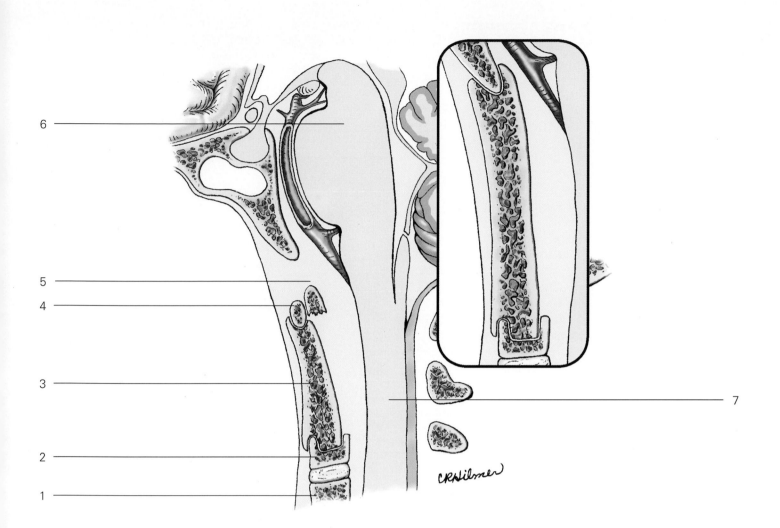

F
Anterior decompression and stabilization is obtained with a
clothespin type strut graft from the clivus to the C3.

1   C4
2   C3
3   Graft
4   C1
5   Odontoid
6   Pons
7   Cord

Postoperative management

If the pharynx or esophagus has been inadvertently entered, a nasogastric tube should be inserted intra-operatively with the wound open under direct vision to ensure that the nasogastric tube bypasses the rent in the pharynx or esophagus. The rent is then closed in two layers with absorbable sutures. Parenteral antibiotics which target the anaerobic oral flora are added to the routine postoperative antibiotic regime. The nasogastric tube is left in place for 7–10 days postoperatively to prevent esophageal or pharyngeal leakage and fistula formation, which can lead to mediastinitis and its associated high mortality rate.

The patient is awakened in the supine position on the operative wedge turning frame and a neurologic examination is performed. The patient is carefully transferred to a bed in the Intensive Care Unit and skull traction is maintained with the head elevated 30° to reduce upper airway edema. Nasal intubation is maintained for 48 hours postoperatively before extubation, and flexible nasopharyngoscopy is used to evaluate upper airway edema at the time of extubation. If it is anticipated that the duration and extent of retraction of soft tissues will prevent extubation within 48 to 72 hours, a tracheostomy should be considered. Skull traction is discontinued and a halo vest is secured approximately 2–4 days postoperatively.

Patients typically remain in a halo for approximately 3 months. The need for a halo may be modified for individual cases, such as those in which there is already a solid posterior associated fusion that has been confirmed intraoperatively. If an anterior strut graft has been performed, it should be thought of as only providing stability to compression. The spine may be unstable to such a point that posterior stabilization may be indicated. This can be done in a one stage combined anterior/posterior procedure.

Complications

In the series reported by McAfee et al (1987), there were no postoperative infections. No patient had a respiratory arrest or required an emergency tracheostomy. The anterior bone grafts may loosen as well as the halo rings, and one may encounter neuropraxia to the hypoglossal nerve as well as the marginal mandibular branch of the facial nerve. Most of these problems resolved within 3 months. There is also the possibility of inadvertent injury to the pharynx or esophagus. There were no iatrogenic neurologic deficits of the spinal cord or nonunions of the arthrodesis. There were no deaths due to the procedure.

Conclusions

The anterior retropharyngeal approach to the upper cervical spine has several advantages over transmucosal approaches or the lateral Whitesides approach that make it the preferred approach for most upper cervical procedures. The transmucosal approach should be reserved mainly for biopsies and drainage of infections. The lateral retropharyngeal approach has the disadvantages that: (1) the anterior decompression of the spinal cord is more difficult and does not provide a direct anterior visualization of the vertebral bodies; (2) the narrow interval makes it more difficult to insert long strut grafts; and (3) the approach does not allow visualization of and access to both vertebral arteries and the approach remains very close to the ipsilateral vertebral artery if an anterior decompression of the spine is performed. Nevertheless, Whitesides' experience with the lateral retropharyngeal approach is very impressive.

Bibliography

Fang HSY, Ong GB (1962) Direct anterior approach to the upper cervical spine. *J Bone Joint Surg* **44A**:1588–1604

Hall JE, Denis F, Murray J (1977) Exposure of the upper cervical spine. *J Bone Joint Surg* **59A**:121–3

McAfee PC, Bohlman HH, Riley LH et al (1987) The anterior retropharyngeal approach to the upper part of the cervical spine. *J Bone Joint Surg* **69A**:1371–83

Riley LH (1973) Surgical approaches to the anterior structures of the cervical spine. *Clin Orthop* **91**:16–20

Southwick WO, Robinson RA (1957) Surgical approaches to the vertebral bodies in the cervical and lumbar regions. *J Bone Joint Surg* **39A**:631–44

Whitesides TE (1983) Lateral retropharyngeal approach to the upper cervical spine. In: The Cervical Spine Research Society, *The Cervical Spine*, pp517–27. Philadelphia, Lippincott

5

Anterior exposures of the lower cervical spine and fusion techniques

Howard S An

Introduction

The Smith–Robinson approach is most commonly used for the exposure of the middle and lower cervical spine, but other approaches may be useful in special circumstances. In addition to surgical exposure of the anterior aspect of the cervical spine, techniques of discectomy and corpectomy and stabilization with different types of bone grafts will be described in this chapter.

Anatomy

The anterior approaches to the cervical spine involve dissections of related vital structures around the neck. The anatomic knowledge of these structures is obviously important in preventing injuries during exposure.

The carotid sheath is an investment of the internal and common carotid arteries, the internal jugular vein, and the vagus nerve. It is adherent to the thyroid sheath and the fascia under the sternocleidomastoid. The carotid artery in the sheath can be palpated for pulsation and retracted but should not be entered during the anterior exposure of the cervical spine.

During the left side approach to the lower cervical spine, the thoracic duct may be encountered. The thoracic duct lies behind the left common carotid artery, internal jugular vein, and vagus nerve, and terminates at the junction of the left internal jugular and subclavian veins. The thoracic duct lies ventral to the subclavian artery, vertebral artery, thyrocervical trunk and the prevertebral fascia, which separates the duct from the phrenic nerve and anterior scalene muscle.

The phrenic nerve lies on the ventral surface of the anterior scalene muscle and is crossed by the inferior belly of the omohyoid muscle and the transverse cervical and suprascapular arteries, and passes between the subclavian artery and vein to reach the thorax. The spinal accessory nerve emerges under the posterior aspect of the sternocleidomastoid muscle between the lesser and greater auricular nerves. The spinal accessory nerve and the cervical plexus innervate the sternocleidomastoid and trapezius muscles. Both the spinal accessory nerve and the phrenic nerve are at risk of injury during anterolateral approach to the cervical spine.

The larynx is an important structure for respiration and vocalization. The cricothyroid muscle is innervated by the external laryngeal branch of the superior laryngeal nerve of the vagus nerve, and the other intrinsic muscles of the larynx are innervated by the recurrent laryngeal nerve. For surgical landmarks, the anterior thyroid cartilage is located at C4–C5, and the cricoid cartilagenous ring is located at C6 (Fig. 5.1A). The superior laryngeal nerve is a branch of the inferior ganglion of the vagus nerve and travels along with the superior thyroid artery. The inferior laryngeal nerve is a recurrent branch of the vagus nerve which innervates all laryngeal muscles except the cricothyroid. On the left side, the recurrent laryngeal nerve loops under the arch of the aorta and is protected in the left tracheoesophageal groove. On the right side, the recurrent nerve travels around the subclavian artery, passing dorsomedial to the side of the trachea and esophagus. It is vulnerable as it passes from the subclavian artery to the right tracheo-esophageal groove. The recurrent laryngeal nerve should be located when working from C6 downward. The best guideline to its location is the inferior thyroid artery. The nerve usually enters the tracheoe-sophageal groove where the inferior thyroid artery enters the lower pole of the thyroid. It is also more common for the right inferior laryngeal nerve to be non-recurrent where it travels directly from the vagus nerve and carotid sheath to the larynx.

Indications

1   Anterior discectomy and fusion for herniated disc or osteophyte
2   Anterior corpectomy and fusion for burst fractures, cervical spondylotic myelopathy, kyphosis, neoplasm, infection
3   Anterolateral approach for vertebral artery exposure, neoplasm.

Surgical technique

Exposure

The patient is positioned supine with Gardner–Wells traction to the head. The reverse Trendelenburg position allows venous drainage and less bleeding during surgery. The cervical spine is extended and slightly rotated toward the opposite side. In order to minimize injury to the recurrent laryngeal nerve, the lower cervical spine is approached from the left. The anatomic landmarks include the hyoid bone overlying C3, the thyroid cartilage overlying the C4–5 interver-tebral disc and the cricoid ring at C6 (Fig. 5.1A). A horizontal incision is used in the majority of cases, but a vertical incision anterior to the sternocleidomastoid may be used for the exposure of multiple levels. A transverse incision in line with the skin crease is made from the midline beyond the anterior aspect of the sternocleidomastoid muscle. The skin and subcuta-neous tissue are undermined slightly and division of the platysma muscle is completed (Fig. 5.1B). The platysma muscle may be divided either horizontally or vertically. Retraction of the divided muscle exposes the sternocleidomastoid muscle laterally and strap muscles medially. The deep cervical fascia is divided between the sternocleidomastoid muscle and strap muscles, and blunt finger dissection is done through the pretracheal fascia while palpating and retracting the carotid sheath laterally (Fig. 5.1C). The omohyoid muscle may be divided if necessary. A self-retaining retractor is then positioned to expose the preverte-bral fascia and longus colli muscles (Fig. 5.1D). A sharp self-retaining retractor should be avoided to prevent perforation of the esophagus medially. It is also important to check for the temporal arterial pulse when the retractor is spread, as prolonged occlusion of the carotid artery may cause brain ischemia and stroke. The superior thyroid artery is encountered above C4 and the inferior thyroid artery is seen below C6. These vessels should be identified and ligated as necessary. One should also be aware of the thoracic duct below C7 during the leftsided approach. The prevertebral fascia is divided longitudinally to expose the disc and vertebral body (Fig. 5.1E). The longus colli muscles are mobilized laterally with a Cobb elevator or curet. The self-retaining retractors are repositioned under the longus colli muscles (Fig. 5.1F). The disc margins are prominent and the verte-bral bodies are concave. A bent 18 gauge needle is placed in the disc space and a lateral radiograph is taken to confirm the correct level (Fig 5.1G).

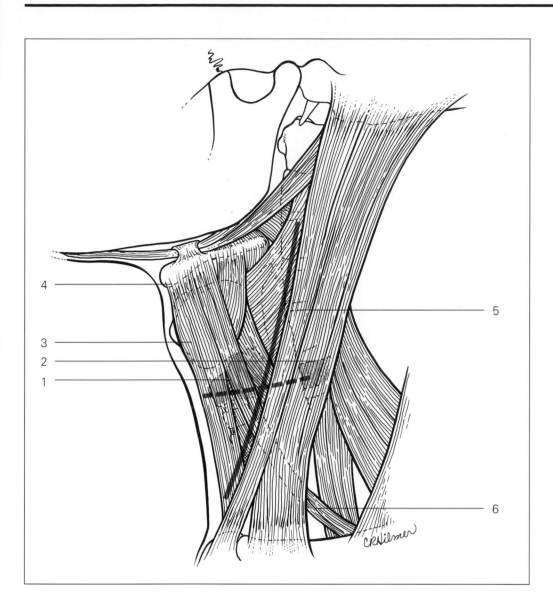

Contd

Figure 5.1

Anteromedial approach to the cervical spine.

A
The anatomic landmarks include the hyoid bone overlying C3, the thyroid cartilage overlying the C4–5 intervertebral disc and the cricoid ring at C6. A horizontal incision or vertical incision anterior to the sternocleidomastoid may be used.·

1   Cricoid ring
2   C6
3   Thyroid cartilage
4   Hyoid bone
5   Sternocleidomastoid m.
6   Omohyoid m.

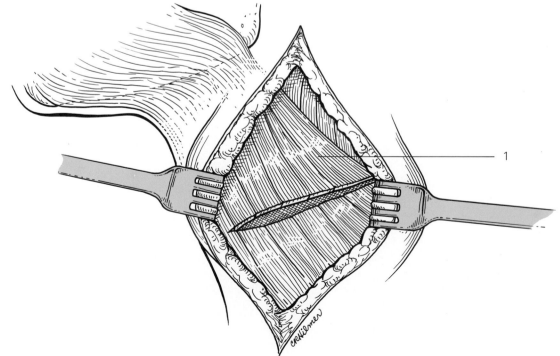

B
A transverse (or vertical) incision in line with the skin crease is made from the midline beyond the anterior aspect of the sternocleidomastoid muscle. The skin and subcutaneous tissue are undermined slightly and division of the platysma muscle is completed.

1   Platysma m.

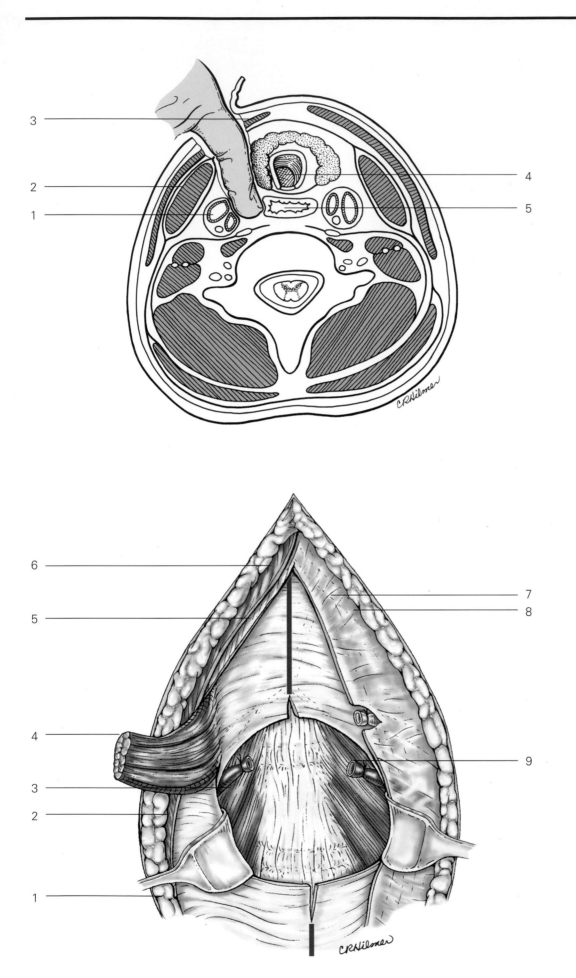

Figure 5.1 *(Contd)*

C
The deep cervical fascia is divided between the sternocleidomastoid muscle and strap muscles, and blunt finger dissection is done through the pretracheal fascia while palpating and retracting the carotid sheath laterally.

1   Carotid contents
2   Sternocleidomastoid m.
3   Platysma m.
4   Trachea
5   Esophagus

D
The omohyoid muscle may be divided if necessary. A self-retaining retractor is then positioned to expose the prevertebral fascia and longus colli muscles.

1   Ant. jugular
2   Cervical fascia
3   Longus colli m.
4   Cut omohyoid m.
5   Cervical fascia
6   Platysma m.
7   Sternocleidomastoid m.
8   Ext. jugular
9   Inf. thyroid a.

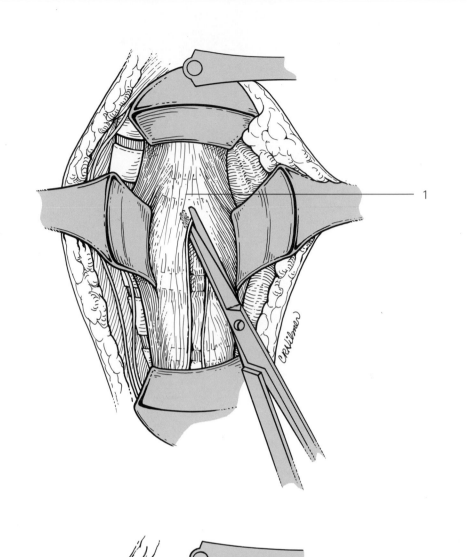

E
The prevertebral fascia is divided longitudinally to expose the disc and vertebral body.

1   Prevertebral fascia

F
The longus colli muscles are mobilized laterally with a Cobb elevator or curet. The self-retaining retractors are repositioned under the longus colli muscles.

1   Longus colli m.

Contd

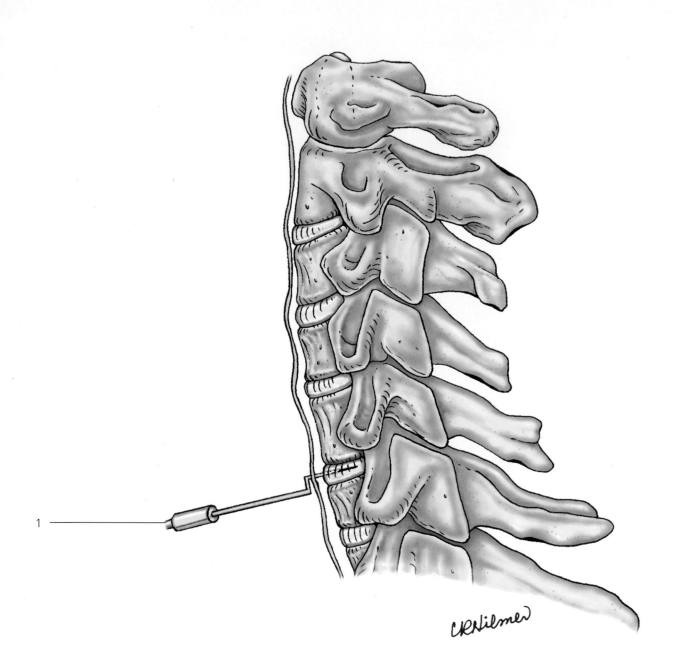

Figure 5.1 *(Contd)*

G

The disc margins are prominent and the vertebral bodies are concave. A bent 18 gauge needle is placed for radiographic localization.

1   Needle

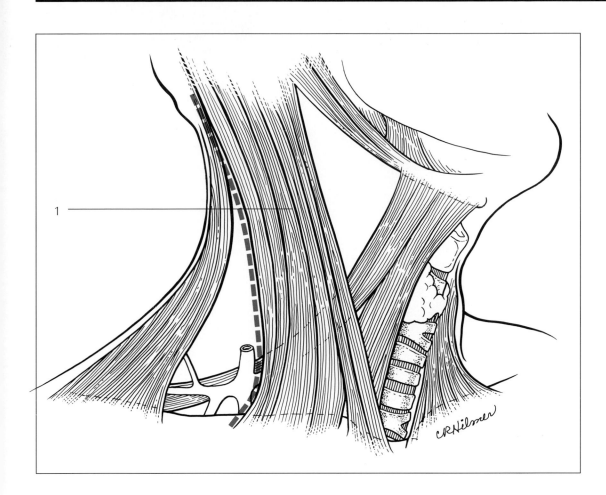

1

Figure 5.2

Alternative approaches
to the cervical spine

A
Anterolateral approach
by Hodgson and King. A
tranverse or oblique skin
incision is made
posterior to the
sternocleidomastoid
muscle.

1   Sternocleidomastoid
m.

Contd

This anteromedial approach to the cervical spine is utilized in the majority of cases. However, in special circumstances, lateral approaches described by Hodgson and King (1956), Henry (1959) and Verbiest (1969) may be used. Hodgson described an approach to the lower cervical spine, dissecting posterior to the carotid sheath to expose the anterior and lateral aspect of the cervical spine. A tranverse or oblique skin incision is made from the right side (Fig. 5.2A). The subcutaneous tissue and the platysma muscle are divided, and the branches of the external jugular vein are ligated, but the cutaneous nerves should be protected. The posterior border of the sternocleidomastoid muscle is identified, and blunt dissection should follow the fat pad through the posterior triangle of the cervical spine. The dissection should stay anterior to the anterior scalene muscle and anterior to the anterior tubercle of the transverse process to avoid injuries to the vertebral artery or nerve root. If retraction of the sternocleidomastoid muscle is difficult, the posterior third of this muscle can be divided to enhance exposure. The inferior belly of the omohy-oid muscle may be divided as necessary (Fig. 5.2B). The cervical sympathetic plexus on the lateral aspect of the prevertebral musculature should be identified and protected. The prevertebral fascia and longus colli muscle are incised in the midline for subperiosteal exposure of the cervical spine. This approach may be extended cephalad to expose the upper cervical spine as described by Whitesides and Kelley (1966) (Fig. 5.2C). Verbiest modified the original approach for exposure of the vertebral artery by Henry: this involves dissecting anterior to the carotid sheath and exposing the vertebral artery and nerve roots posterior to the transverse processes. The dissection is similar to the anteromedial approach by Smith–Robinson initially. After palpation of the anterior tubercle of the transverse process, the anterior tubercle is removed, and the vertebral artery and venous plexus are exposed. The spinal nerve is approached posterior to the vertebral artery. These lateral approaches may be better in cases where the lesion is localized more laterally or if the vertebral artery must be exposed (Fig. 5.2D).

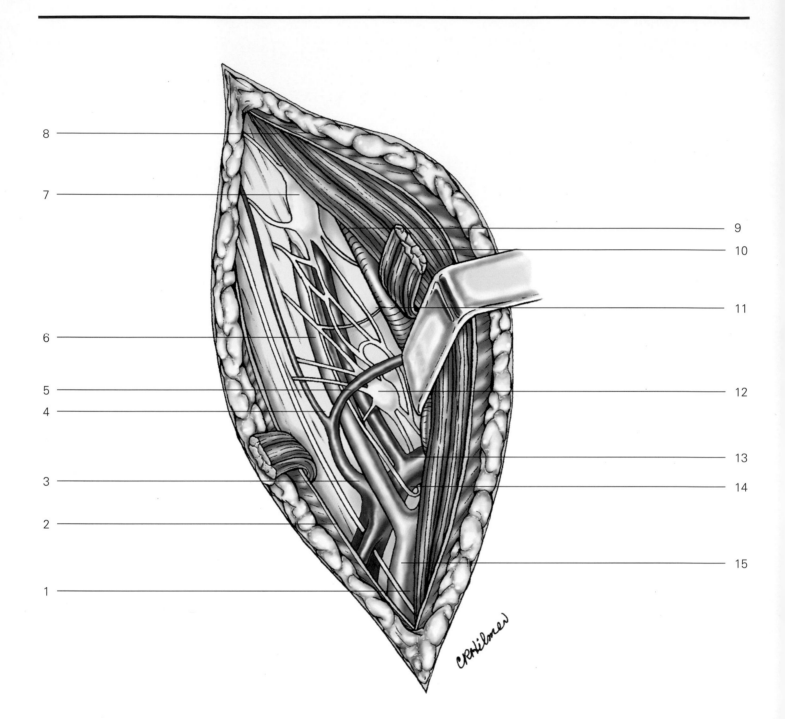

Figure 5.2 *(contd)*

B

The subcutaneous tissue and the platysma muscle are divided. The posterior border of the sternocleidomastoid muscle is identified and blunt dissection should follow the fat pad through the posterior triangle of the cervical spine. Neurovascular structures in the posterior triangle are shown. The inferior belly of the omohyoid muscle may be divided as necessary.

1   Phrenic n.
2   Platysma m.
3   Thyrocervical trunk
4   Ascending cervical a.
5   Inf. thyroid a.
6   Ext. jugular v.
7   Middle cervical ganglion
8   Sternocleidomastoid m.
9   Int. jugular v.
10   Omohyoid m.
11   Inf. thyroid n.
12   Inf. cervical ganglion
13   Subclavian a.
14   Ansa subclavia
15   Subclavian v.

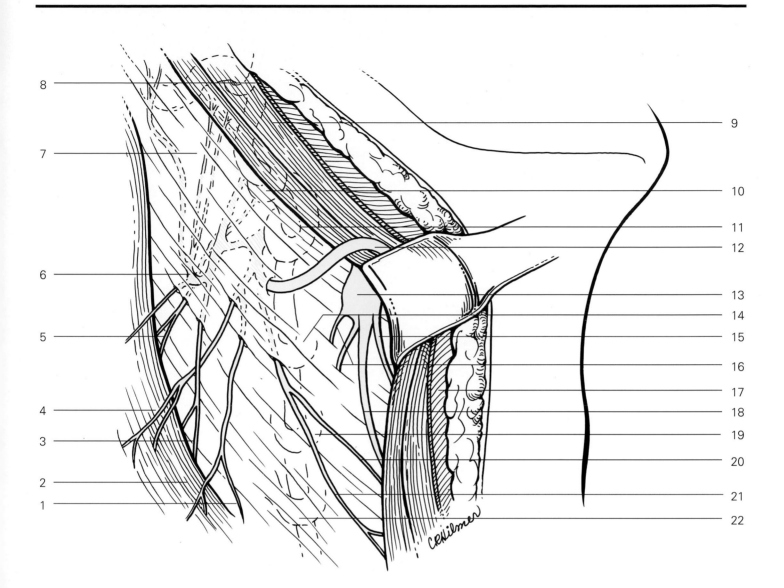

C
This approach may be extended cephalad to expose the
upper cervical spine as described by Whitesides and Kelley.

1 Intermediate supraclavicular n.
2 Trapezius m.
3 Lat. supraclavicular n.
4 Branch to trapezius
5 Spinal accessory n.
6 Lesser occipital n.
7 Prevertebral layer of cervical fascia
8 C1
9 Sternocleidomastoid m.
10 C2
11 C3
12 Great auricular n.
13 Sup. cervical ganglion
14 C4
15 Cardiac branch of sup. cervical ganglion
16 Rami communicantes
17 Platysma m.
18 Sympathetic trunk
19 C5
20 Phrenic n.
21 Med. supraclavicular n.
22 C6

Contd

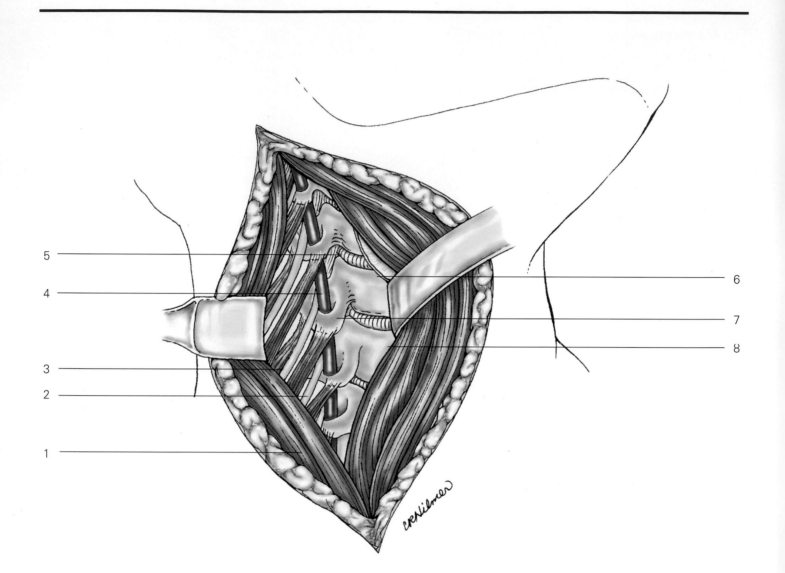

Figure 5.2 *(contd)*

D
The anterolateral approach by Verbiest involves dissecting
anterior to the carotid sheath and exposing the vertebral
artery and nerve roots posterior to the transverse processes.

1   Sternocleidomastoid m.
2   C5 nerve root
3   C4 nerve root
4   Vertebral a.
5   Uncovertebral joint C3–C4
6   C4
7   Ant. tubercle of transverse process
8   C5

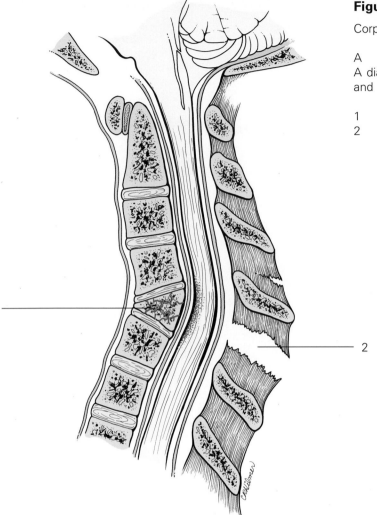

Figure 5.3

Corpectomy for spinal cord decompression.

A

A diagram showing a burst fracture with kyphotic deformity and posterior ligamentous disruption.

1   Burst fracture
2   Ligament disruption

Contd

Anterior discectomy and corpectomy

The proper technique of discectomy and corpectomy cannot be overemphasized, as neurological consequences may be devastating.

Proper lighting and loupe magnification of the surgical field are essential during discectomy. The anulus fibrosus is incised sharply and removed with a rongeur. The nucleus pulposus is removed using curets and rongeur (Fig. 5.3B). All of the disc material is removed down to the posterior longitudinal ligament. If the posterior longitudinal ligament is perforated by the offending disc material, further decompression should be performed on the dural margin. Use of an operating microscope and microsurgical instruments is important during dissection around the posterior longitudinal ligament and the dura. For burst fractures, cervical spondylotic myelopathic cases, or tumors, corpectomy is performed. Following discectomy above and below the vertebra, corpectomy is initiated with a rongeur (Fig. 5.3C). The posterior margin of the vertebral body is thinned with a power burr (Fig. 5.3D). The posterior shell is then removed with an angled curet away from the dura. Traction or distraction may be applied in the corpectomy defect to restore cervical lordosis (Fig. 5.3F).

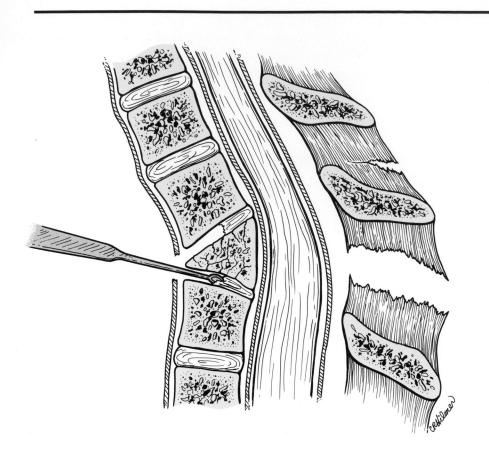

Figure 5.3 *(contd)*

B
The anulus fibrosus is incised sharply and removed with a rongeur. The nucleus pulposus is removed using curets and rongeur.

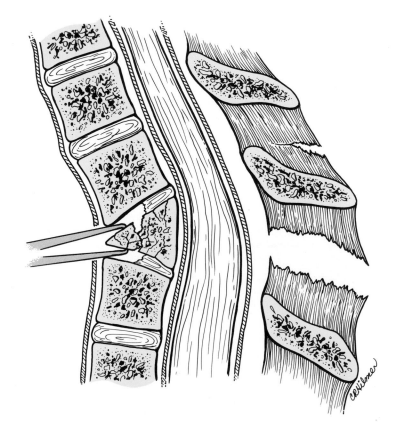

C
Following discectomy above and below the vertebra, corpectomy is initiated with a rongeur.

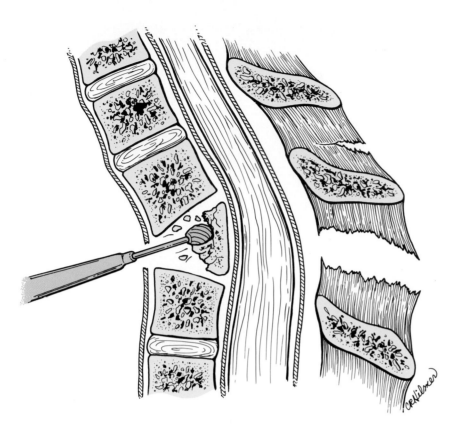

D
The posterior margin of the vertebral body is thinned with a power burr.

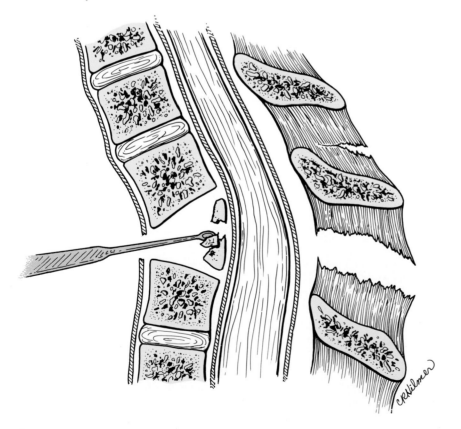

E
The posterior shell is then removed with an angled curet away from the dura.

Contd

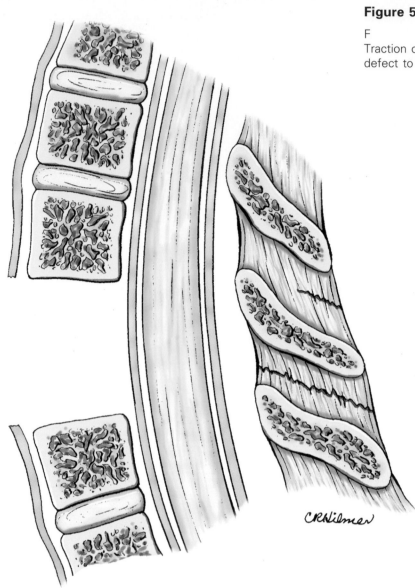

Figure 5.3 *(contd)*

F
Traction or distraction may be applied in the corpectomy defect to restore cervical lordosis.

Anterior cervical fusion techniques

There are several techniques of anterior fusion of the cervical spine. Following discectomy, the Smith–Robinson interbody fusion is preferred by the author (Fig. 5.4A). The graft height should be about 2 mm greater than the degenerated disc space, or at least 5 mm to obtain adequate compressive strength and to enlarge the neural foramina. Overdistraction of the intervertebral space may result in graft collapse and pseudarthrosis. The distraction of the disc space may be achieved by skull traction, laminar spreader or vertebral screws. Traction using the Gardner–Wells tongs is temporarily increased to 30–40 lb. Either a laminar spreader or a vertebral screw distractor are placed for further distraction.

The endplates in the disc space should be burred to create flat surfaces on both sides. Additionally,

small holes may be created in the endplate to promote vascularization of the graft. After measuring the depth and width of the disc space, the tricortical graft is obtained from the anterior iliac crest region. The graft is gently placed 2 mm under the anterior cortical margin of the vertebral body (Fig. 5.4A). The tricortical graft may be reversed so that the cortical margin is placed posteriorly. The traction is then reduced to 5 lb and the laminar spreader is removed. The graft should be stable with compression forces from the endplates. Additional cancellous chips may be inserted into defects in the disc space. Simmons et al. reported on the keystone technique of anterior cervical graft. This technique involves the removal of the endplate and exposure of the cancellous bone for greater potential of graft healing. However, there is a theoretical concern for inadequate maintenance of disc space distraction with this technique (Fig. 5.4B).

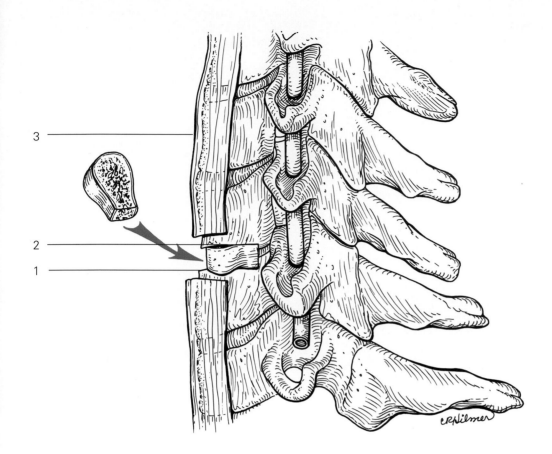

3 —————————————

2 —————————————
1 —————————————

Figure 5.4

Anterior discectomy and
interbody fusion

A
The Smith–Robinson
technique: the tricortical graft
is inserted between the
flattened endplates with 2 mm
distraction and 2 mm
posterior to the anterior
margin of the vertebral body.

1   2 mm countersunk
2   Flattened endplates
3   Ant. longitudinal lig.

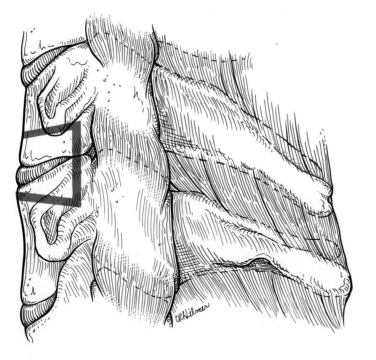

B
The keystone technique by
Simmons: the inferior
endplate of the superior
vertebral body and superior
endplate of the inferior
vertebral body are removed in
a keystone shape, followed by
insertion of a keystone-shaped
graft.

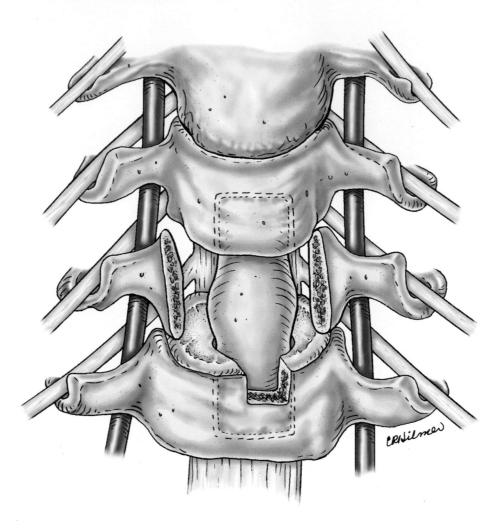

Following corpectomy, strut grafting is performed. The source of the strut graft is mostly from the iliac crest bone, but the fibula may be utilized for multiple level reconstruction cases. A strut graft must be countersunk in order to prevent graft dislodgement. The bone graft may be placed between the inferior endplate of the superior vertebra and the superior endplate of the inferior vertebra, particularly if anterior plating is planned. A longer strut graft that is slotted between the superior endplate of the superior vertebra and the inferior endplate of the inferior vertebra provides greater stability. The slots are created in the vertebral bodies using the power burr and curets. A correctly sized tricortical bone graft is obtained from the iliac crest. The anterior wall of the inferior vertebra is notched to create a window defect (Fig. 5.5A). The graft is inserted into the slot in the superior vertebra first and the graft is placed into the window in the inferior vertebra. While interspace distraction is being applied, the graft is then rotated and tapped into the slot in the inferior vertebra. The distraction is discontinued and the graft should be stable with compression forces from the superior

Figure 5.5

Strut grafting techniques following corpectomy.

A

A strut graft that may be slotted between the superior endplate of the superior vertebra and the inferior endplate of the inferior vertebra. The slots are created in the vertebral bodies using the power burr and curets. A correctly sized tricortical bone graft is obtained from the iliac crest. The anterior wall of the inferior vertebra is notched to create a window defect. The graft is inserted into the slot in the superior vertebra first and the graft is placed into the window in the inferior vertebra. While interspace distraction is being applied, the graft is then rotated and tapped into the slot in the inferior vertebra.

endplate of the superior vertebra and the inferior endplate of the inferior vertebra (Fig. 5.5B). A similar technique may be used to insert a longer fibular strut graft (Fig. 5.5C).

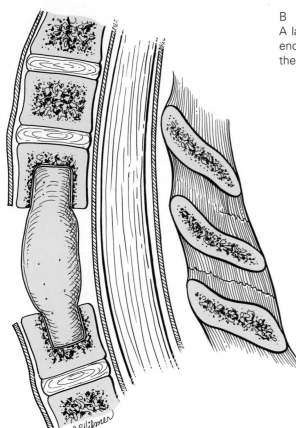

B
A lateral view showing the graft spanning from the superior endplate of the superior vertebra and the inferior endplate of the inferior vertebra.

C
A similar technique may be used to insert a longer fibular strut graft.

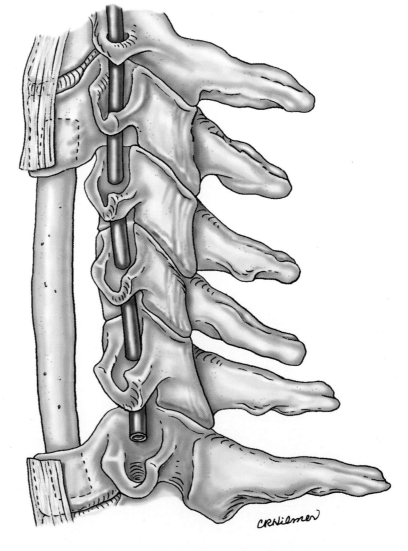

Bibliography

An HS (1992) Surgical exposure and fusion techniques of the spine. In: HS An, JM Cotler (eds), *Spinal Instrumentation*. Baltimore, Williams & Wilkins

An HS, Simpson JM (1994) *Surgery of the Cervical Spine*. London and Baltimore, Martin Dunitz and Williams & Wilkins

An HS, Evanich C, Nowicki B et al (1993) Ideal thickness of Smith–Robinson anterior cervical interbody graft. *Spine* **18**:2043–7

Bohlman HH (1979) Acute fractures and dislocations of the cervical spine: An analysis of 300 hospitalized patients and review of the the literature. *J Bone Joint Surg* **61A**:1119–42

Henry AK (1959) *Extensile Exposure*. Baltimore, Williams & Wilkins

Hodgson AR, King FE (1956) Anterior spinal fusion. A preliminary communication on the radical treatment of Pott's disease and Pott's paraplegia. *Br J Surg* **44**:266.

Robinson RA, Southwick WO (1960) Surgical approaches to the cervical spine. In: The American Academy of Orthopaedic Surgeons, *Instructional Course Lectures*, Vol XVII. St Louis, C. V. Mosby

Simmons EH, Bhalla SK (1969) Anterior cervical discectomy and fusion. A clinical and biomechanical study with eight-year follow-up. *J Bone Joint Surg* **51B**:225–32

Verbiest H (1969) Anterolateral operations for fractures and dislocations in the middle and lower parts of the cervical spine. *J Bone Joint Surg* **51A**:1489–1530

Whitesides TE Jr, Kelley RP (1966) Lateral approach to the upper cervical spine for anterior fusion. *South Med J* **59**:879–83

6

Anterior instrumentations of the cervical spine

Howard S An

Introduction

Recently, several devices have been developed and implemented for osteosynthesis of the anterior cervical spine. The most common indication for anterior cervical surgery remains degenerative conditions. Techniques such as Smith–Robinson fusions have been widely accepted and successful for degenerative conditions. However, in a traumatic unstable cervical spine, bone graft alone may not offer sufficient stability. Additional methods and techniques for augmentation of cervical stabilization have been employed. These methods include concomitant posterior arthrodesis, prolonged immobilization in a halo-vest device or other external cervical orthosis, and prolonged bed rest with cranial tong traction. Anterior decompressive procedures followed by stabilized reconstructive techniques potentially offer a sufficient stability through a single surgical approach and minimize patient morbidity. In this chapter, techniques of anterior screw stabilization of the odontoid and anterior plate–screw stabilization of the lower cervical spine will be illustrated.

Anterior screw stabilization of the odontoid

Indications

The traditional approach for the treatment of odontoid fractures is conservative management through halo immobilization, as a large percentage of these fractures heal uneventfully. However, for widely displaced Type II fractures, early surgical stabilization may be contemplated to enhance the potential for fracture healing and the patient's functional recovery. The rationale for direct anterior fixation is the preservation of the C1–C2 rotation, while providing rigid internal fixation without the requirement for restrictive bracing and avoiding the additional complications associated with bone grafting techniques.

The indications for this technically demanding procedure may include displaced odontoid fractures that cannot be reduced adequately through skeletal traction or use of a halo device. Also, patients with fractures of the odontoid associated with a concomitant C1 ring fracture are also good candidates for this operative technique.

Surgical technique

The patient is positioned supine with the neck hyperextended. Halter traction may help positioning the head. Before initiating the actual surgery, time must be taken to obtain sufficient radiographic imaging in both anteroposterior and lateral planes. The use of biplanar fluoroscopy facilitates the imaging of the position of the odontoid. Reduction of the fracture may be completed by closed means through application of skeletal traction and gentle manipulation of the head. Once reduction of the odontoid process is complete, surgical exposure and stabilization is performed.

The surgical approach utilizes a standard anteromedial approach to the cervical spine. A rightsided, transverse incision is made at the C5–C6 level (Fig. 6.1A). The platysma muscle is split in a longitudinal fashion at the medial border of the sternocleidomas-

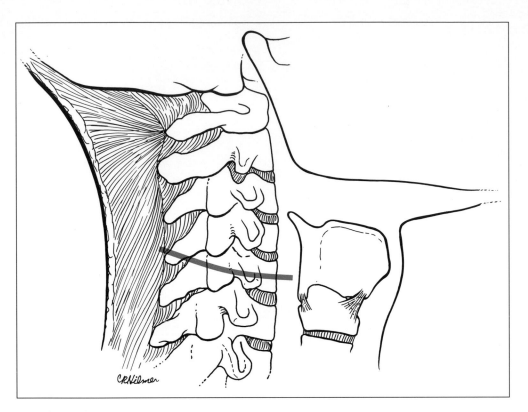

Figure 6.1

Odontoid screw fixation.

A
A rightsided, transverse incision is made at the C5–6 level.

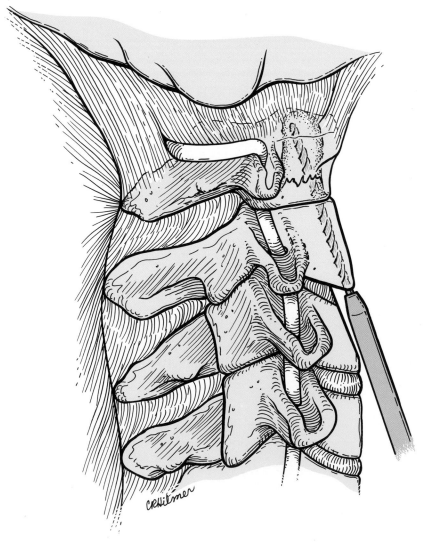

B
The anterior inferior border of the C2 body is the starting point for drilling.

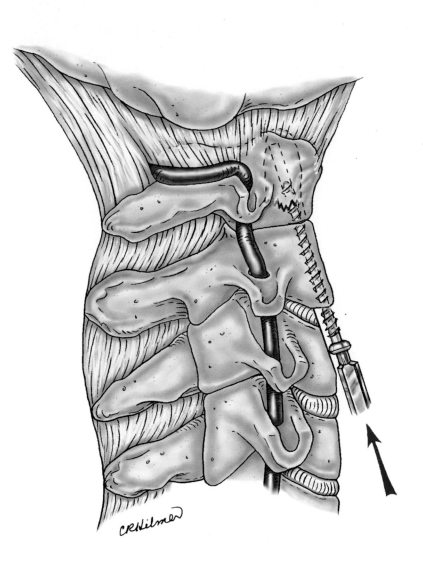

C
Lateral view, showing screw insertion into the drilled hole.

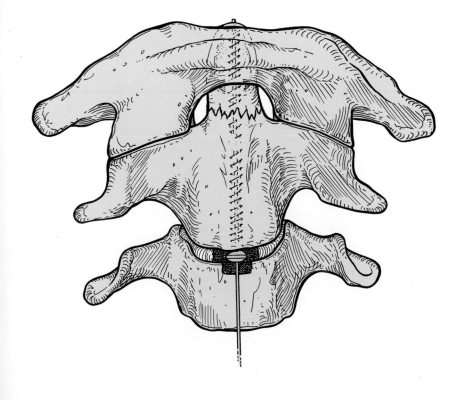

D
Anterior view, showing the screw inserted over the Kirschner guide wire.

Contd

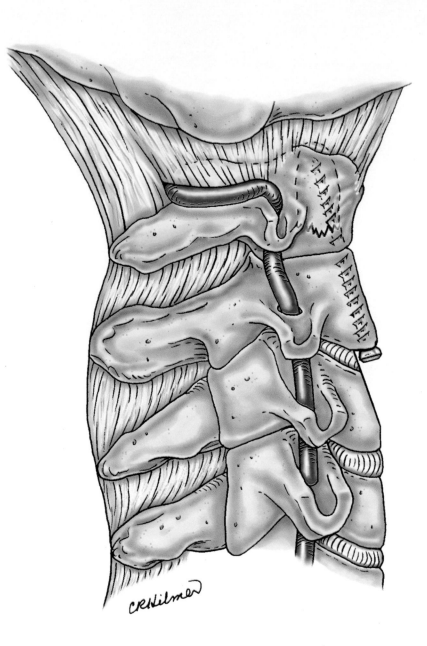

Figure 6.1 *(contd)*

E
Lateral view of the final position of
the screw.

toid muscle. The contents of the carotid sheath are identified, and the retropharyngeal space is then accessed just medial to the palpable carotid pulse. Blunt finger dissection is then continued to the pre-vertebral fascia and anterior longitudinal ligament. Self-retaining retractors are positioned. The anterior tubercle of the atlas is palpably identified. The prevertebral fascia and anterior longitudinal ligament are then split to expose the C2–C3 junction. Exposure of the C2 body will allow placement of Kirschner wires and screws up into the odontoid using biplanar fluoroscopy. The anterior inferior border of the C2 body is the starting point for drilling.

The author prefers using a K-wire, which is placed under image intensification through the body of C2 into the odontoid process. The anterior superior edge of the C3 vertebral body and part of the annulus are overdrilled to accommodate the drill (Fig. 6.1B). Once it is secured in this position, the hole is tapped, and a 3.5 mm screw is placed (Fig. 6.1C–E). The average length of the screw usually approximates 40 mm. One screw fixation may be sufficient, but two screws are recommended to improve rotational stability if the size of the odontoid allows space for two screws. Postoperatively, either a Philadelphia collar or a cervi-cothoracic orthosis is utilized for 2 months.

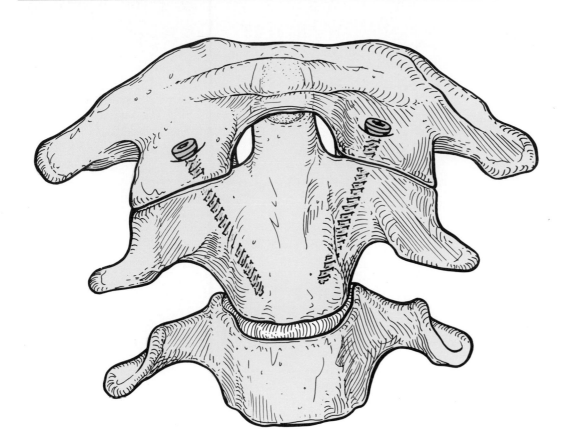

Figure 6.2

Starting 5–6 mm above the joint line, the drilling is performed 15° posteriorly and 25° medially for a distance of 20–25 mm. A malleolar lag screw or cortical screw is inserted.

Anterior C1–C2 screw stabilization

Anterior C1-C2 screw stabilization can be attempted for C1-C2 instability and fractures. This procedure is rarely performed, as most C1-C2 problems can be better approached posteriorly. It may be useful in patients with deficient posterior elements or failed posterior attempts. Either transoral or bilateral lateral retropharyngeal approaches may be utilized. Following exposure, the articular surfaces of the atlantoaxial joints are cleared of cartilage, and cancellous bone chips are packed into the joints. Starting 5-6 mm above the joint line, the drilling is performed 15° posteriorly and 25° medially for a distance of 20-25 mm. A malleolar lag screw or cortical screw is inserted (Fig. 6.2). Through the transoral approach, a special plate may be utilized to stabilize the C1-C2 joint.

Anterior plating of the lower cervical spine

Indications

1   Reconstruction of the spine after corpectomy for tumor, fracture, or spondylosis
2   Multiple level interbody fusions after excision of the intervertebral disc.

Techniques

The surgical approach for most conditions includes a standard anteromedial Smith-Robinson technique. A transverse incision generally suffices, although a longitudinal incision along the anterior border of the sternocleidomastoid may be required in some cases. Once exposure and decompression are complete, fusion and instrumentation are performed. The grafting technique is extremely important, as poor grafting technique will

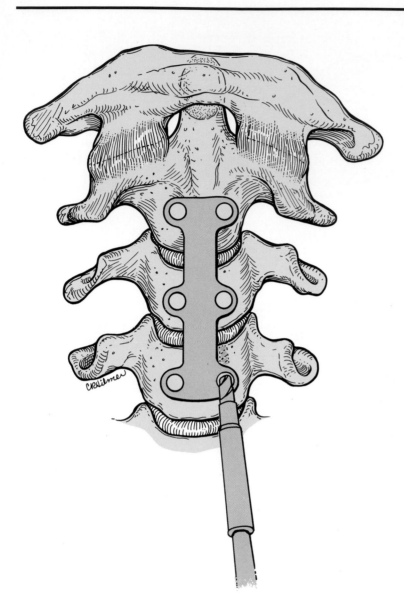

Figure 6.3

Anterior plating of the lower cervical spine.

A

Drilling is performed after the plate is centered. The directions and depth of drilling vary depending on the types of implant used.

result in graft dislodgement, graft collapse, or instrumentation failure.

Once the graft is inserted, the process of instrumentation is started with selection of an appropriately sized cervical plate, which must extend from the middle or proximal portion of the superior uninvolved vertebrae to the middle or distal portion of the adjacent inferior uninvolved vertebrae. The plate is then contoured to the anterolateral surfaces of the cervical spine, maximizing contact to the plate. When osteophytes are present on the vertebral bodies, their removal with a power burr or rongeur is required to maximize bony contact to the plate and thus enhance stability of the construct. At this point, the plate is stabilized with screws implanted at the proximal and distal poles of the plate (Fig. 6.3A). With the Caspar

or AO-Orozco systems, these holes may be drilled manually or with an air-driven adjustable drill guide. It is important to measure the anterior–posterior depth, and correct sized screws are inserted (Fig. 6.3B). With the plate stabilized, the hole is drilled through a drill guide, allowing no more than 16–18 mm of penetration. The drilling should parallel the endplates of the vertebral body, and be directed slightly toward the midline. Bicortical screws are used for the AO-Orozco or Caspar plates. Tapping is done to the known depth (Fig. 6.3C).

The plate should be contoured into cervical lordosis and to the convexity of the vertebral body to maximize the contact between the plate and the bone (Fig. 6.3D). Once the hole is completed, it is then tapped with a 3.5 mm cortical tap through both the

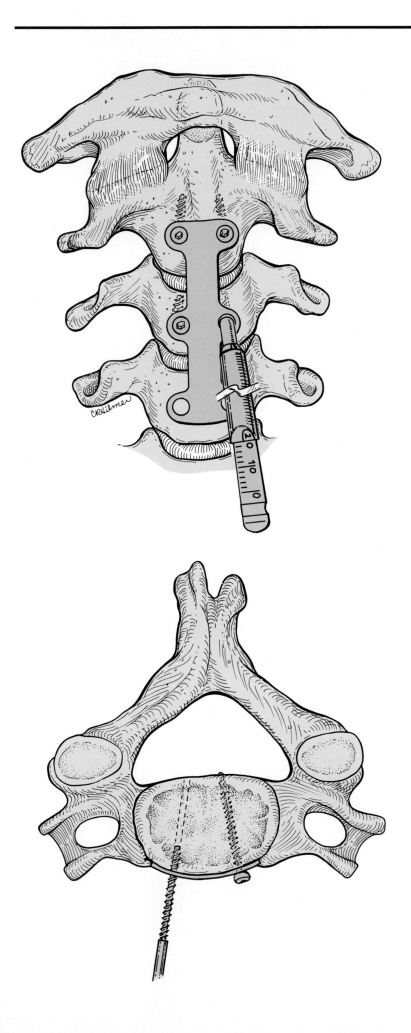

B
The depth is measured using a depth gauge.

C
Bicortical screws are used for the AO-Orozco or
Caspar plates. Tapping is done to the known depth.

Contd

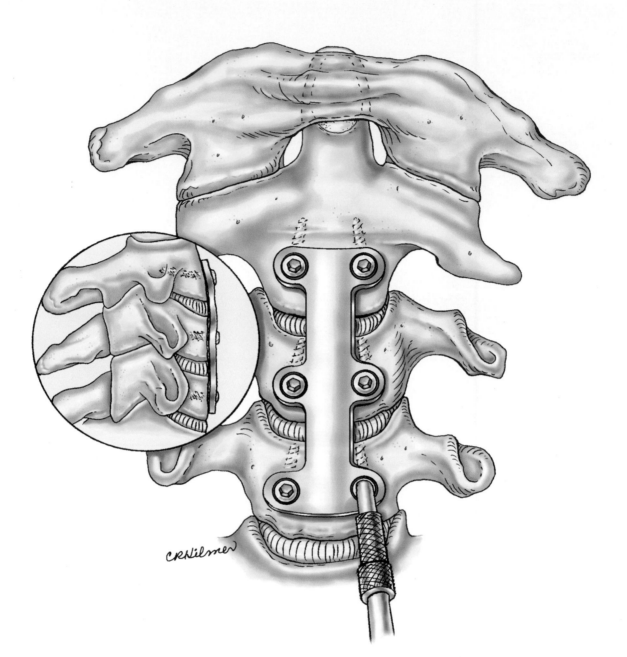

Figure 6.3 *(contd)*

D

The plate should be contoured into cervical lordosis and to the convexity of the vertebral body to maximize the contact between the plate and the bone. Tapping is done to the known depth.

anterior and posterior vertebral walls. A 3.5 mm cortical screw is then inserted, and only lightly tightened until the remaining screws are placed.

The Caspar and AO-Orozco plate systems are composed of stainless steel. These plates come in various sizes. The AO-Orozco plate is available in sizes from 5 holes to 20 holes, and ranges in length from 23 mm to 133 mm. Screw hole placement is also variable, and ranges from 16 mm to 21 mm in each of the various lengths. These plates can be cut and contoured easily to the surfaces of the anterior cervical

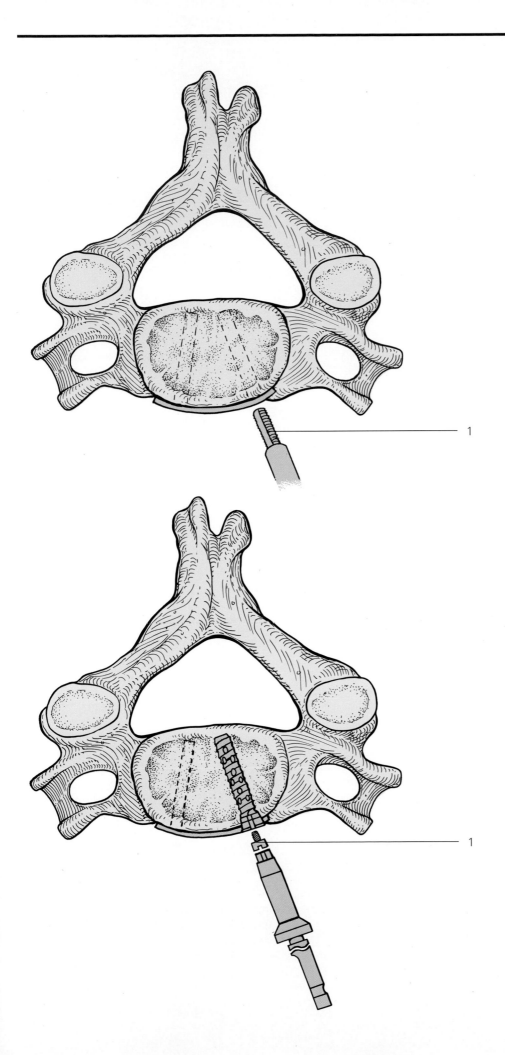

E
For the AO-Morscher or Orion titanium cervical plates, unicortical screws are used.

1   Tap

F
The AO-Morscher plate with expansion locking head screw.

1   Expanding screw head

Contd

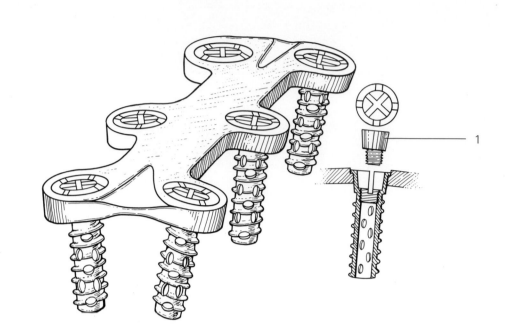

Figure 6.3 *(contd)*

G
The expansion screw fits into the hollowed out cylindrical portion of the expansion head screw, and with tightening, widens the shoulder of the expansion head screw, locking it to the cervical plate.

1   Expanding locking screw head

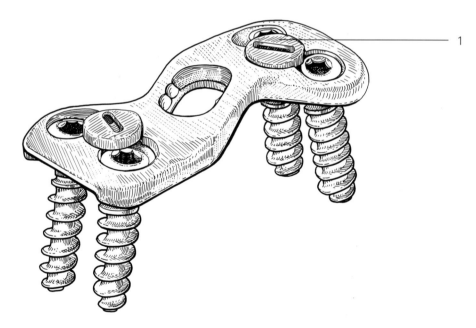

H
Orion plate screws with locking screws. The screws are inserted in a divergent manner in the superior–inferior plane.

1   Locking screw

spine. This system utilizes 3.5 mm screws, and allows variable placement of the screws through the holes of the plate up to 45°.

The AO-Morscher pure titanium cervical plate is available in 5 and 8 hole configurations with length varying from 24 mm to 63 mm (Fig. 6.3E–G). Hole spacing is also variable from 16 mm to 55 mm. At one end of the plate, screw direction is set at a 12°

angle to facilitate insertion of the screw where the anatomy does not allow right angle application. There are several screws available for application with this plate. A standard 3.5 mm titanium screw is available for conventional bicortical purchase, as described earlier. However, the most commonly utilized screw with this plate is the 14 mm expansion head screw, which comes in a 4 mm diameter. This expansion head screw comes in perforated and non-perforated forms. The proximal portion of the screw is hollowed out and has an expansile shoulder. Once the 4 mm diameter expansion head screw is placed through the plate and into the vertebral body, it is then locked to the plate with use of the smaller expansion screw (Fig. 6.3F). The expansion screw fits into the hollowed out cylindrical portion of the expansion head screw, and with tightening, widens the shoulder of the expansion head screw, locking it to the cervical plate. The benefits of this screw are primarily related to the fact that bicortical purchase is not required. The stability of this configuration, however, is dependent on the unity of the screw to the plate and the quality of the bone. Similarly, Orion plates utilize unicortical screws and have locking screw heads (Fig. 6.3H). The screws are divergent in the superior–inferior plane so that the plate spans from the middle of the superior vertebral body to the middle of the inferior vertebral body.

cation that should be recognized intraoperatively. Radiographs should be obtained once the screws are placed for placement confirmation. With penetration into a disc space, one can be relatively assured that eventual loosening of the screw can occur, due to movement across that particular motion segment. These screws should be removed and redirected. Another severe complication associated with anterior instrumentation of the cervical spine is that of hardware loosening and subsequent injury to surrounding vital structures and organs. Esophageal erosion secondary to screw or plate loosening can be disastrous. Hardware loosening may be the result of osteoporosis with insufficient bony purchase, technical difficulties where multiple attempts at insertion lead to inadequate purchase, and finally, improper postoperative immobilization of the patient. Anterior cervical plate fixation should be avoided in the osteoporotic patient.

Complications

Any of the complications inherent in the anterior cervical approach, such as neurologic injury, esophageal tears, recurrent laryngeal nerve injury, injuries to the carotid or vertebral artery, and Horner's syndrome, still apply with attempts at anterior cervical instrumentation. Meticulous technique during surgical exposure, without undue pressure on the vital structures of this region, will avoid these complications. Bone grafting complications such as graft collapse, graft extrusion, and pseudarthrosis may result. Potential complications directly referrable to anterior instrumentation are multiple. Certainly the most feared complication is that of iatrogenic neurologic injury. This would be most often encountered with use of excessively long screws, which penetrate the posterior cortex and directly injure the dura and underlying neurologic structures. Such an injury may also occur during the drilling process. It is important to use a drill guide that prevents inadvertent posterior penetration. Another complication is misplacement of the screw into the adjacent disc space. This is a compli-

Bibliography

Aebi M, Zuber K, Marchesi D (1991) Treatment of cervical spine injuries with anterior plating. *Spine* **16**:S38

An HS, Cotler JM (1992) *Spinal Instrumentation.* Baltimore, Williams & Wilkins

An HS, Simpson JM (1994) *Surgery of the Cervical Spine.* London and Baltimore, Martin Dunitz and Williams & Wilkins

Böhler J (1982) Anterior stabilization of acute fractures and non-unions of the dens. *J Bone Joint Surg* **64A**:18

Caspar W, Barbier DD, Klara PM (1989) Anterior cervical fusion and Caspar plate stabilization for cervical trauma. *Neurosurg* **25**:491–501

Ripa DR, Dowall MG, Meyer PR et al (1991) Series of 92 traumatic cervical spine injuries stabilized with anterior ASIF plate fusion technique. *Spine* **16**:S46–S55

Simmons EH, DuToit G (1978) Lateral atlanto-axial arthrodesis. *Orthop Clin North Am* **9**:1101–14

7

Anterior exposures of the cervicothoracic junction

Alexander R Vaccaro
Howard S An

Introduction

Anterior exposure of the cervicothoracic junction (C7–T2) is a challenging surgical exercise because of the overlying clavicle and sternum and the close proximity of the great vessels. Pathologic processes requiring decompression and stabilization in this region may include deformities, tumors, infections, and traumatic spinal cord compression after trauma. Spinal deformities at the cervicothoracic junction may be associated with a significant kyphotic deformity, particularly in patients who underwent previous laminectomy. Traditional approaches using the high anterior transthoracic route tend to give no or poor access to the lower cervical spine, while the antero-medial cervical approach limits the exposure distal to T1.

Three methods of anterior approaches to the cervicothoracic junction for the purpose of vertebral decompression and reconstruction are described in this chapter. These methods comprise the: (1) transthoracic, (2) low cervical and high transthoracic, and (3) anterior clavicular/clavicular manubrium or sternal splitting approaches.

Anatomy

The thoracic inlet is bounded by the manubrium and two clavicles anteriorly, the upper thoracic vertebrae posteriorly and the first thoracic ribs on both sides of the upper thoracic spine. Beneath the subcutaneous fat lies the thin platysma muscle, which extends distally to the second or third rib. Deep to this in the supraclavicular region is the deep cervical fascia, which invests both the anteriorly situated sternoclei-domastoid muscle and the posteriorly situated trapez-ius muscle. The next fascial layer encountered deep to the deep cervical fascia is the pretracheal fascia, extending from its hyoid bone attachment superiorly into the chest below. The pretracheal fascia invests the medially situated strap muscles (sternohyoid, sternothyroid and omohyoid muscles) and laterally is continuous with the carotid sheath, which encloses the vagus nerve, the internal jugular vein and the common carotid artery. The deepest layer of fascia, the prevertebral fascia, covers the right and left longus colli muscles, the so-called prevertebral muscles of the anterior cervical spine. These muscles extend distally as far as the level of T3. The cervical sympathetic trunks lie along the surface of the prevertebral fascia at the level of the cervical transverse processes. The inferior thyroid artery, a branch of the subclavian or thyrocervical trunk, lies on the left side of the neck at the superior portion of the cervicothoracic junction. This vessel crosses the surgical field before supplying the thyroid gland. This may need to be ligated to obtain good exposure of this region of the spine. The stellate ganglion of the sympathetic nervous system is located at or near the C7–T1 level, lateral to the longus colli muscle, with the vertebral artery and vein lying just lateral to it. The thoracic duct is found on the left side caudal to the stellate ganglion and courses anteriorly to the subclavian vessels and posterior to the common carotid artery, before opening into the region marking the union of the internal jugular, subclavian and left innominate veins. The apex of the lung lies approximately at the T1 level and is situated between the longus colli muscle and the subclavian artery. The great vessels in this region include the left brachiocephalic vein, the aortic arch and its junction with the brachiocephalic trunk, the left common carotid artery, and the left subclavian artery.

When possible, surgeons may prefer to approach the cervicothoracic junction from the left side because of the varying and unpredictable course of the right recurrent laryngeal nerve. The left recurrent laryngeal nerve descends into the thorax within the carotid sheath and then curves around the aorta to lie between the trachea and esophagus before supplying the larynx. The right recurrent laryngeal nerve departs from the vagus nerve at differing levels before circling around the right subclavian artery, making it vulnerable to injury during rightsided approaches. As it ascends into the neck, the right recurrent laryngeal nerve courses obliquely from lateral to medial before lying along the junction of the esophagus and trachea. Occasionally, the right recurrent laryngeal nerve may pass ventral to the inferior thyroid artery instead of caudad to it, again making it vulnerable to injury during rightsided exposures.

Indications
1   Spinal tumors
2   Spinal infections
3   Thoracic disc herniation
4   Spinal cord compression after trauma
5   Kyphoscoliosis.

Surgical techniques

The high transthoracic approach

In general, the choice of approaching the upper thoracic spine on the left or right is primarily dictated by the presenting pathology. In patients with scoliosis, one would approach on the side of the spinal convexity. If one can choose, the rightsided approach is usually preferable for the midthoracic spine because this approach avoids manipulation and retraction of the aorta. This is less of a problem in the upper thoracic spine, when the exposure is cephalad to the great arch of the aorta.

The patient is placed in the left lateral decubitus position with a bean bag contoured to the shape of the body for stable positioning. A kidney rest may be utilized for elevation to add some extension to the operative site. The patient's arm on the side of the surgical approach is elevated above his/her head as high as possible and supported on an airplane splint, protecting all bony protuberances and neurovascular structures. An axillary roll is placed to prevent compression of the axillary artery and vein.

A periscapular J-shaped incision is made approximately 2.5 cm (1 inch) medial to the superior angle of the scapula and continued down around its inferior angle (Fig. 7.1A). Dissection continues in the line of the incision through the subcutaneous fat to the level of the superficial muscles of the back. The trapezius is divided close to the spinous processes and parallel to the direction of the skin incision so as to avoid injuring the spinal accessory nerve. The latissimus dorsi muscle is next divided as medially as possible for adequate retraction and to avoid injuring its nerve supply, the thoracodorsal nerve (Fig. 7.1B). Next, the deeper lying rhomboideus major muscle is divided near its insertion into the scapula. Lying inferiorly and laterally, the serratus anterior muscle is divided as caudally as possible to avoid injuring its nerve supply, the long thoracic nerve (Fig. 7.1C). The scapula can now be retracted superolaterally after protecting its medial surface with a saline-soaked sponge, thus exposing the third and fourth ribs. The periosteum on the third rib is incised along the longitudinal axis of the rib parallel to its course and sharply dissected off with use of an elevator and a Doyen raspatory (Fig. 7.1D). The rib is divided posteriorly approximately 1–2 cm from its attachment to the transverse process and anteriorly at its junction with the costal cartilage. The deeper periosteum is then incised along the direction of the rib bed, allowing one to proceed in either a retropleural or an intrapleural direction for subsequent exposure of the cervicothoracic junction.

Exposure through the intrapleural cavity involves making a transverse incision into the parietal pleura and retracting the dome of the lung inferiorly to expose the anterior surface of the spine. The parietal pleura overlying the upper thoracic vertebrae is then carefully incised to avoid injuring the right superior intercostal vein and artery and the sympathetic trunk and ganglion. Malleable retractors are positioned around the spine (Fig. 7.1E). The longus colli muscles can now be visualized down to their insertion into the first, second, and third thoracic vertebrae. In order to visualize C7, bluntly dissect the fascia (Sibson's) above the pleural dome along the longus colli muscles. The right superior intercostal artery and vein as well as the upper intercostal vessels may be ligated at this time to obtain better exposure.

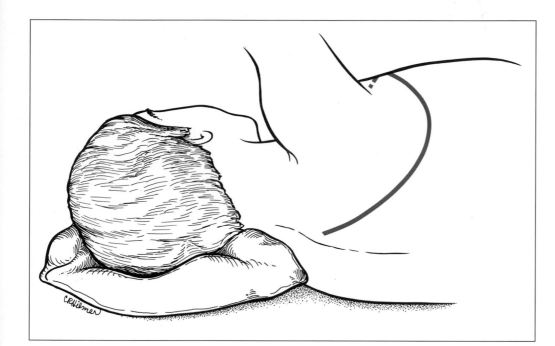

Figure 7.1

High transthoracic approach to the upper cervical spine.

A

A periscapular **J**-shaped incision is made approximately 2.5 cm (1 inch) medial to the superior angle of the scapula and continued down around its inferior angle.

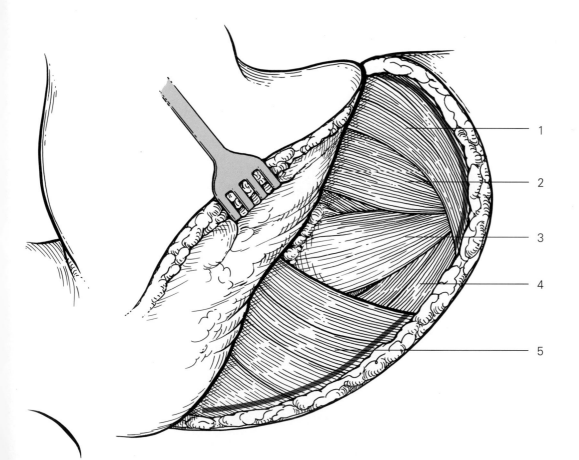

B

The trapezius muscle is divided close to the spinous processes and parallel to the direction of the skin incision so as to avoid injuring the spinal accessory nerve, and the latissimus dorsi muscle is next divided as medially as possible for adequate retraction and to avoid injuring its nerve supply, the thoracodorsal nerve.

1   Latissimus dorsi m.
2   teres major m.
3   Infraspinous m.
4   Rhomboideus major m.
5   Trapezius m.

Contd

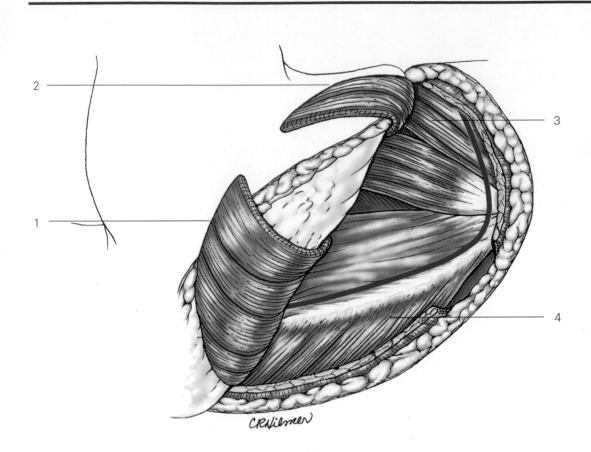

Figure 7.1 *(contd)*

C
Deeply, the rhomboideus major muscle is divided near its insertion into the scapula, and the serratus anterior muscle is divided as caudally as possible to avoid injuring its nerve supply, the long thoracic nerve.

1   Trapezius m.
2   Latissimus dorsi m.
3   Serratus anterior m.
4   Rhomboideus major m.

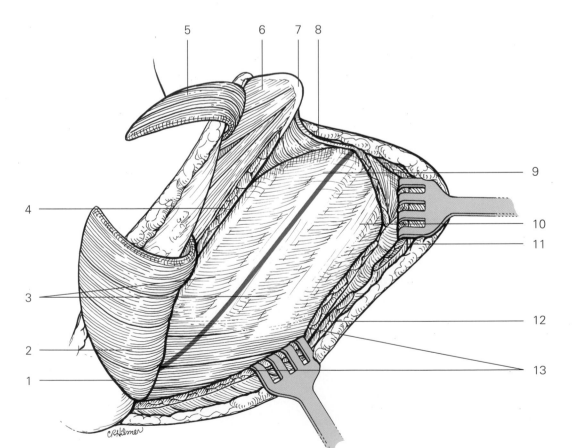

D
The scapula can then be retracted superolaterally, and the periosteum on the third rib is removed.

1   Iliocostal m.
2   Trapezius m.
3   Ext. intercostal m.
4   Cut edge of rhomboideus major m.
5   Latissimus dorsi m.
6   Teres major m.
7   Inf. angle of scapula
8   Serratus anterior m.
9   Third rib
10   Fourth rib
11   Latissimus dorsi m.
12   Trapezius m.
13   Rhomboideus major m.

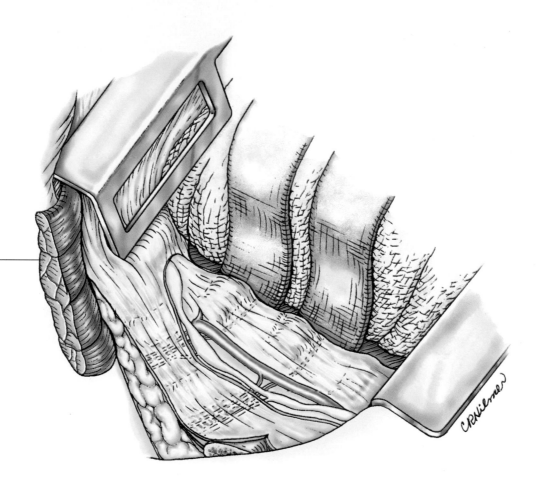

1

For wound closure, a drain is placed and a rib approximator applied followed by a running closure of the pleura, the rib periosteum and the intercostal musculature. The superficial muscles are then closed in layers with interrupted or running sutures.

Potential complications associated with this approach include atelectasis, pleural effusion, pneumonia, an empyema and the possibility of creating a cerebrospinal fluid fistula by surgically invading the dural sheath. The shoulder girdle function is compromised for months following this procedure.

E
Retractors are positioned and the upper thoracic region is exposed.

1   Trapezius m.

The sternal splitting approach

The patient is placed in the supine position with a small bump beneath the shoulders to hyperextend the neck slightly. The head is turned slightly to the right to allow a leftsided approach to the lower cervical spine because of the unpredictable course of the right recurrent laryngeal nerve. The longitudinal skin incision begins superiorly in the upper cervical spine and follows the anterior border of the sternocleidomastoid muscle and courses inferiorly over the midline of the manubrium and sternum to the inferior tip of the xiphoid process (Fig 7.2A). Dissection then proceeds sharply through the subcutaneous tissue and fascial covering of the platysma muscle in line with the skin incision. The platysma is then divided longitudinally with either finger dissection, forceps or a cautery knife to the level of the deep cervical fascia which invests the anterior border of the sternocleidomastoid muscle in the cervical spine, or to the level of the bony sternum in the thorax. The deep cervical fascia is divided sharply, allowing the sternocleidomastoid muscle to be retracted laterally (Fig. 7.2B). At this point, using the tips of the index and middle fingers, palpate the laterally placed carotid artery within its carotid sheath.

With one's fingers protecting the carotid sheath laterally, the pretracheal fascia is divided sharply by spreading it with the blunt tips of a forceps, allowing the carotid sheath to be taken laterally and the strap muscles of the neck and the underlying trachea and esophagus to be taken medially. This allows exposure of the prevertebral fascia below, which invests the longus colli muscles on both sides of the cervical spine.

The soft tissue aponeurosis investing the superior border of the sternal notch is released next and blunt finger dissection or cotton applicators are used to clear the underlying retrosternal adipose tissue and thymus remnants from the undersurface of the manubrium. The muscular aponeurotic soft tissue attachments to the inferior xiphoid process are released sharply and the retrosternal fatty tissue, underlying mediastinum and pleura is separated bluntly from its undersurface and from that of the sternum in preparation for their division with a Gigli saw, sternotomy, or a sternotomy saw. Once the sternotomy is completed and periosteal bleeding is controlled, a gently placed thoracic retractor is used to open the thoracic rib cage carefully so as to avoid injury to the underlying pleura and mediastinal structures. At this point the strap muscles of the neck (sternohyoid, sternothyroid and omohyoid muscles) are visualized, undermined and divided (Fig. 7.2C). Dissection is now continued from the previously exposed cervical spine with further caudal dissection of the pretracheal fascia to the level of the left innominate or brachiocephalic vein (Fig. 7.2D). This vein can be ligated, if necessary, along with the inferior thyroid artery, which crosses the field of exposure obliquely. To complete the exposure of the prevertebral fascia, the esophagus, trachea and brachiocephalic trunk are retracted gently to the right using flexible spatulas, while the thoracic duct, the cupola of the pleura, and the left common carotid artery are retracted to the left (Fig. 7.2E).

The prevertebral fascia overlying the longus colli muscles is then divided in the midline to allow subperiosteal dissection of these muscles to the base of the transverse processes or to the costovertebral joints. This approach allows excellent exposure from C4 through to T4.

Wound closure consists of reapproximating the split sternum with transosseous wire sutures followed by the reattachment of the strap muscles to their aponeurotic insertions into the undersurface of the sternum using interrupted sutures. The platysma muscle is closed tightly with interrupted absorbable sutures in order to remove tension from the skin, which improves wound healing.

Potential complications associated with this approach include injury to the pleura and underlying mediastinum as well as injury to the left recurrent laryngeal nerve and the great vessels during retraction.

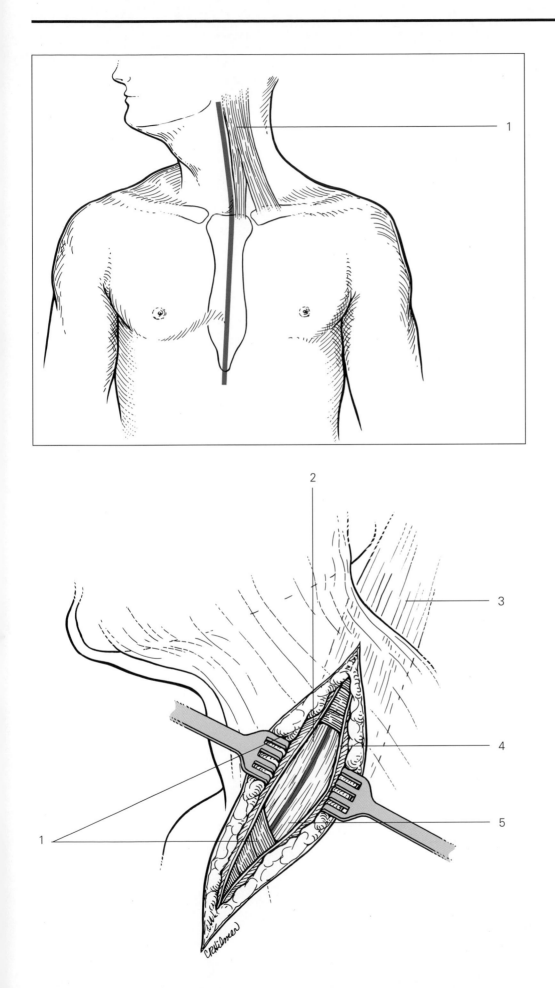

Figure 7.2

Sternal splitting approach.

A
The longitudinal skin incision begins superiorly in the upper cervical spine, follows the anterior border of the sternocleidomastoid muscle, and courses inferiorly over the midline of the manubrium and sternum to the inferior tip of the xiphoid process.

1   Sternocleidomastoid m.

B
After division of the platysma muscle, the deep cervical fascia is divided sharply, allowing the sternocleidomastoid muscle to be retracted laterally and the strap muscle medially.

1   Platysma m.
2   Strap m.
3   Sternocleidomastoid m.
4   Fascia over platysma m.
5   Deep cervical fascia over sternocleidomastoid m.

C
Retractors are positioned and the
omohyoid muscle is divided
along with the traversing inferior
thyroid artery.

1   Strap m.
2   Sternocleidomastoid m.

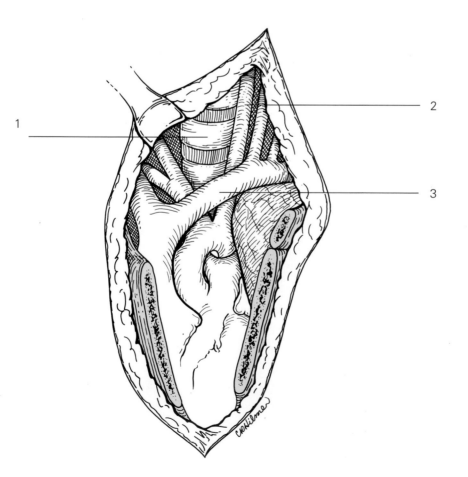

D
Sternotomy connects the
dissection to the previously
exposed cervical spine, with
further caudal dissection of the
pretracheal fascia to the level of
the left innominate or
brachiocephalic vein.

1   Trachea
2   Common carotid a.
3   L. brachiocephalic v.

E
To complete the exposure, the esophagus, trachea and brachiocephalic trunk are retracted gently to the right, using flexible spatulas, while the thoracic duct, the cupola of the pleura, and the left common carotid artery are retracted to the left.

1   Trachea
2   L. common carotid a.
3   Brachial plexus
4   Sympathetic chain
5   Dura mater

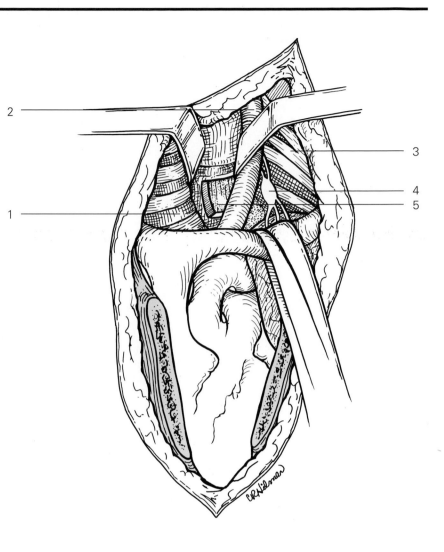

Partial manubrial splitting or clavicular approaches

A similar but less aggressive version of the sternal splitting approach is the surgical approach described by Sundaresan et al (1984). In this approach, a T-shaped incision is made with the vertical limb overlying the manubrium and upper portion of the sternum and the horizontal limb of the incision overlying the base of the neck from approximately 1 cm above the clavicle and extending to the point of the lateral margins of the sternocleidomastoid muscles on each side (Fig. 7.3A). Dissection is carried down to the level of the bony manubrium and upper sternum along the vertical incision and along the transverse incision to the level of the clavicle on the side of the approach. The platysma muscle is divided in line with the skin incision. The superficial anterior veins may be ligated, while the ipsilateral internal and external jugular veins, as well as the medial supraclavicular nerve, should be retracted if possible to prevent their sacrifice (Fig. 7.3B). The sternal and clavicular heads of the sternocleidomastoid muscle on the side of the approach are detached at the level of the manubrium and clavicle and retracted. The strap muscles on the ipsilateral side of the approach are detached below the level of the clavicle and retracted medially (Fig. 7.3C). After clearing the fatty and areolar tissues in the suprasternal space, the sternal origin of the pectoralis major is stripped laterally. The medial half of the clavicle is then stripped subperiosteally and its medial third (ipsilateral side) removed with a Gigli saw. The sternoclavicular joint is disarticulated sharply and curetted. A rectangular piece of manubrium, along with its posterior periosteum, is removed, using power drill holes and heavy scissors (Fig. 7.3D). Great care must be taken to then protect the underlying left innominate and subclavian veins, which lie posterior and inferior to the undersurface of the clavicle (Fig. 7.3E). If further retraction is believed needed inferiorly, the thyroid vein may be ligated. The remainder of this approach is similar to that described for the sternal splitting approach.

Closure is performed in the routine fashion without reattachment of the resected bony manubrium and clavicle, both of which may be used for additional bone graft material. The strap muscles are reattached with interrupted sutures and the sternocleidomastoid aponeurosis is reattached to the remaining clavicular periosteum.

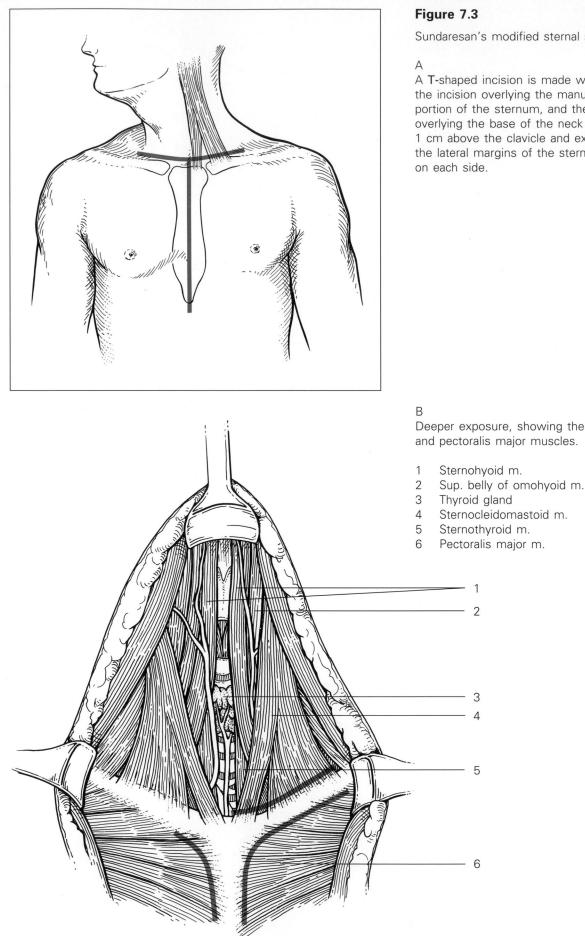

Figure 7.3

Sundaresan's modified sternal splitting approach

A

A **T**-shaped incision is made with the vertical limb of the incision overlying the manubrium and the upper portion of the sternum, and the horizontal limb overlying the base of the neck from approximately 1 cm above the clavicle and extending to the point of the lateral margins of the sternocleidomastoid muscles on each side.

B

Deeper exposure, showing the sternocleidomastoid and pectoralis major muscles.

1   Sternohyoid m.
2   Sup. belly of omohyoid m.
3   Thyroid gland
4   Sternocleidomastoid m.
5   Sternothyroid m.
6   Pectoralis major m.

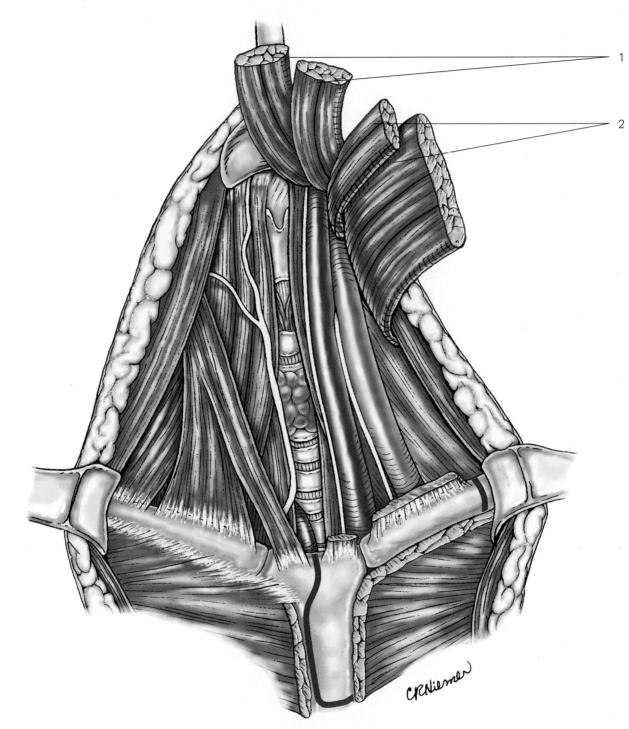

C

The sternal and clavicular heads of the sternocleidomastoid muscle on the side of the approach are detached at the level of the manubrium and clavicle and retracted. The strap muscles on the ipsilateral side of the approach are detached below the level of the clavicle and retracted medially.

1   Strap m.
2   Sternocleidomastoid m.

Contd

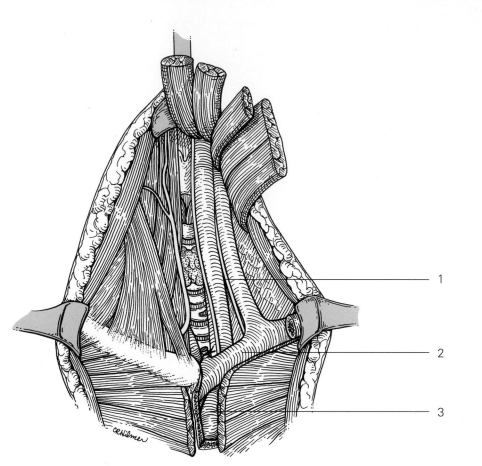

Figure 7.3 *(contd)*

D
The medial third of the clavicle and a rectangular piece of manubrium are removed.

1   Vagus n.
2   L. brachiocephalic a.
3   Aortic arch

E
Retraction of vessels and the trachea exposes the cervicothoracic junction.

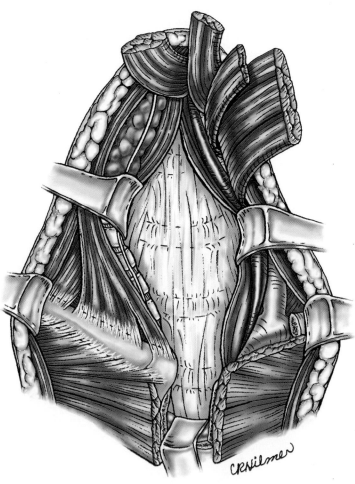

LeSoin et al (1986) modified this approach by leaving the sternocleidomastoid muscle attachments to the manubrium and clavicles in place, and by resecting the medial third of both clavicles as well as the superior portion of the manubrium in order to lift the central sternal clavicular complex as a unit (Fig. 7.4A–C). A benefit associated with this approach is to allow the supporting muscles of respiration, the sternocleidomastoid and strap muscles, to remain firmly attached to their clavicular insertion, with a possible decrease in the degree of associated pulmonary impairment. LeSoin also advocated a curved horizontal incision rather than a T-shaped incision, claiming better wound healing. The clavicle in this instance may be reattached with 2.7 or 3.5 AO reconstruction plates and the manubrium reapproximated with wire sutures.

Kurz, Pursel and Herkowitz (1991) modified the anterior approach to the cervicothoracic junction by resecting only the ipsilateral medial third of the clavicle without disturbing the bony manubrium. They report successful exposure to the level of T4 using this approach (Fig. 7.5).

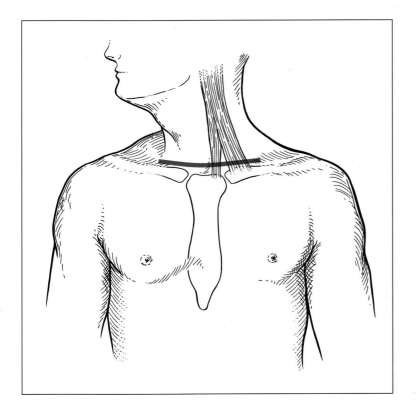

Figure 7.4

LeSoin's exposure of the cervicothoracic junction.

A
The incision is made 1 cm above the clavicle to the edge of the sternocleidomastoid muscle.

Figure 7.4 *(contd)*

B
Deeper dissection, showing the clavicular attachments of the sternocleidomastoid and pectoralis major muscles.

1   Sternocleidomastoid m.
2   Pectoralis major m.

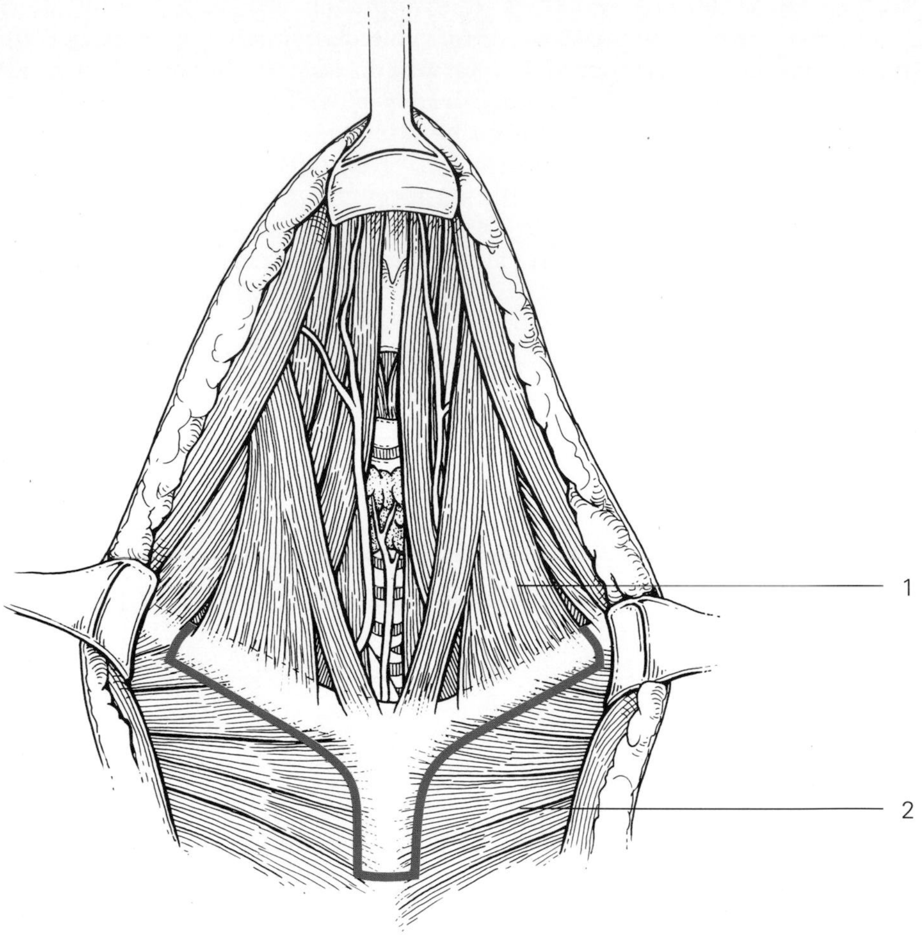

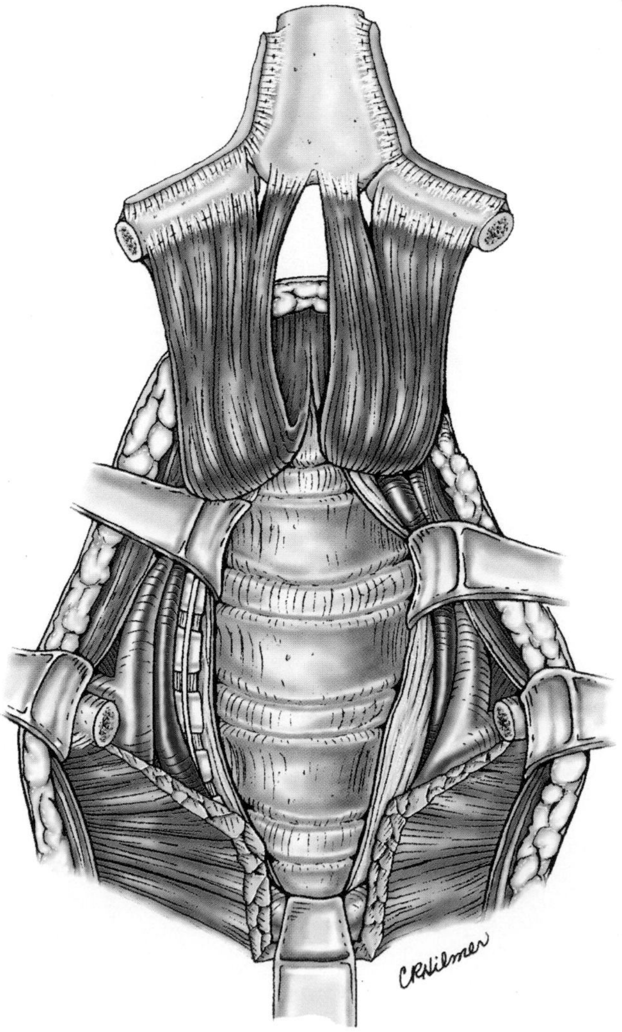

C
The manubrium and clavicles are resected and lifted superiorly as a unit, and later reattached with plates.

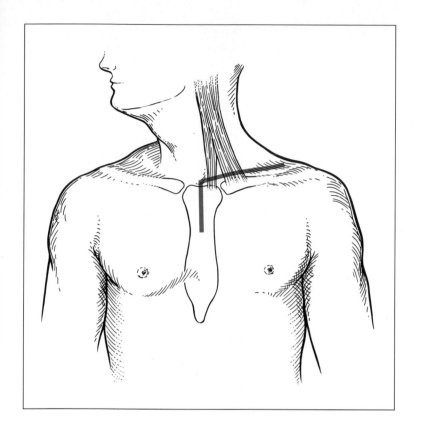

Figure 7.5

Exposure of the cervicothoracic junction by Kurz, Pursel and Herkowitz: the incision is placed over the clavicle unilaterally and curved toward the manubrium. The ipsilateral third of the clavicle is resected only, without disturbing the bony manubrium.

The combined cervical and thoracic approach to the cervicothoracic spine

Micheli and Hood (1983) described the combined cervical and thoracic anterior approach to the cervical thoracic spine. This approach is particularly useful in patients with kyphoscoliosis. The patient is positioned in the left lateral decubitus position with the right upper extremity draped free for easy manipulation within the sterile field during the surgical exposure. An oblique cervical incision is made parallel to the clavicle, with division of the platysma muscle in line with the incision, and a high thoracic incision is made around the scapula (Fig. 7.6A). For the cervical incision, the deep cervical fascia along the anterior medial border of the sternocleidomastoid muscle is incised, allowing rotation and retraction of this muscle laterally to expose its deep surface. The carotid sheath is now retracted anteriorly, following gentle blunt exposure of its posterior border. The inferior thyroid artery is ligated as it courses posterior to the carotid sheath to obtain better exposure. The transverse processes of the cervical vertebrae, covered by the longus colli muscle between the sternocleidomastoid laterally and the carotid sheath medially, can now be palpated and visualized. The cervical wound is packed before proceeding to the transthoracic approach to the upper thoracic spine. The thoracic incision curves around the scapula, and, by retracting the scapula superiorly, the upper thoracic ribs can be approached (Fig. 7.6B). The transthoracic approach to the upper thoracic spine has been described earlier in this chapter. The cervicothoracic junction is then approached from both the cervical and the thoracotomy dissections (Fig. 7.6C).

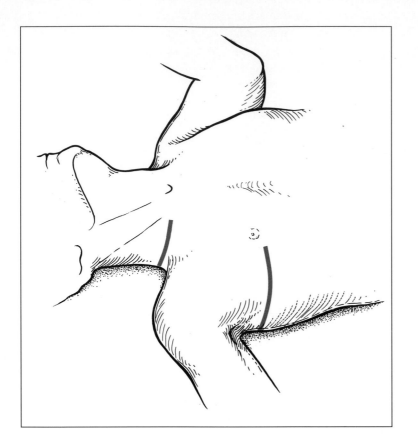

Figure 7.6

Combined cervical and thoracic approach to the cervicothoracic spine

A
The cervical incision is over the clavicle and the thoracic incision is around the scapula.

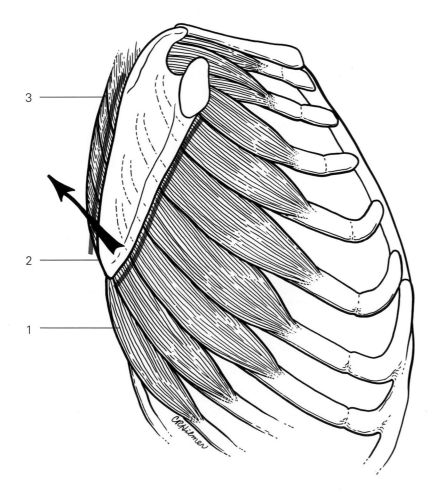

B
Transthoracic dissection includes division of the rhomboid and serratus anterior muscles and retraction of the scapula superiorly.

1   Serratus anterior m.
2   Scapula
3   Rhomboid m.

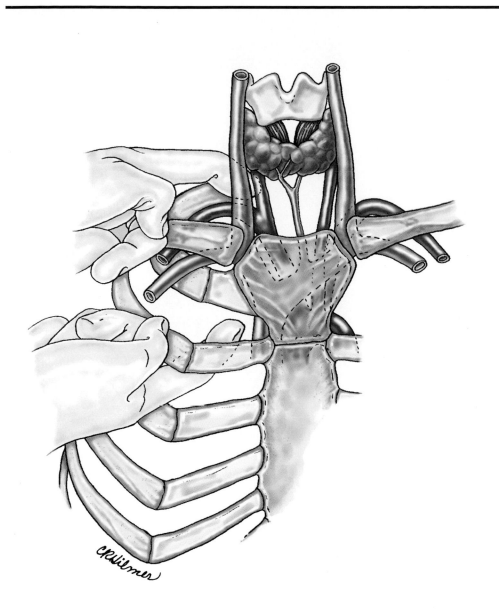

C
The cervicothoracic junction is approached from both cervical and thoracotomy approaches.

Conclusion

A number of surgical approaches have been described for exposing the lower cervical and upper thoracic spine. It is important, regardless of the approach selected, that adequate visualization be attained before attempting surgical decompression in this region, because of the potential for catastrophic neurologic and great vessel injury. The surgeon should be familiar with the anatomy of this region as well as the various methods of reconstruction available before undertaking this technically challenging surgical exercise.

Bibliography

An HS, Vaccaro A, Cotler JM et al (1994) Spinal disorders at the cervicothoracic junction. *Spine* **15**:2557–64

Bauer R, Kerschbaumer F, Poisel S (1987) Cervical spine and cervicothoracic junction. In: R Bauer, F Kerschbaumer, S Poisel (eds), *Operative Approaches in Orthopaedic Surgery and Traumatology*, pp2–16. New York, Thieme Medical

Cauchoix J, Binet J (1957) Anterior surgical approaches to the spine. *Ann R Coll Surg Engl* **27**:237–43

Chou SN, Selkeskog EL (1973) Alternative surgical approaches to the cervical spine. *Clin Neurosurg* **20**:306–21

Dohn DF (1981) Thoracic spinal cord decompression: Alternative surgical approaches and basis of choice. *Clin Neurosurg* **27**:611–23

Fang HSY, Ong BG, Hodgson AR (1964) Anterior spinal fusion. The operative approaches. *Clin Orthop* **35**:16–33

Hodgson AR, Stock FE, Fang HSY et al (1960) Anterior spinal fusion: The operative approach and pathologic findings in 412 patients with Pott's disease of the spine. *Br J Surg* **48**:172–8

Hoppenfeld S, De Boer P (1984) The spine. In: S Hoppenfeld, P de Boer (eds), *Surgical Exposures in Orthopaedics. The Anatomic Approach,* pp209–300. Philadelphia, Lippincott

Kirkaldy-Willis WH, Allen PBR, Rostrup O et al (1966) Surgical approaches to the anterior elements of the spine: Indications and techniques. *Canad J Surg* **9**:294–308

Kurz LT, Pursel SE, Herkowitz HN (1991) Modified anterior approach to the cervicothoracic junction. *Spine* **16**:542–7

LeSoin F, Thomas CE III, Autrieque A et al (1986) A transitional biclavicular approach to the upper anterior thoracic spine. *Surg Neurol* **26**:253–6

Micheli LJ, Hood RW (1983) Anterior exposure of the cervicothoracic spine using a combined cervical and thoracic approach. *J Bone Joint Surg* **65A**:992–7

Sundaresan N, Shah J, Foley KM et al (1984) An anterior surgical approach to the upper thoracic vertebrae. *J Neurosurg* **61**:686–90

8

Posterior exposures of the thoracic spine

J Michael Simpson
Howard S An

Introduction

Posterior surgical exposures of the thoracic spine are commonly used for a variety of pathologic conditions. The direct posterior approach is safe and allows full exposure of the posterior vertebral elements with minimal potential for neurovascular injury. This surgical approach is used routinely in scoliosis surgery and for fractures of the thoracic and thoracolumbar spine. The posterolateral (costotransversectomy) and transpedicular approaches expand the surgeon's access to anterior vertebral elements. These exposures are less commonly employed but remain valuable for posterolateral spinal cord decompression. Additional indications for these techniques may include vertebral body biopsy, treatment of infections, tumor resection and deformity. The classic posterolateral approach was developed for drainage of tuberculous abscesses in the thoracic spine, its major advantage being to avoid contamination of the thoracic cavity while allowing adequate drainage and decompression. The posterolateral and transpedicular exposures offer limited access to the anterior vertebral elements when compared to a formal thoracotomy, but may avoid the associated morbidity of the former technique. The anatomy of the posterolateral and transpedicular approaches is not as familiar or safe as the direct posterior approach. Potential does exist for injury to various neurovascular structures, and therefore appreciation of the anatomy in three dimensions is required.

Anatomy

The muscular anatomy of the posterior thoracic spine must be understood, and is somewhat variable, depending on the particular vertebral level. The musculature can be described as having three distinct layers: superficial, intermediate and deep. The superficial muscle layer consists of the trapezius, latissimus dorsi and rhomboids. The trapezius is most superficial, has its origin from the spinous process of C2–T12, and inserts onto the clavicle, acromion and spine of the scapula. The latissimus dorsi, like the trapezius, is a broad muscle with origin from the posterior part of the iliac crest, the lumbar fascia, and the spines of the lower six thoracic vertebrae just deep to the trapezius. The tendinous portion of this muscle wraps around the lower border of the teres major and inserts onto the bicipital groove of the humerus. Just deep to the trapezius in the upper aspects of the thoracic spine are the rhomboid muscles. The rhomboid minor has its origin from the lower aspect of the ligamentum nuchae in the spines of C7 and TI vertebrae. Rhomboid major has its origin from the spines of T2 to T5 and the corresponding supraspinous ligament. Both rhomboid muscles insert onto the medial border of the scapula.

Classically, the intermediate muscular layer is described as consisting of the serratus posterior muscles. The serratus posterior superior and serratus posterior inferior muscles represent very thin flat muscles that arise from the spines throughout the thoracic and lumbar spine, inserting onto the ribs. The deep muscles of the back form a broad, thick column of muscle tissue which occupies the hollow on each side of the spinous processes. The muscles in this group include the sacrospinalis, semispinalis, the multifidi and the rotator muscles.

The nerve supply to the superficial and intermediate layers is unaffected by posterior surgical dissection. However, the muscles of the deep layer are segmentally supplied by the posterior rami, and far lateral dissection beyond the transverse processes may lead to denervation. The bony anatomy on the thoracic spine deserves some attention. The vertebral foramen is relatively small throughout the thoracic spine and is circular in formation. The spinous processes are long and inclined in a caudal direction, tending to overlap the vertebrae below. As opposed to the cervical and lumbar regions of the spine the vertebral bodies of the spine have articulations for the ribs. The head of the rib is wedge-shaped and presents two articular facets for articulation with the numerically corresponding vertebrae and the vertebrae superior to it. These facets are separated by the crest of the head, which is joined to the intervertebral disc. The facet of the numerically corresponding vertebrae is located at the base of its pedicle. The relationship of the rib for given disc space in the thoracic spine must be remembered. For example, access to the disc between T8 and T9 through a costotransversectomy is best accomplished with resection of the ninth rib. The facet joints into the thoracic spine are largely located in a coronal plane. The orientation of the joint does change in the lower thoracic spine to a more sagittal plane orientation, which is typical of the lumbar spine.

With the costotransversectomy approach the surgeon must be aware of the intercostal nerves and blood vessels. These structures are found at the interior aspect of the rib and can be damaged with stripping of the rib. Additionally, the parietal pleura is encountered just underneath the rib upon its resection. Care must be taken during the approach not to damage the pleura and create a pneumothorax.

The blood supply to the spinal cord must also be given consideration with any surgical approach. The segmental blood supply to the thoracic cord is considered tenuous. The artery of Adamkiewicz, which is the major segmental contributing to the anterior spinal artery, most often (80 per cent of cases) has its origin on the left side between T9 and T12. The operating surgeon must have concern for injury to this important segmental artery and subsequent medullary ischemia. By avoiding injury to the structures of the neural foramen such a complication should be avoided.

Indications

1. Scoliosis
2. Kyphosis
3. Fractures
4. Tumors
5. Osteomyelitis.

Surgical techniques

The posterior surgical approach of the thoracic spine

The patient is placed in a prone position on the operating table. The surgeon has the option of utilizing supportive cushions under the chest and both iliac crests or utilization of specialized frames such as the Relton–Hall frame. Care is taken with patient positioning not to compress the abdomen so as to prevent venous reflux and consequent increase in venous bleeding. It is equally important that the anterior chest wall clears the operating table so that adequate chest expansion can occur during the surgical procedure. Once the patient has been carefully positioned, the incision is made in the midline directly over the spinous processes. In cases of scoliosis, a plumbline is created from the spinous process of C7 to the gluteal cleft (Fig. 8.1A). A straight incision is then made over the operative segments. Sharp dissection is carried through the subcutaneous tissues to the fascia. A certain amount of undermining at the junction of the fascia and subcutaneous tissues will be necessary in cases of scoliosis to identify the tips of the spinous processes (Fig. 8.1B). In children and adolescents, the cartilaginous spinous process apophyses are split in the midline with a sharp knife together with the interspinal ligaments. A Cobb elevator then can be used to strip the apophyses with the adherent periosteum along the spinous process to the vertebral arches. In adult patients, the fascia is stripped near the bone with electrocautery on both sides of the spinous processes (Fig. 8.1C). In a continuous fashion the paraspinal muscles are stripped from the spinous processes and partially from the laminae by subperiosteal dissection. The surgeon has a choice of sharp Cobb dissection versus electrocautery. In the thoracic spine it is best to work in a distal to proximal fashion, which is in the direction of the muscle fibers (Fig. 8.1D). For most deformity cases the dissection is carried out laterally to expose the transverse processes. A Cobb elevator and sponge are used to retract the muscles laterally to the tips of the transverse processes (Fig. 8.1E). Deep retraction is maintained with a series of self retaining retractors. A radiograph can be taken to identify the operative level. Optionally, particularly when the surgeon is exposing both the thoracic and lumbar spine, identification of the twelfth rib and transverse process of L1 can be completed.

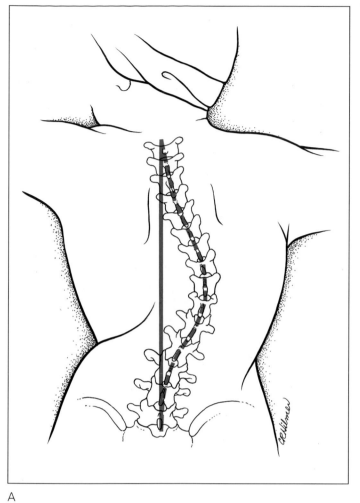

A

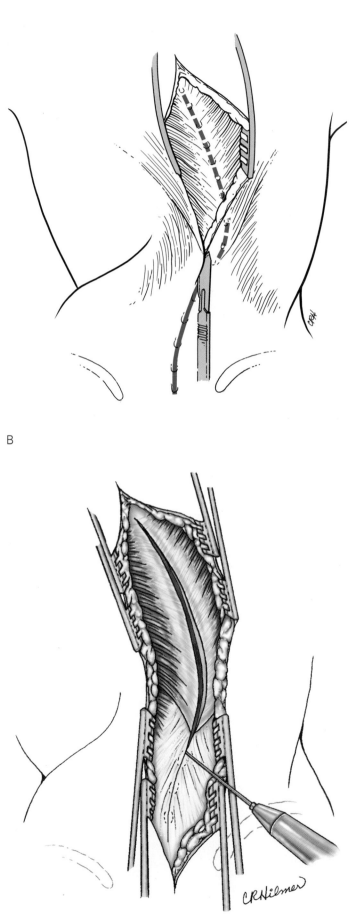

B

Figure 8.1

Posterior approach to the thoracic spine.

A The incision is made in the midline directly over the spinous processes for the posterior approach; but in cases of scoliosis, a plumbline is created from the spinous process of C7 to the gluteal cleft so that the incision is over the midline after correction of deformity.

B Sharp dissection is carried through the subcutaneous tissues, and the fascia is divided over the spinous processes.

C The fascia is stripped near the bone with electrocautery on both sides of the spinous processes.

Contd

C

Figure 8.1 *(contd)*

D The paraspinal muscles are stripped from the spinous
processes and from the laminae by subperiosteal
dissection. Self retaining retractors are progressively
seated deeply, and further dissection of the muscles is
accomplished with a combination of electrocautery and
Cobb elevator.

E A cross-section diagram showing the subperiosteal
dissection of muscles to the tip of the transverse
processes using the Cobb elevator and a sponge.

D

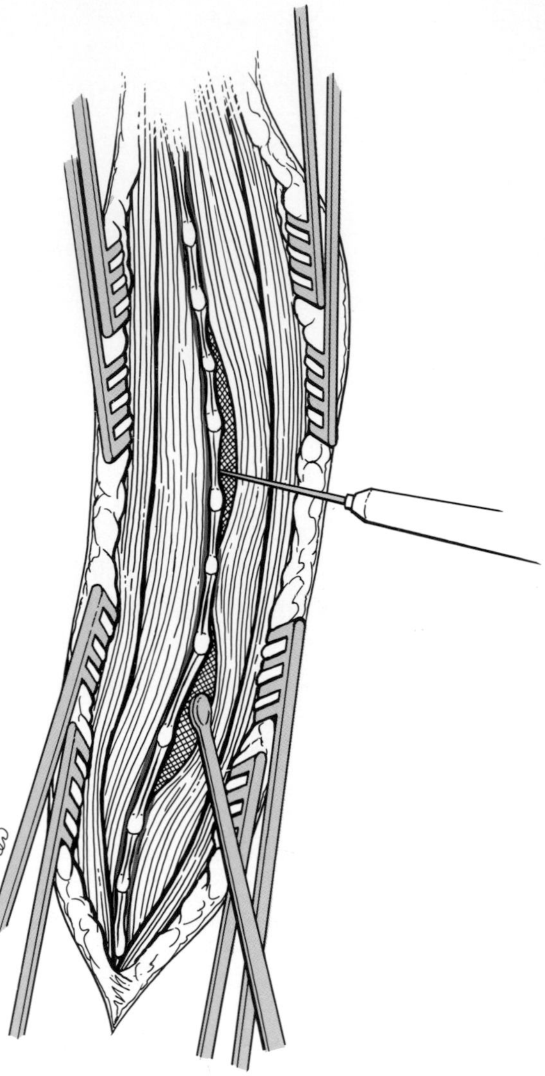

E

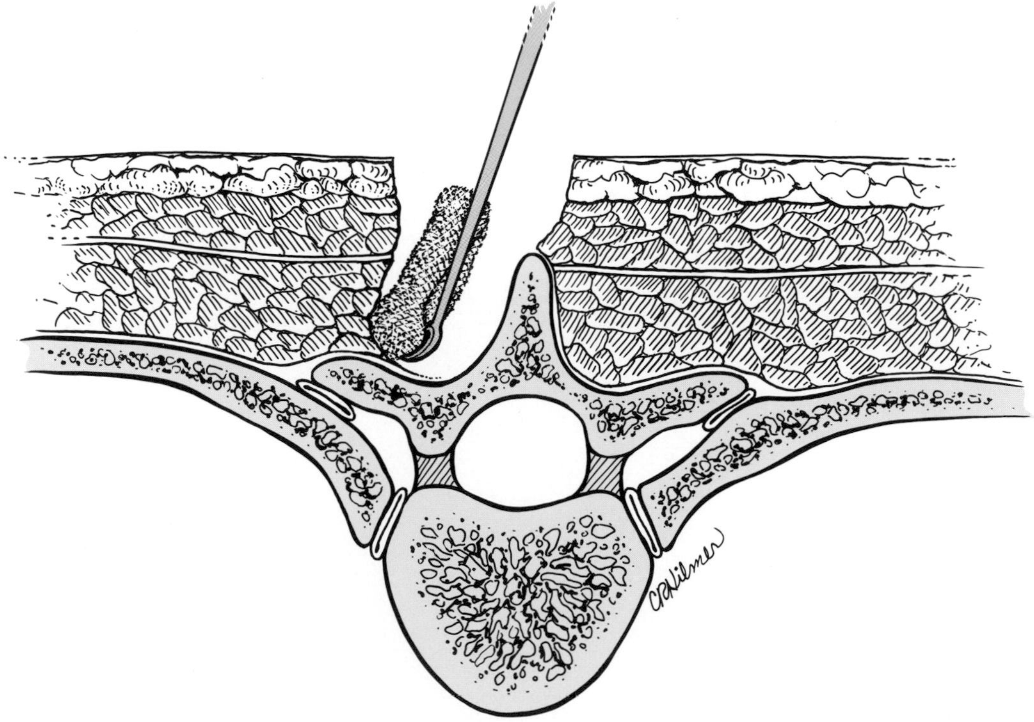

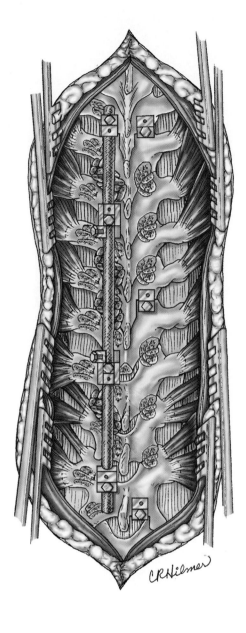

F

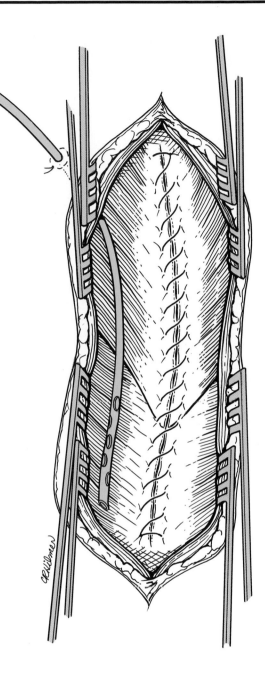

G

F After exposure of the posterior bony elements, decortication, fusion, and instrumentation are performed as necessary.

G Following the completion of the procedure, the fascia is closed first, followed by subcutaneous tissues and the skin. A drain is inserted deep to the fascia and occasionally in the subcutaneous tissue.

Remaining soft tissues in the intralaminar space are then cleared with a series of large curetes and rongeurs. Regardless of the specific diagnosis, the common goal with most posterior exposures of the thoracic spine is to decompress neural structures and/or to stabilize through instrumentation and fusion. For most stabilization procedures, hook and rod constructs are utilized (Fig. 8.1F). Presently, there are a multitude of such devices available. Following the completion of the procedure, the fascia is closed first, followed by subcutaneous tissues and the skin. A drain is inserted deep to the fascia and occasionally in the subcutaneous tissue (Fig. 8.1G).

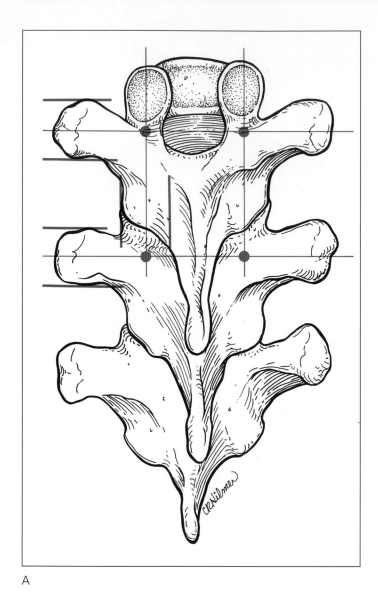

A

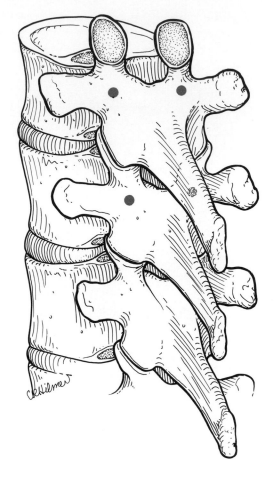

B

Although not in common use, the thoracic pedicle can serve as a site of internal fixation. Like the lumbar spine, the entry to the thoracic pedicle is identified by creating a horizontal line through the midportion of the transverse processes and a vertical line through the midportion of the facet joint (Figs. 8.2A and B). The thoracic pedicle is oriented in a posterolateral to anteromedial direction by approximately 10° along most of the thoracic spine, with a slight anterior and lateral angulation at T12 (Fig. 8.2C). Sagittal plane orientation of the thoracic pedicle is slightly cephalad. Care must be taken to place screws parallel to the vertebral endplates (Fig. 8.2D).

The transpedicular approach is best accomplished with a midline incision over the pathologic segment. A midline incision is made directly over the spinous process for a distance of approximately 6 to 8 cm. It is often advisable to take a preoperative radiograph with a skin marker to identify an approximate level. The dissection of the subcutaneous tissues as well as the muscle is then carried out in a manner identical

Figure 8.2

Transpedicular approach to the thoracic spine.

A   The entry to the thoracic pedicle is identified by creating a horizontal line through the midportion of the transverse processes and a vertical line through the midportion of the facet joint.

B   Oblique view of the spine showing the pedicle entry sites.

to that used in the posterior approach to the spine. This approach, however, is often made unilaterally, as dictated by the pathology. The dissection is carried out laterally to the tips of the transverse processes and a self-retaining retractor is then placed.

This exposure is largely used for decompressive procedures such as a herniated thoracic disc. It is also a useful procedure in biopsy of the anterior vertebral elements. For the purposes of biopsy, a high speed burr is best used to create a small cortical window into the pedicle using the previously described landmarks. Once this cortical window has been created, a probe may then be placed into the pedicle slowly under fluoroscopic guidance to ensure proper positioning. Through this entry portal into the thoracic vertebrae, a Craig needle or similar biopsy instrument may be used to obtain tissue for diagnostic purposes. In transpedicular decompressions, a burr may also be utilized in removing the pedicle in a piecemeal fashion. A partial hemilaminectomy may also be completed, essentially creating a gutter for access to either the vertebral body or the intervertebral disc. The thoracic pedicle is quite dense bone. Use of a high speed burr with adequate irrigation and visualization is usually a safe procedure. Potential pitfalls of this technique include injury to the thoracic cord given its proximity, inadequate exposure of the pathology and potential damage to the facet joint. Given these potential difficulties and limitations, this is not the preferred technique for most cases when compared to either a formal thoracotomy or a costotransversectomy.

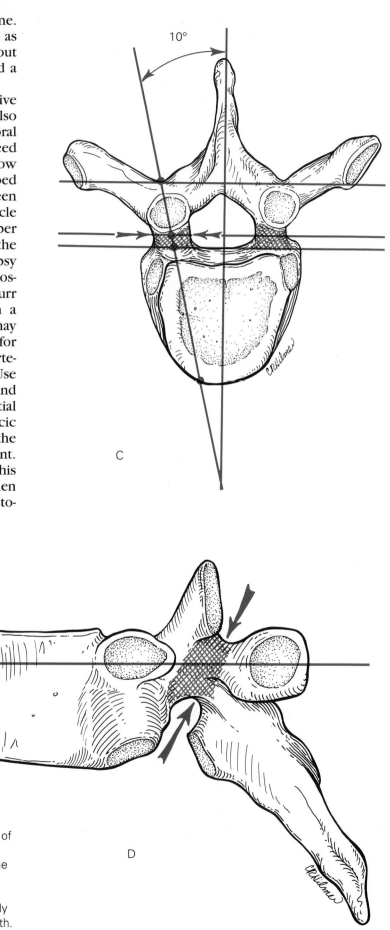

C The thoracic pedicle is oriented in a posterolateral to anteromedial direction by approximately 10° along most of the thoracic spine, with a slight anterior and lateral angulation at T12. The depth, width and angulation of the pedicle must be determined with imaging studies preoperatively.

D Sagittal plane orientation of the thoracic pedicle is slightly cephalad, and the pedicle height is greater than the width.

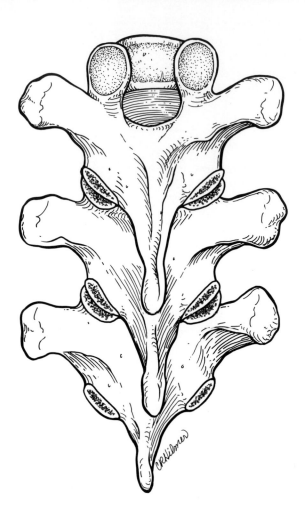

A

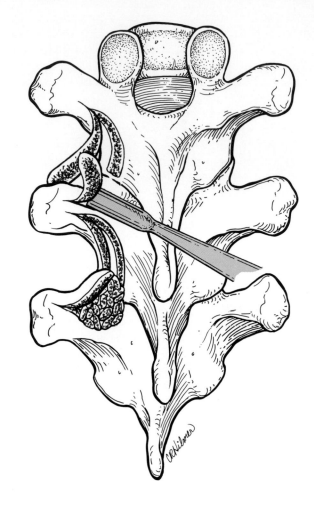

B

When performing any stabilization procedure proper preparation of the bony spine is necessary to achieve fusion. Facet joints must be resected, and the cartilage in the joint is thoroughly removed (Fig. 8.3A). Decortication must be completed over the involved laminae and spinous and transverse processes (Fig. 8.3B). This process may be completed with a high speed burr, osteotome or gouge. Cancellous bone is then packed about the facet joint and other decorticated surfaces (Figs. 8.3C, 8.4D).

Thoracic laminectomies are rarely performed in decompression of the thoracic spinal cord, but may still be required in treatment of some spinal cord tumors or epidural hematoma, or in conjunction with stabilization procedures. Laminectomies in this region of the spine for fractures should be avoided, as unacceptably high rates of progressive neurologic loss and deformity have been reported.

Figure 8.3

Posterior fusion technique of the thoracic spine.

A Facet joints must be resected, and the cartilage in the joint is thoroughly removed.

B Decortication is completed over the involved laminae, spinous and transverse processes with a gouge, osteotome or power burr.

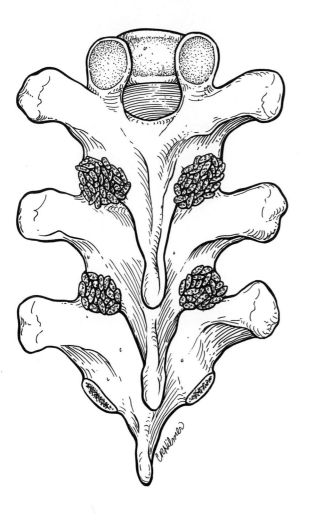

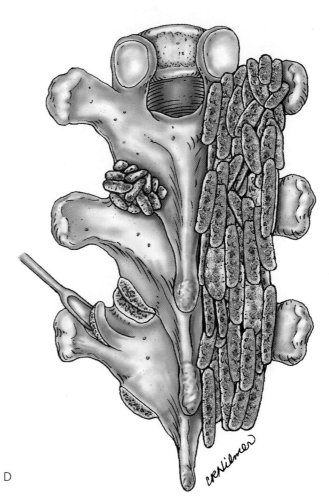

C Cancellous bone is then packed into the joint for facet fusion.

D Strips of bone graft are laid along the transverse processes and laminae for posterolateral fusion.

Posterolateral approach to the thoracic spine (costotransversectomy)

The costotransversectomy is a surgical approach to the thoracic spine that can be made in one of two positions, either prone or in the lateral decubitus position, with the patient being tilted anteriorly approximately 20 to 30°. In the prone position the patient should be placed on cushioned bolsters to allow for adequate chest expansion. In the lateral decubitus position the sandbag is best utilized. For approaches to the upper region of the thoracic spine, the arm on the affected side must be maximally elevated to move the scapula away from the midline. Three types of skin incisions have been described. A curvilinear incision approximately 8 cm lateral to the appropriate spinous process and measuring 9 to 14 cm in length is utilized (Fig. 8.4A). The center portion of the incision should be centered over the rib involved in the pathologic process. This is the most commonly used incision. Alternatively, a straight paramedian incision can be utilized. This should be placed approximately three fingers'-breadths (6 cm) from the midline. The length of this incision averages 10 to 12 cm. Finally, a T-shaped incision can be utilized, which gives maximal exposure. This is only utilized when wide, multi-level posterior lateral exposure is required. With this T-shaped incision the longitudinal portion is made in the midline directly over the spinous processes and measures approximately 15 cm in length. The transverse limb of the incision is made at the level of the vertebrae to be exposed. It is wise to take an intraoperative radiograph to verify the level prior to making this portion of the incision.

For the purposes of biopsy and exposure of an intervertebral disc or a vertebral body, the prone position with either a straight paramedian or a curved linear incision is generally recommended. For complete resection of a vertebral body and an intervertebral disc followed by strut graft reconstruction, a wider exposure is required. It is generally recommended that the semilateral decubitus position be utilized either with a curved linear paraspinous skin incision or the T-shaped incision as described above.

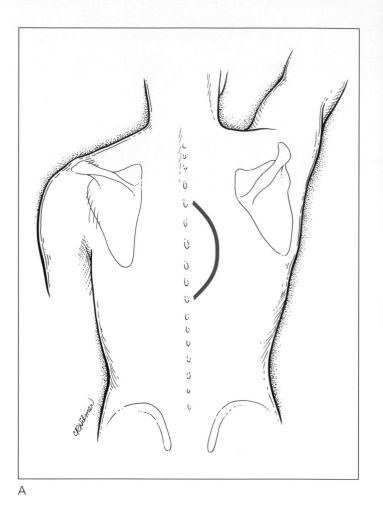

A

Figure 8.4

Costotransversectomy.

A A curvilinear incision approximately 8 cm lateral to the appropriate spinous process and measuring 9–14 cm in length is utilized. The center portion of the incision should be centered over the rib involved in the pathologic process.

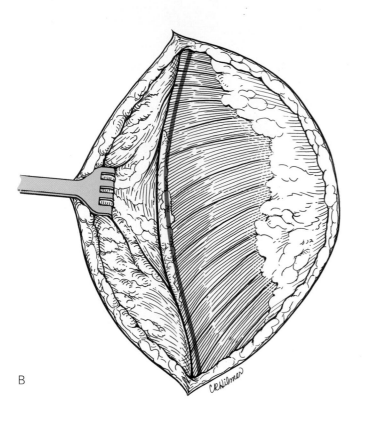

B

After mobilization of the the skin and subcutaneous flap, the trapezius muscle is then identified. The fascia and muscle fibers of the trapezius may be split in line with its fibers, particularly when a limited exposure is required. For wider exposure, the trapezius may be cut transversely (Fig. 8.2B). The trapezius muscle receives its nerve supply cranially from the spinal accessory nerve, and as such is not denervated with either technique. The paraspinal muscles can be retracted medially. Alternatively, they can be cut in a transverse fashion and retracted in a craniocaudal fashion. Since these muscles are innervated segmentally, they are not at risk for denervation. The proper rib to be resected must be identified radiographically. Subperiosteal rib dissection is then completed for a distance of 6 to 10 cm from the costotransverse articulation. Using a rib cutter, the rib is initially divided laterally. The subperiosteal dissection is carried out in a circumferential fashion approximating the costotransverse articulation (Fig. 8.4C). The ligamentous structures about the costotransverse articulation are then resected either with a sharp knife or with electrocautery. Once this joint is freed, the transverse process may preferentially be resected with a bone

B The skin and subcutaneous tissues are mobilized as a flap, and the trapezius muscle is then divided in line with its fibers or vertically if wider exposure is needed.

C The paraspinal muscles are retracted medially or cut in a transverse fashion and retracted in a craniocaudal fashion. The rib is exposed and dissected subperiosteally for a distance of 6–10 cm from the costotransverse articulation. Using a rib cutter, the rib is initially divided laterally, and disarticulated at the costotransverse articulation.

1 Semispinalis m.
2 Transverse process of T8
3 Vertebral column
4 T7
5 T6
6 Longissimus m.
7 Trapezius m.
8 Lung
9 Ext. intercostal m.
10 Iliocostal m.
11 Periosteum of 7th rib
12 Costotransverse lig.

Contd   C

Figure 8.4 *(contd)*

D The resection of the rib and transverse process is followed by exposure of the lateral aspect of the vertebral body.

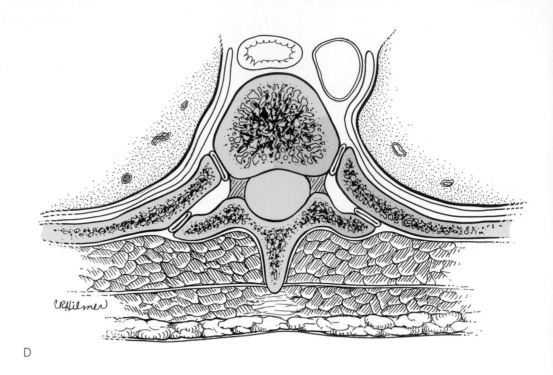

D

E Following retraction of the parietal pleura from the vertebral bodies, malleable retractors are inserted to provide adequate visualization. Sympathetic trunk is preserved, and segmental vessels may be ligated.

1 Sympathetic trunk
2 Communicating branch
3 Iliocostal n.
4 Greater splanchnic n.
5 Lung
6 Iliocostal vessels
7 Intervertebral disc

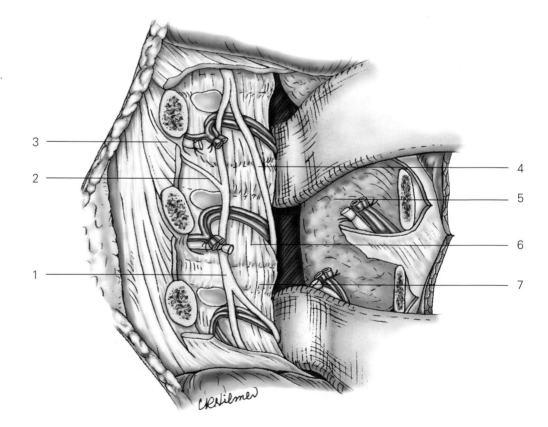

E

rongeur. The rib is then lifted carefully out of the bed. The neurovascular bundle lying at the caudal aspect of the rib should have carefully been separated from the rib itself. Removal of the rib at this point is accomplished with a combination of sharp dissection of the costovertebral joint and rotatory manipulation of the rib. Care must be taken in this region to avoid hemorrhage from the segmental vessels. It should be remembered that the neurovascular bundle courses on the lower edge of the rib, having exited the intervertebral foramen just caudal to the base of the transverse process. Care must be taken when stripping the periosteum over the anterior aspect of the rib to avoid damaging the pleura, which lies immediately under the rib bed. Depending on the extent of the exposure required, multiple rib resections may be completed in this manner.

Sharp dissection is then carried from the base of the transverse process directly onto the pedicle and subsequently the vertebral body. The resection of the rib and transverse process will lead to the exposure of the lateral aspect of the vertebral body (Fig. 8.4D). This portion of dissection is largely completed using a series of sponge sticks. The endothoracic fascia beneath the rib periosteum as well as the parietal pleura is cautiously retracted along the anterior aspect of the vertebrae as well as of the intervertebral disc. Care is generally taken to preserve the neurovascular bundle. If necessary, the intercostal vessels may be ligated and transected. Following retraction of the parietal pleura from the vertebral bodies, malleable retractors may then be inserted to provide adequate visualization (Fig. 8.4E). This approach may be utilized bilaterally in spondylectomy cases for tumor resection. Care must be taken to avoid entry into the pleural cavity. If in fact this occurs the patient will require a chest tube postoperatively. The most common encounter to a problem is either avulsion or transection of one of the intercostal vessels. These must be controlled and carefully ligated. The intercostal nerves should be spared as much as possible. Additional structures at risk include the dura and spinal cord. Care must be taken during any decompression to maintain a three-dimensional mental image of the spinal canal.

Conclusion

The posterior, transpedicular, and posterolateral approaches of the thoracic spine have been included for discussion. The posterior approach to the thoracic spine is a relatively safe technique and is used largely for fracture and deformity cases. The costotransversectomy approach as well as the transpedicular approach represent techniques that are largely used for decompression as well as biopsy of the anterior vertebral elements. The visualizations of these posterolateral techniques certainly are not as broad as the traditional thoracotomy, but hopefully avoid the associated complications of the latter technique in selected cases.

Bibliography

Bohlman HH, Zdeblick TA (1988) Anterior excision of herniated thoracic discs. *J Bone Joint Surg* **70A**:1038–47

Larson SJ, Holst RA, Hemmy DC et al (1976) Lateral extracavity approach to traumatic lesions of the thoracic and lumbar spine. *J Neurosurg* **45**:628–37

Lesoin F, Rousseaux M, Lozes G et al (1986) Posterolateral approach to tumours of the dorsolumbar spine. *Acta Neurochir* (Wien) **81**:40–4

Otani K, Nakai S, Fujimura Y et al (1982) Surgical treatment of thoracic disc herniation using the anterior approach. *J Bone Joint Surg* **64B**:340–3

Patterson RH Jr, Arbit E (1969) A surgical approach through the pedicle to protruded thoracic discs. *J Neurosurg* **31**:459–61

Perot PL Jr, Munro DD (1969) Transthoracic removal of midline thoracic disc protrusions causing spinal cord compression. *J Neurosurg* **31**:452–8

Ransohoff J, Spencer F, Siew F et al (1969) Transthoracic removal of thoracic disc: Report of three cases. *J Neurosurg* **31**:459–61

Simpson JM, Silveri CP, Simeone FA et al (1993) Thoracic disc herniation. Reevaluation of the posterior approach using a modified costotransversectomy. *Spine* **18**:1872–7

Stener B (1971) Total spondylectomy in chondrosarcoma arising from the seventh thoracic vertebra. *J Bone Joint Surg* **53B**:288–95

9

Anterior exposure and fusion of the thoracic spine

Lee H Riley III

Introduction

Robinson was the first to describe thoracotomy and partial lobectomy for the treatment of bronchiectasis (1917). Reinhoff (1933) demonstrated that a pneumonectomy could be performed safely. Widespread use of the thoracotomy approach, however, began much later, when more advanced life support techniques to reduce perioperative mortality were developed and widely used. Hodgson and Stock (1956) demonstrated its usefulness in spine surgery, using the technique to perform an anterior vertebral body debridement and bone grafting for a tuberculous abscess. Since 1956, the anterior approach to the thoracic spine through a thoracotomy incision has been used for a wide variety of procedures.

Indications

1. Anterior release for fixed deformity such as scoliosis and kyphosis
2. Epiphysiodesis for congenital bars and hemivertebrae
3. Anterior decompression for fractures, tumor, infection and disc herniations
4. Fusion
5. Biopsy.

Surgical techniques

The thoracic spine can be reached using either a right or left sided thoracotomy. An approach through the right chest is easier to perform and is more commonly used because it avoids the thoracic aorta, which courses through the left chest. A left sided approach is used when the pathology is predominantly located on the left side, such as a thoracic scoliosis with a left apex or a left sided thoracic tumor or disc. A left sided approach may also be preferable in the lower thoracic spine, when conversion into a thoracoabdominal approach may be necessary, since the liver can limit the distal extent of the dissection if a right sided approach is chosen.

The operation is performed in the lateral decubitus position with the patient's upper leg and knee flexed to help maintain the position. Exposure can be improved by placing the patient over the break in the table, so that the rib interspace is widened when the table is flexed and better visualization of the operative field is obtained. Care should also be taken to position the patient securely in the direct lateral position. Knowing the location of the spinal canal relative to the plane of the table is critical during the course of the operation, when anatomic landmarks have been resected or obscured. A bean bag, rolled blankets, water bags, tape, and other devices can all be used to position, pad, and secure the patient to the operating table.

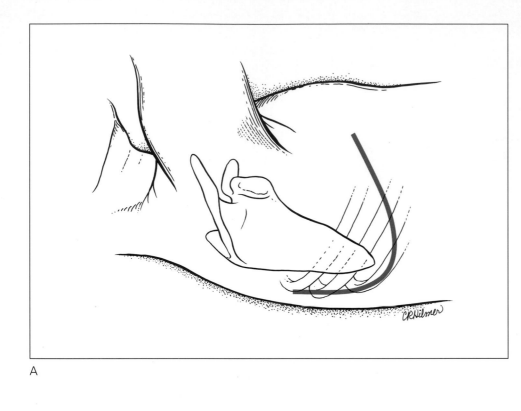

A

Figure 9.1

High transthoracic anterior thoracotomy.

A
The curved incision for high thoracic thoracotomy is made below the tip of the scapula.

The incision is made two ribs higher than the center of the lesion. Four or five vertebral bodies can usually be reached. Because the ribs slope caudally and the lower ribs are floating, caudal dissection is easier than cranial dissection. The amount of exposure possible depends upon the level entered, the mobility and slope of the surrounding ribs, and the nature of the thoracic deformity. If further cranial exposure is needed, an osteotomy or partial resection of the posterior aspect of one or two adjacent cranial ribs will often allow an additional one or two vertebrae to be reached. A second thoracotomy incision and approach can also be performed.

High transthoracic anterior thoracotomy

A curved skin incision is made below the tip of the scapula (Fig. 9.1A). This is carried down to the latissimus dorsi muscle (Fig. 9.1B), which is incised using electrocautery, leaving a cuff of muscle attached to the

scapula to allow for an adequate repair (Fig. 9.1C). The scapula can then be retracted superiorly. For added exposure, the anterior aspect of the trapezius muscle can also be undermined and incised. Rib resection is then performed by first incising the overlying periosteum in the mid portion of the rib using electrocautery (Fig. 9.1D). Once the rib has been exposed, it is divided anteriorly, elevated and resected as far posteriorly as the exposure will allow. This rib can then be saved for bone grafting.

The chest is then sharply entered in the center of the rib bed, a Finochetto retractor is placed, and the lung is retracted anteriorly and inferiorly. The pleura overlying the vertebral bodies is then incised and the segmental vessels are ligated as needed in the middle of the vertebral bodies. Blunt dissection with a kitner is then performed, beginning over the disc spaces, and then developed over the vertebral bodies. A moist laparotomy pad and a malleable retractor are placed to the opposite side of the vertebral body to retract and protect the great vessels and esophagus (Fig. 9.1E).

B
The incision is carried down to the latissimus dorsi muscle.

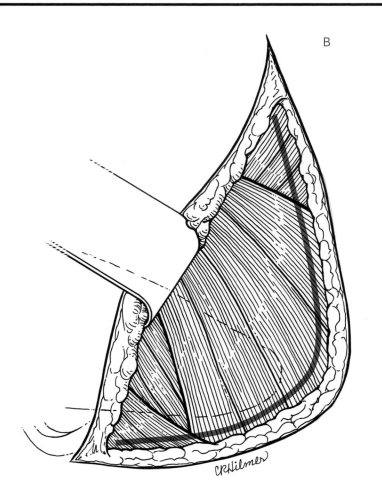

C
A cuff of muscle is left attached to the scapula for an adequate repair.

1 Trapezius m.
2 Serratus ant. m.
3 Latissimus m.
4 Inf. angle of scapula

Contd

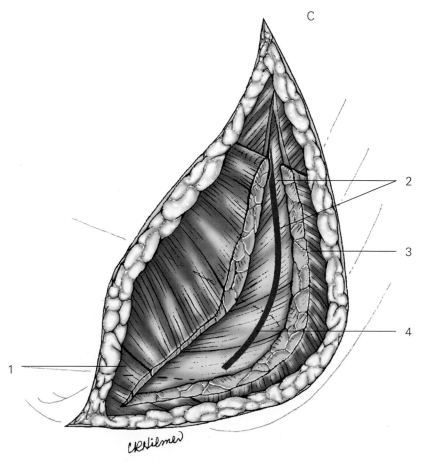

Figure 9.1 *(contd)*

D
The periosteum is incised over the middle of the rib to be removed.

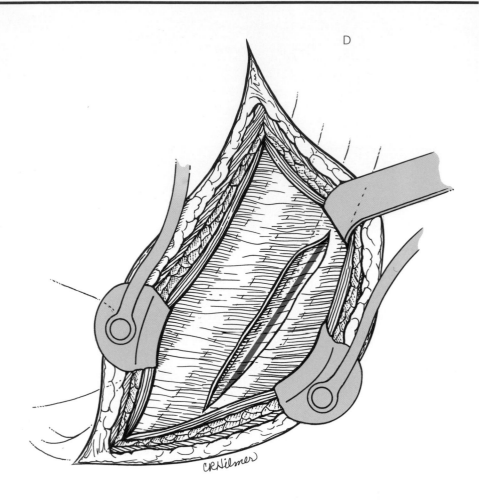

E
Final exposure prior to placement of a laparotomy pad and malleable retractors to protect the great vessels and the esophagus.

1 Reflected tongue of pleura
2 Medial end of rib
3 Azygos v. ligated
4 Reflected tongue of pleura
5 Esophagus, retracted off spine
6 Aorta
7 Ant. longitudinal lig. over thoracic spine
8 Pleura
9 Ext. surface of retracted rib

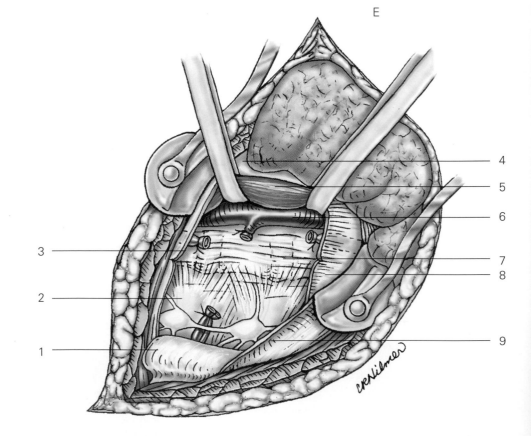

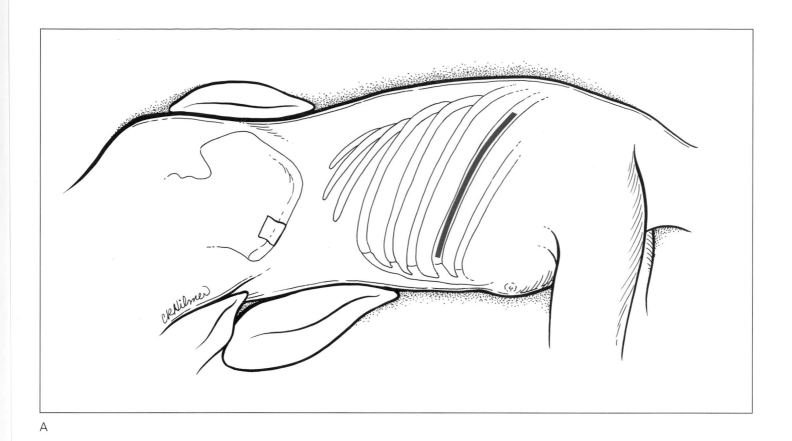

A

Figure 9.2

Transthoracic anterior thoracotomy.

A

Skin incision extending from the anterior border of the latissimus muscle to the costochondral junction.

Contd

Transthoracic anterior thoracotomy

The skin incision is made along the rib intended for removal from the anterior margin of the latissimus muscle anteriorly to the costochondral junction (Fig. 9.2A). The anterior aspect of the latissimus muscle can be undermined or minimally incised (Fig. 9.2B). Rib resection is then performed by first incising the overlying periosteum in the mid portion of the rib using electrocautery. A rib stripper is then used to dissect off the intercostal musculature (Fig. 9.2C). Along the superior margin of the rib the intercostal musculature is stripped from posterior to anterior, and along the inferior rib margin it is stripped anterior to posterior. Care is taken to not damage the neurovascular bundle that travels along the inferior margin of the rib. Once the rib has been exposed, it is divided at the costochondral junction anteriorly, elevated and resected as far posteriorly as the exposure will allow (Fig. 9.2D). This rib can then be saved for bone grafting. The chest is then sharply entered in the center of the rib bed, a Finochetto retractor is placed and the lung is retracted anteriorly and inferiorly. The pleura overlying the vertebral bodies is then incised and the segmental vessels are ligated as needed in the middle of the vertebral bodies. A blunt dissection with a kitner is then performed beginning over the disc

Figure 9.2 *(contd)*

F
Extrapleural dissection is best performed manually or with a sponge stick on the delicate pleura.

F

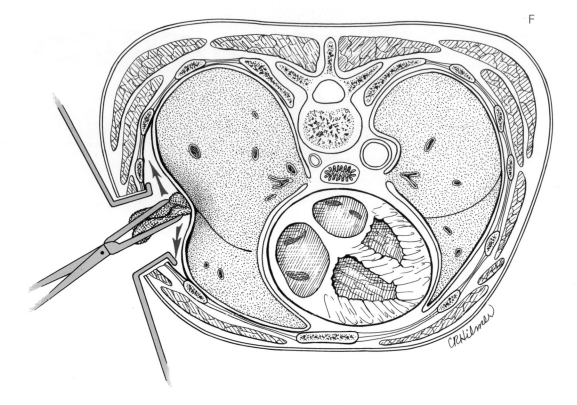

G
Retraction of the lung and the placement of a retractor provides the exposure of the anterolateral aspect of the vertebral body

G

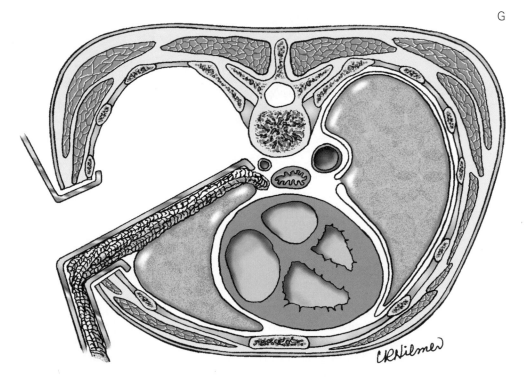

Excision of thoracic disc herniation

A standard anterior thoracotomy approach is used. The rib below the disc herniation is followed to the neural foramen and the disc is identified and exposed by incising the paravertebral tissue longitudinally. Segmental vessels are ligated as necessary. The rib head is removed and portions of the pedicle above and below are drilled out to provide access to the interspace (Fig. 9.3A). The nerve can be traced to the intervertebral foramen to identify the lateral margin of the dura. The interspace is entered through a large incision as close to the posterior longitudinal ligament as possible. Decompression proceeds from as far across the interspace as possible and towards the exposed side, so that the process of decompression does not compromise exposure as the dura expands anteriorly (Fig. 9.3B). Disc material is brought into this created space so that further neural compression does not occur during the process of decompression. Once the decompression is complete, a fusion can be performed if substantial destabilization has occurred, using portions of the excised rib or iliac crest bone (Fig. 9.3C).

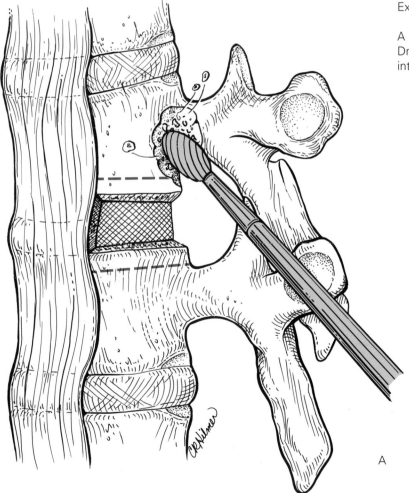

Figure 9.3

Excision of thoracic disc herniation.

A

Drilling of the pedicle to gain access to the interspace.

Contd.

Figure 9.3 *(contd)*

B
Exposure is best maintained by beginning the decompression as far across the interspace as possible and proceeding to the ipsilateral side.

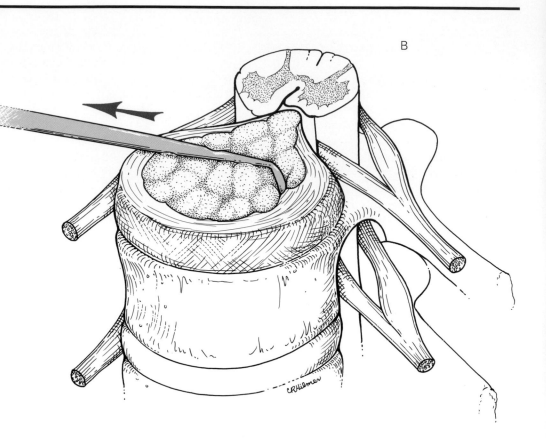

C
Pieces of the removed rib can be used for reconstruction. This should not constrict the spinal canal.

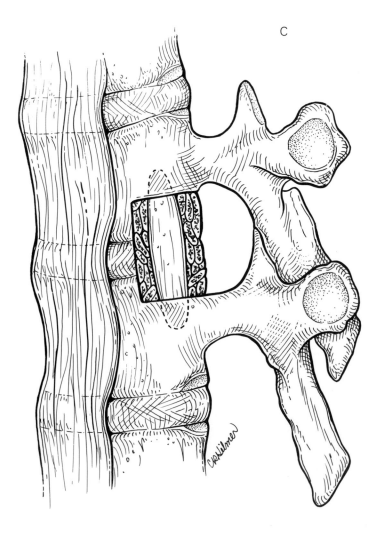

Anterior fusion techniques

Vascularized rib graft

This procedure may be indicated for severe kyphosis or a compromised vascular bed. The thoracotomy is made through the rib at the level intended for fusion. The segmental vessels are not ligated. For fusion of a kyphosis with an apex between T2 and T5 the rib two to three levels below the apex is used. For a kyphosis with an apex at T6 or distal the rib two or three levels above the apex is rotated. The intercostal musculature is divided above the rib intended for rotation. The intercostal musculature caudal to the rib is then divided 4 mm below the rib to preserve the neurovascular bundle. This is continued to the costal angle, where a subperiosteal exposure preserving the neurovascular bundle is performed and the rib cut. The neurovascular bundle is then followed to the intervertebral foramen. Distally the rib is cut and the segmental vessel ligated at the length necessary to span the desired distance (Fig. 9.4A). The rib is then rotated and the ends are driven into the anchoring holes (Fig. 9.4B).

Anterior rib and fibula strut graft for kyphosis

A high speed burr or chisel is used to prepare the anchoring holes in the anterior aspect of the vertebral

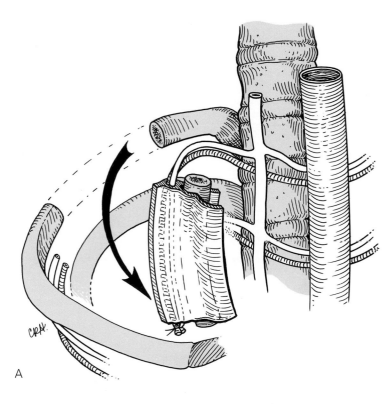

A

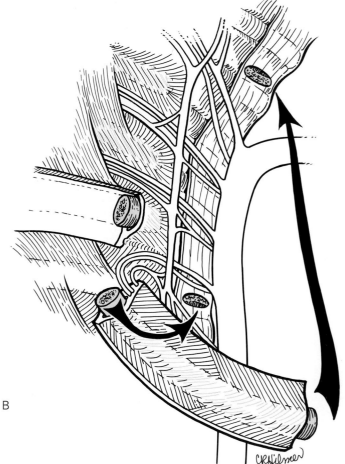

B

Figure 9.4

Anterior fusion techniques.

A
The neurovascular bundle is preserved proximally and ligated distally. The rib is cut proximally and distally to its desired length.

B
The rib is rotated around its vascular pedicle and inserted into anchoring holes in the vertebral bodies.

Contd

bodies of the end vertebrae and intervening vertebrae. The most structurally sound strut graft is used to span the end vertebrae and the less structurally sound strut graft is used for the intervening segments. Morsellized cancellous graft is placed in the intervening disc spaces (Fig. 9.4C).

Anterior tricortical strut graft

A high speed burr or curved curet is used to create anchoring holes in the mid portion of the adjacent end plates. Tricortical iliac crest or other structural allograft bone is fashioned into the shape of a fat 'T' using bone rongeurs. A tip of the bone graft is then impacted into an anchoring hole and either the opposite end is pressed into the anchoring hole by distracting the intervening segment or a small trough in the lateral cortex is made to allow keying of the graft into the opposite anchoring hole (Fig. 9.4D). The graft spans from the superior endplate of the proximal vertebra to the inferior endplate of the lower vertebra. The construct is then assessed for stability and bone graft packed into the adjacent dead space. If anterior instrumentation is to be utilized, the graft should span from the lower endplate of the proximal vertebra to the superior endplate of the lower vertebra so that screws can be inserted into the vertebral bodies.

C

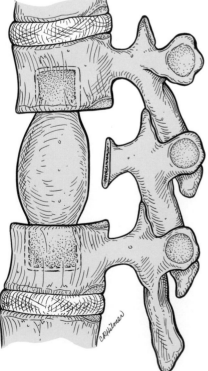

Figure 9.4 *contd*

C
Structural strut grafts are placed into anchoring holes in the vertebral bodies. Cancellous bone graft is then placed in the intervening disc spaces.

D
A structural graft can be placed between the superior endplate of the proximal vertebra and the inferior endplate of the lower vertebra.

D

Bibliography

Bohlman HH, Zdeblick TA (1988) Anterior excision of herniated thoracic discs. *J Bone Joint Surg* **70A**:1038–47

Crafoord C, Hiertonn T, Lindblom K et al (1958) Spinal cord compression caused by a protruded thoracic disc: Report of a case treated with anterolateral fenestration of the disc. *Acta Orthop Scand* **28**:103–7

Dwyer AF, Schafer MF (1974) Anterior approach to scoliosis: Results of treatment in fifty-one cases. *J Bone Joint Surg* **56B**:218–44

Hodgson AR (1965) Correction of fixed spinal curves. A preliminary communication. *J Bone Joint Surg* **47A**:1221–7

Hodgson AR, Stock FE (1956) Anterior spinal fusion, a preliminary communication on the radical treatment of Pott's disease and Pott's paraplegia. *Br J Surg* **44**:266–75

Martin NS, Williamson J (1970) The role of surgery in the treatment of malignant tumors of the spine. *J Bone Joint Surg* **52B**:227–37

Reinhoff WJ (1933) Pneumonectomy. Preliminary report of the operative technique in two successful cases. *Bull Johns Hopkins Hosp* **53**:390–3

Robinson S (1917) The surgery of bronchiectasis: Including a report of five complete resections of the lower lobe of the lung with one death. *Surg Gynecol Obstet* **24**:194–215

10

Posterior instrumentation of the thoracolumbar spine

Lee H Riley III
Harry L Shufflebarger

Introduction

The modern era of spinal instrumentation began in the late 1950s with the development of an instrumentation system that allowed deformity reduction and immediate stability under normal loading conditions by Paul Harrington (Harrington 1960). Although there has been a rapid evolution in methods and instrumentation types, the fundamental functions of instrumentation remain the same. Many of the more recent advances in instrumentation allow the surgeon to achieve reduction and stabilization more efficiently with less disturbance to normal structures and function. This chapter will review segmental spinal fixation techniques for scoliosis and kyphosis, sublaminar wiring, and spinous process wiring using Drummond buttons.

Indications

1. Scoliosis
2. Kyphosis
3. Instability associated with tumor, infection and fracture.

Segmental hook–rod systems

In the late 1970s and early 1980s the concept of multiple hook sites on a single rod was pioneered by Cotrel and Dubousset. This system type has seen widespread acceptance and modification since its inception. These systems provide the ability to correct deformity in multiple planes. Multiple purchase points also provide secure fixation, allowing many patients to forgo bracing postoperatively without loss of fixation. Regardless of manufacturer, all segmental hook-rod systems contain multiple hook designs which allow secure fixation to the lamina, transverse process or pedicle with minimal penetration of the spinal canal (Figs. 10.1A–D). The main difference between systems is the connection mechanism between the hooks and the rod (Fig. 10.1E). Some systems allow the use of sublaminar wires in addition to hooks (Fig. 10.1F). Familiarity with the hook types, sizes, and the associated instrumentation of the system to be used is an important part of preoperative planning to minimize operative time and instrument associated complications.

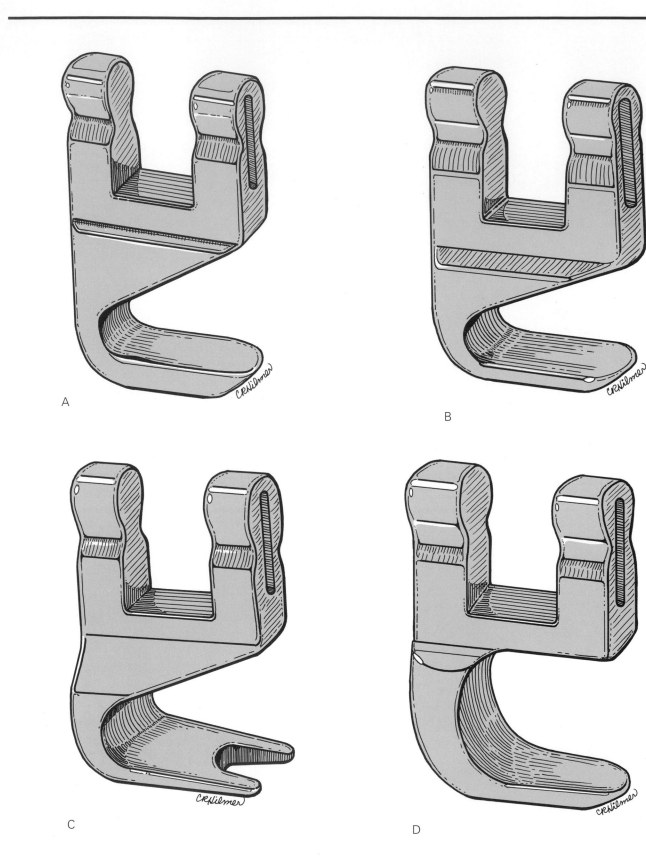

Figure 10.1

Types of hooks for the thoracolumbar spine.Thoracic laminar
(A,B), thoracic pedicle (C), and lumbar laminar hooks (D) are
designed to provide a secure purchase with minimal
penetration into the spinal canal.

E   F

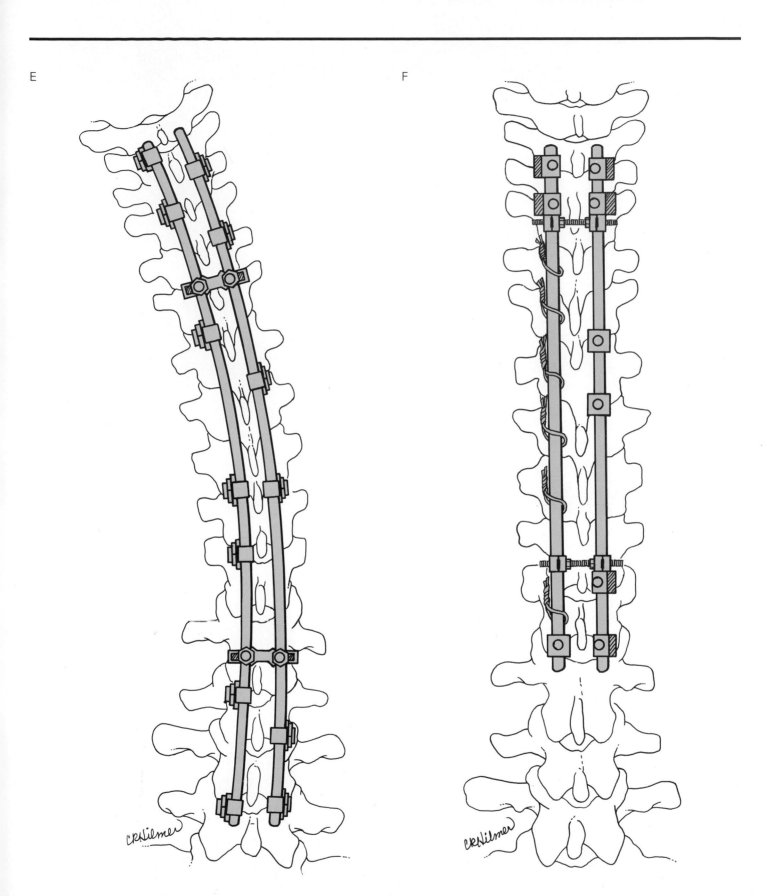

E
An illustration of the Texas Scottish Rite Hospital (TSRH)™
(Acromed Inc, Cleveland, Ohio) system.
F
An illustration of ISOLA™ (Danek Inc, Memphis, Tennessee)
instrumentation with sublaminar wires.

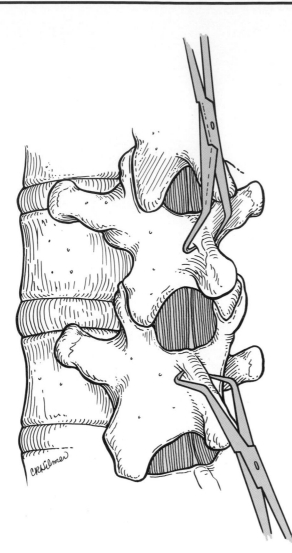

A

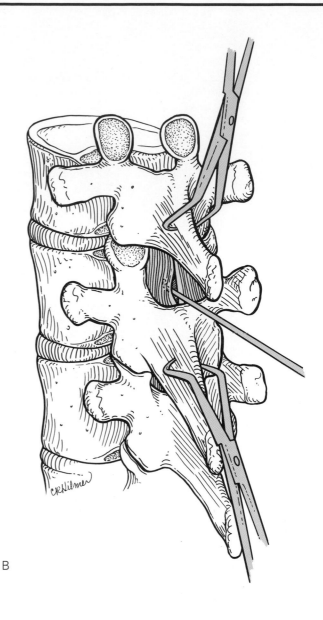

B

Figure 10.2

The supralaminar hook insertion technique.

A
The spinous process is removed and the ligamentum flavum is exposed. Towel clips may be used to widen the space during the insertion of the hook.

B
The midline raphe of the ligamentum flavum is identified and the ligamentum is removed at the hook site to allow for hook placement.

Hook insertion techniques

Supralaminar hook

With any hooks, meticulous exposure of the bony anatomy is important. For the supralaminar hook, the ligamentum flavum is exposed by removing the overlying spinous process and separating the laminae with towel clips (Fig. 10.2A). The laminotomy performed for the supralaminar hook site should remove little or no bone from the superior lamina and as little bone as possible from the superior aspect of the lamina above, to maximize its mechanical strength and minimize the likelihood of the hook plunging into the spinal canal. Placement of a supralaminar hook can be facilitated by removing the cranial spinous process down to its base. This is not advisable at the end of a rigid construct, since this weakens the

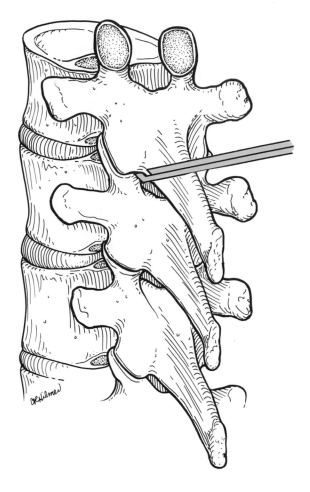

C

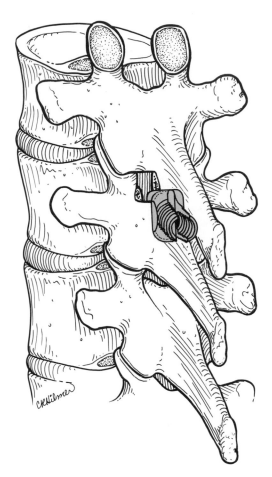

D

adjacent segment and can contribute to future adjacent segment problems.

The midline raphe of the ligamentum flavum is identified (Fig. 10.2B) and the ligamentum flavum removed using a Kerrison punch, which is also used to perform a minimal laminotomy (Fig. 10.2C). The hook is then inserted using a hook holder. Towel clips or a small lamina spreader can be used to widen the laminotomy temporarily during hook insertion. The hook should fit snugly under the lamina with minimal anterior-posterior play (Fig. 10.2D).

C
A minimal laminotomy removing little or none of the superior aspect of the lamina is performed.

D
The hook should have minimal anterior–posterior play after placement under the lamina. The laminotomy should allow insertion of the hook, but be sufficiently small to prevent inadvertent hook intrusion into the spinal canal. (A Moss–Miami hook is illustrated.)

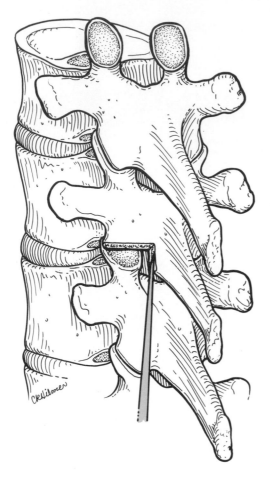

A

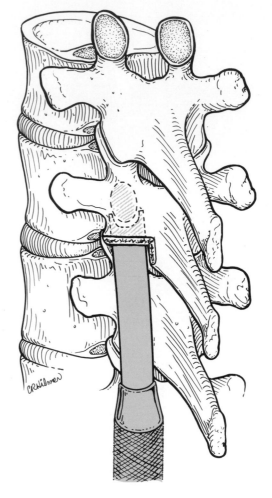

B

Figure 10.3

The pedicle hook insertion technique.

A
The vertical cut is made with an osteotome, beginning at the junction of the convexity of the superior facet with the concavity of the base of the spinous process. The osteotome should be angled so that it cannot plunge into the spinal canal.

B
The pedicle finder is used to delineate clearly the orientation of the facet joint and the location of the pedicle.

Pedicle hook

Pedicle hooks can be placed in the thoracic spine reliably from T1 to T9 and in some instances as far caudad as T11. The caudal extent is determined by the anatomy of the patient. A portion of the inferior facet is removed so that the bifid portion of the blade grips the inferior aspect of the pedicle and the blade itself maximally contacts the inferior aspect of the lamina. This is accomplished by creating a notch in the inferior aspect of the lamina using an osteotome (Fig. 10.3A). A vertical cut is first made at the base of the spinous process near the medial aspect of the facet joint. The osteotome should be oriented as horizontally as possible to prevent penetration of the canal. The transverse cut is then made about 5 mm inferior to the inferior aspect of the transverse process and is oriented perpendicular to the anticipated direction of the rod. The triangular portion of the inferior facet is removed and the articular cartilage of the superior facet joint is curetted.

A pedicle finder is then used to identify the narrow facet joint and pedicle (Fig. 10.3B). It is important to

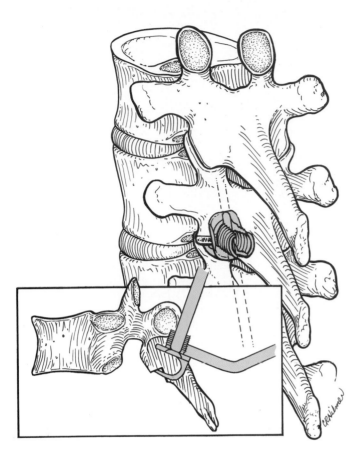

C

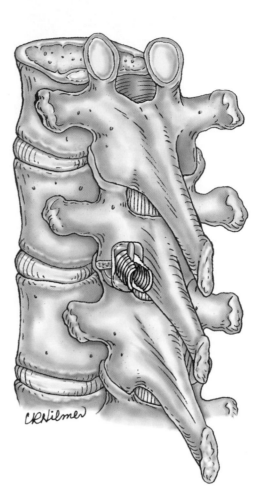

D

insert this instrument gently into the joint, with minimal force directed toward the canal. Another common mistake is to scive shallow to the joint surface and penetrate between the cortices of the inferior facet. Unicortical purchase often leads to laminar fracture and hook pullout.

A hook is then inserted manually using a hook holder (Fig. 10.3C). The hook is initially directed cephalad and anteriorly so that it enters the joint space instead of sciving superficial to it. As it enters the joint space further the angle of the blade and the orientation of the joint space will cause the hook to level out into its final position seated against the pedicle (Fig. 10.3D). If the hook does not glide easily into position it is often useful to remove the hook and use the pedicle finder again to identify the joint space and pedicle before reinserting the pedicle hook. A portion of the caudal transverse process may also need to be removed using a Lexcel rongeur if it blocks proper hook seating.

C

The tip of the hook should initially be directed cephalad and anteriorly so that it slides along the surface of the superior facet. This will facilitate the hook blade entering the joint space instead of sciving superficially into the inferior facet.

D

The hook in its final position should maximally engage the lamina and the bifid end of the blade should contact and straddle the pedicle.

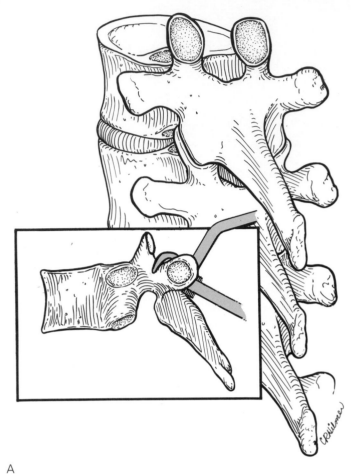

A

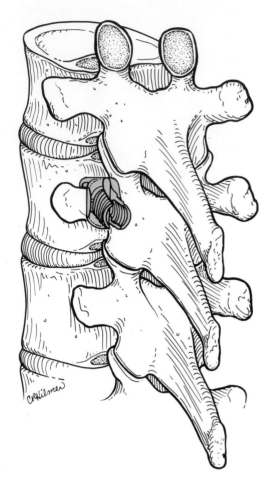

B

Transverse process hook

The superior aspect of the base of the transverse process is identified. A laminar elevator or transverse process elevator is rotated around the base of the transverse process, elevating the ligaments between the rib base and the transverse process. A lumbar laminar hook is then placed using the same motion (Fig. 10.4A). The hook should rest in the vertical position in line with a pedicle hook placed at the same level (Fig. 10.4B).

Figure 10.4

Transverse process hook insertion technique.

A
The hook is rotated into position after the elevator has prepared the hook bed at the base of the spinous process.

B
The transverse process hook should line up with a pedicle hook placed at the same level.

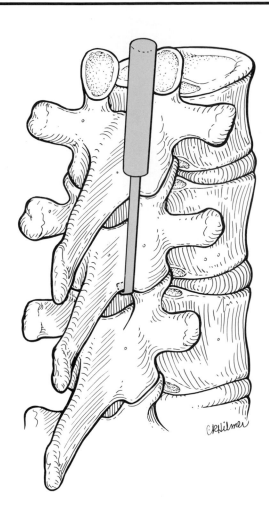

A

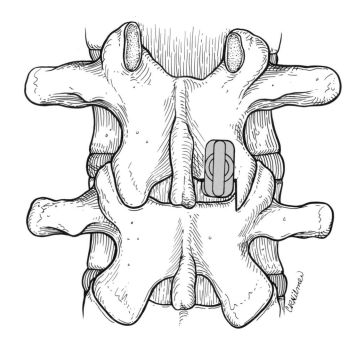

B

Infralaminar hook

Infralaminar hooks are used on the lower end vertebrae on the convex side of scoliotic curves. Hook purchase on the inferior lamina should be maximized by squaring off the inferior aspect of the lamina if necessary to allow for horizontal seating of the hook. Some narrowing of the lamina with a burr or rongeur may be necessary to allow for proper hook purchase, but this should be kept to a minimum. The adjacent capsule should be preserved at ends of constructs.

After squaring off the inferior aspect of the lamina, a lamina elevator is rotated beneath the lamina partially to strip the ligamentum flavum (Fig. 10.5A). The infralaminar hook is then inserted with a hook holder and pushed into place with a hook inserter (Fig. 10.5B).

Figure 10.5

Infralaminar hook insertion technique.

A
The laminar elevator is used to strip the ligamentum flavum from the inferior aspect of the lamina using a rolling motion.

B
The final position of the inferior lamina hook.

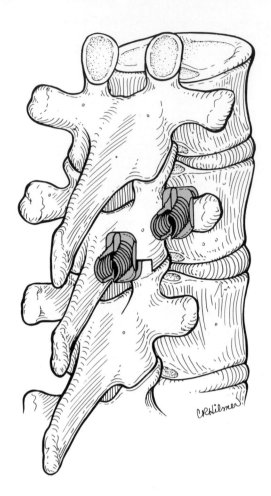

A

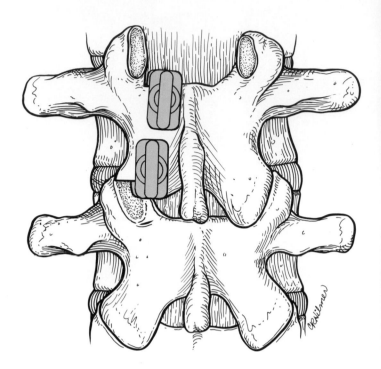

B

Hook combinations

Single level pedicle–transverse process hook claw and pedicle–laminar hook claw

Transverse process hooks are primarily used in conjunction with a pedicle hook at the upper end vertebrae on the convex side of a thoracic curve. This hook combination is also used for kyphosis correction when bone quality is good.

Both hook sites should be prepared before hook insertion. The transverse process hook should be inserted first, followed by the pedicle hook, since the rotation maneuver used to insert the transverse process hook will be blocked if the pedicle hook is inserted first (Fig. 10.6A). A supralaminar hook in combination with the pedicle hook provides a secure single level claw (Fig. 10.6B)

Figure 10.6

Single level pedicle–transverse process hook claw and pedicle–laminar hook claw.

A
Single level pedicle–transverse process hook claw: the transverse process hook should be inserted before the pedicle hook.

B
Single level pedicle–supralaminar hook claw.

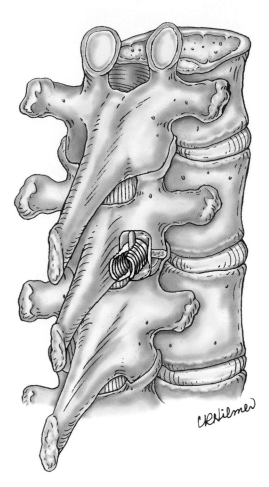

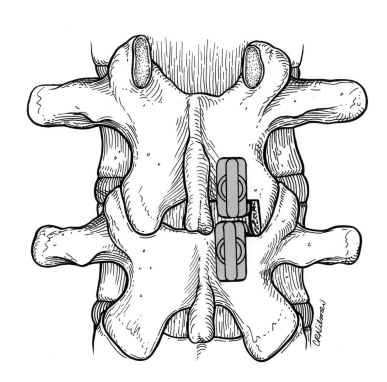

Two level pedicle – supralaminar claw

This is a sequence that can be used in kyphosis and fracture fixation (Fig. 10.7). One or more claws can be applied to distribute force over a larger area. Compression can be applied to each claw construct by locking the supralaminar hook to the rod, placing a rod holder below the pedicle hook, distracting between the rod holder and the pedicle hook and locking the pedicle hook in place once adequate compression has been achieved. The ideal amount of compression applied will depend upon bone quality.

Back to back lumbar hooks

This hook combination (Fig. 10.8) can be used in the lower concave portion of a double major thoracic and lumbar curve to open up an inclined disc space to save a fusion level. It is used in combination with an infralaminar–supralaminar hook combination on the opposite side.

Figure 10.7 *(left)*

Supralaminar–pedicle claw.

Figure 10.8 *(right)*

Back to back lumbar hooks used to level an inclined disc space.

Basic hook patterns for scoliosis

Basic hook patterns for scoliosis attempt to correct the deformity in all planes. Distraction across the concavity of a curve will tend to straighten the curve and increase kyphosis. Compression across the convexity of a curve will straighten the curve and increase lordosis (Fig. 10.9A–E). All structural components of the deformity need to be included in the instrumentation.

A

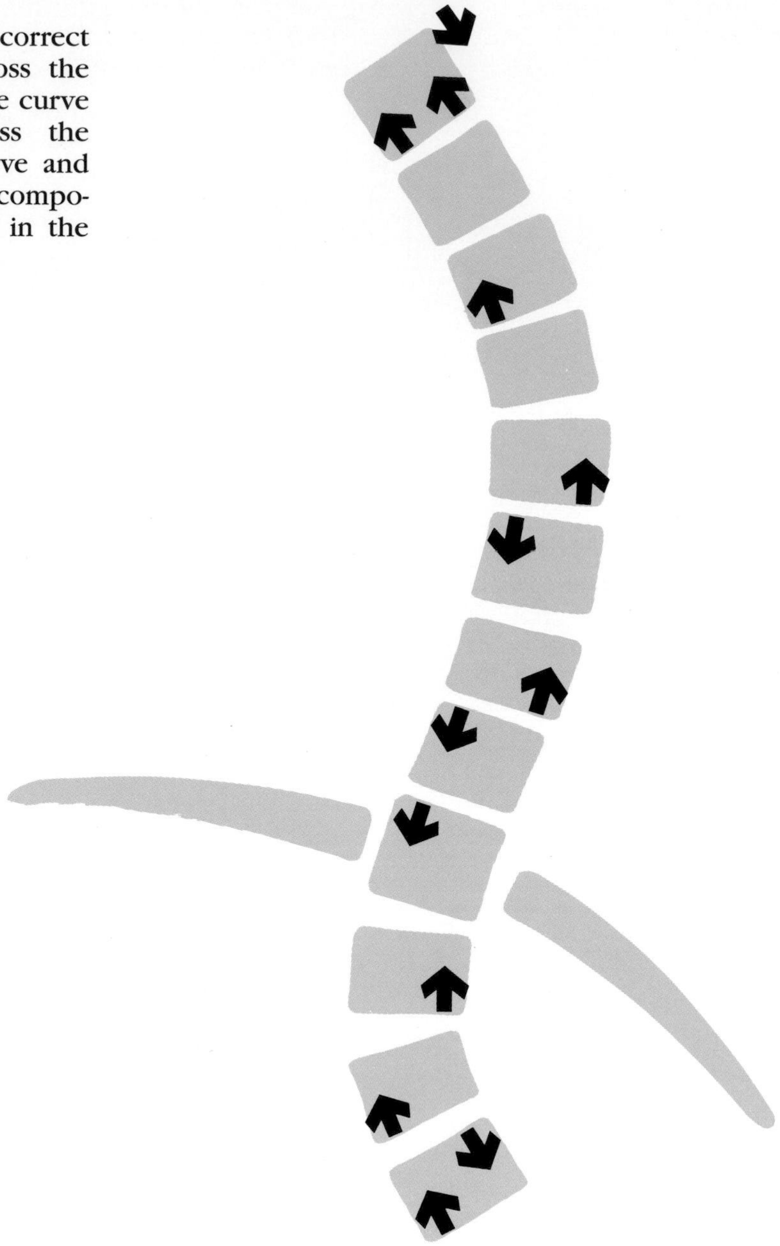

Figure 10.9

Basic hook patterns commonly used for scoliosis curve correction. The exact hook position will vary depending on the nature of the specific deformity.
A
King type I curve: segmental fixation of both thoracic and lumbar curves with distraction of the concave thoracic side and compression of the convex lumbar side, followed by compression of the convex thoracic side and slight distraction to seat the hooks on the concave lumbar side. A rod rotation maneuver may also be utilized by converting the thoracic scoliosis deformity to a kyphotic posture from the concave thoracic rod. Using the same left side rod, the lumbar scoliosis curve can be rotated into a lordosis position simultaneously.

B

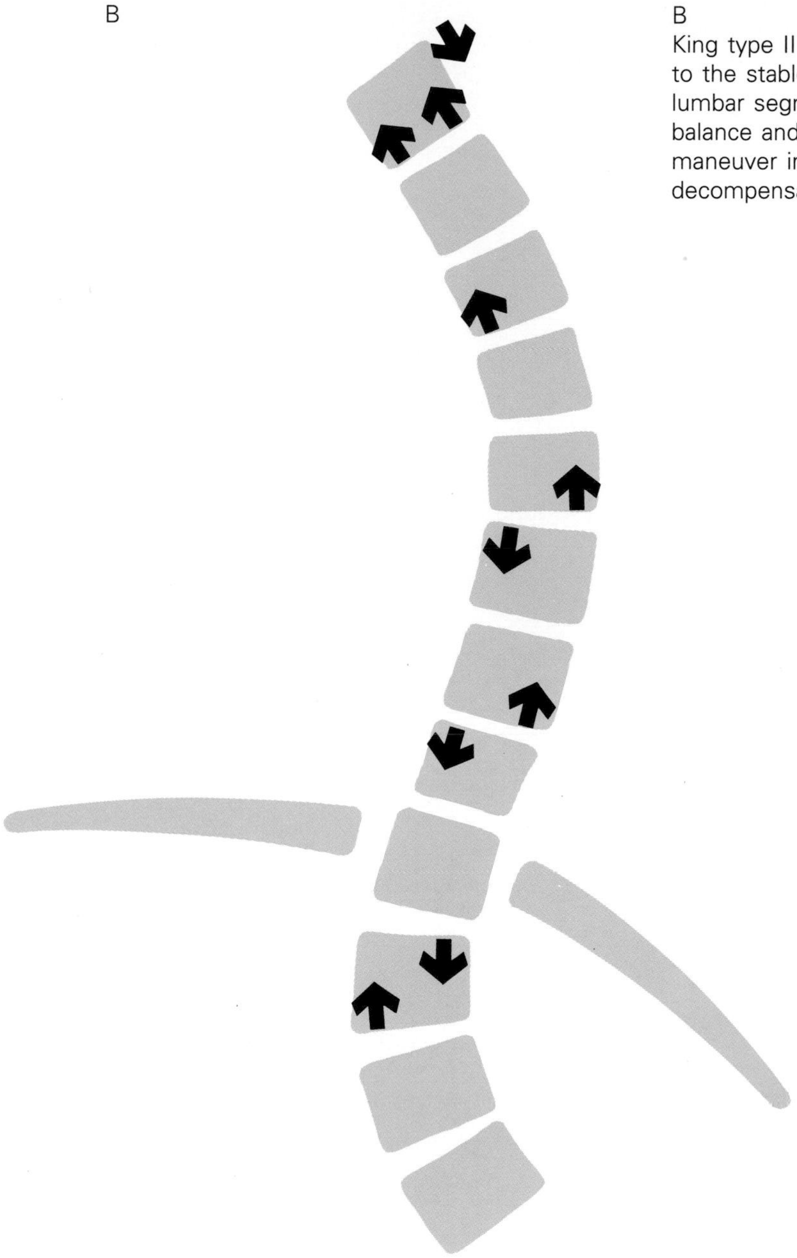

B
King type II curve: segmental fixation of the thoracic curve down to the stable vertebra is performed without fusing the lower lumbar segments. Extension of fusion to L1 may be necessary for balance and to prevent junctional kyphosis. A rod rotation maneuver in this type of curve may frequently result in decompensation of the trunk.

C

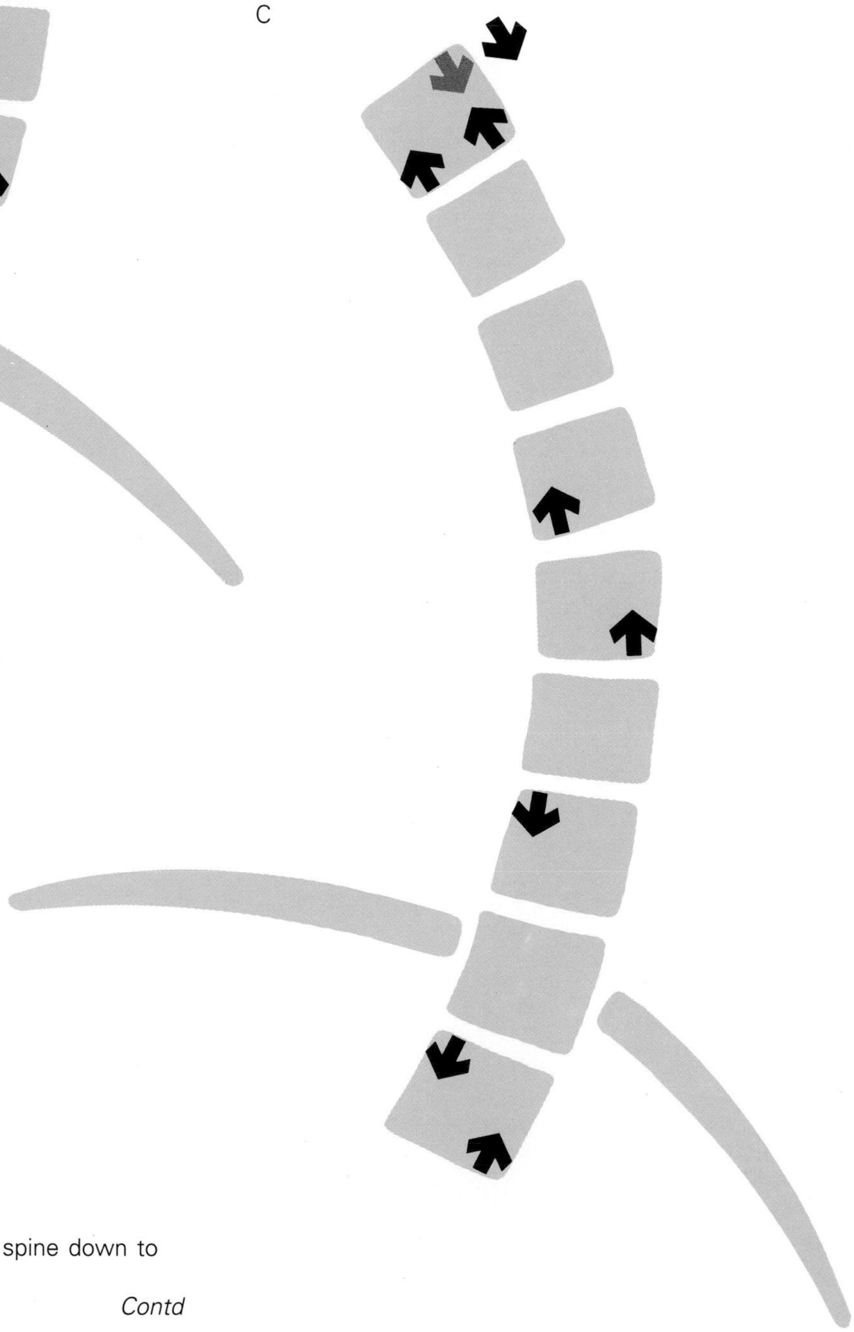

C
King type III curve: instrumentation of the thoracic spine down to the stable vertebra is performed.

Contd

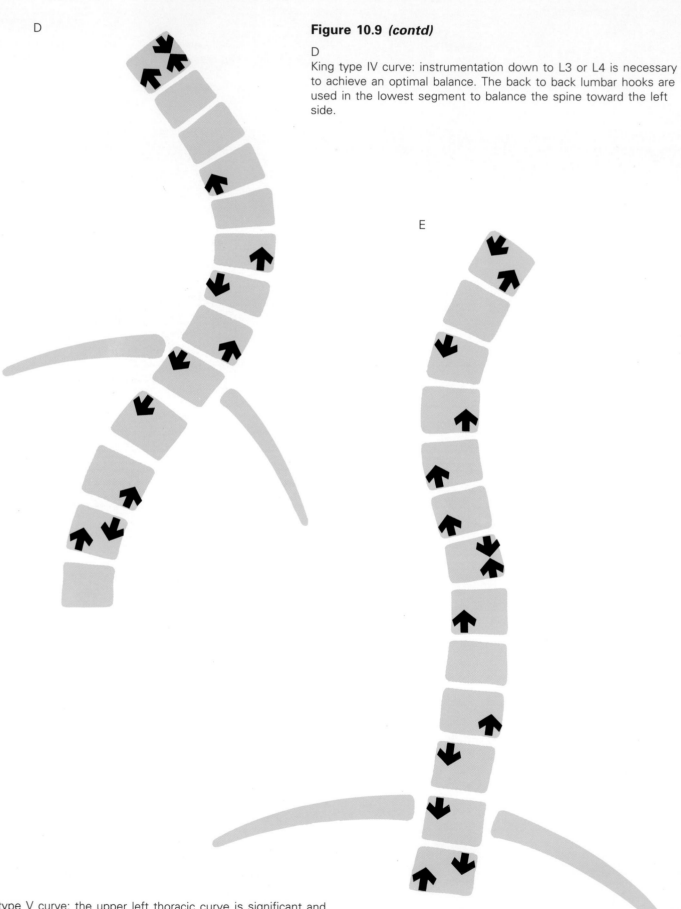

D

Figure 10.9 *(contd)*

D
King type IV curve: instrumentation down to L3 or L4 is necessary to achieve an optimal balance. The back to back lumbar hooks are used in the lowest segment to balance the spine toward the left side.

E

E
King type V curve: the upper left thoracic curve is significant and structural, and fusion and instrumentation is extended to T1 or T2 to balance the shoulders.

Rod rotation maneuver

In lordoscoliosis, rotation of the concave rod accomplishes medial translation of the coronal deformity. The bend in the rod accomplishes posterior angulation of the sagittal plane. These two mechanical effects do not equate with spinal derotation, but only accomplish coronal translation and sagittal angulation. The placement of the second rod in combination with the first accomplishes the en bloc periapical detorsion or derotation; this requires accurate determination of the strategic intermediate implant placement positions in conjunction with a differential bend in the concave and convex rod. The convex rod should be bent less than the concave, providing a three point moment about the long axis of the spine: the combination of posterior pulling on the concave side and anterior pushing on the convex side results in this moment.

Facet fusions on the concave side are performed. For Cotrel–Dubousset instrumentation, the contoured rod is then inserted and blockers placed into the open hooks. C rings can then be applied between the intermediate hooks adjacent to the apex and distraction applied across the apex. The C rings are then locked to maintain distraction, but allow rod rotation. Many surgeons feel that distraction across the intermediate segment will make this segment too stiff and the rod maneuver difficult and dangerous; they therefore do not apply C rings. The rod is then grasped with two rod holders and rotated 90°, with attention focused on the hooks to make sure that adequate seating remains throughout the reduction maneuver (Fig. 10.10A). Hooks are then reseated (Fig. 10.10B). The convex decortication and fusion is then performed to minimize blood loss. The opposite rod is undercontoured to further derotate the spine and inserted in a cranial-to-caudal direction. In the absence of spinal cord monitoring changes and a normal wakeup test, final tightening is performed and DTTs are applied at both ends of the construct (Fig. 10.10C).

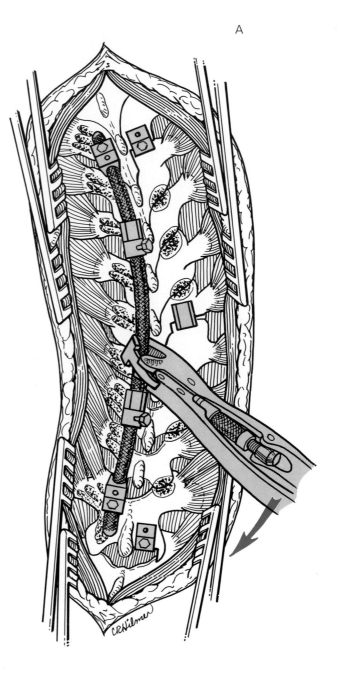

A

Figure 10.10

Rod rotation maneuver for Cotrel–Dubousset instrumentation.

A
After concave rod placement and hook seating, the rod is grasped and rotated into its final position.

Contd

B

C

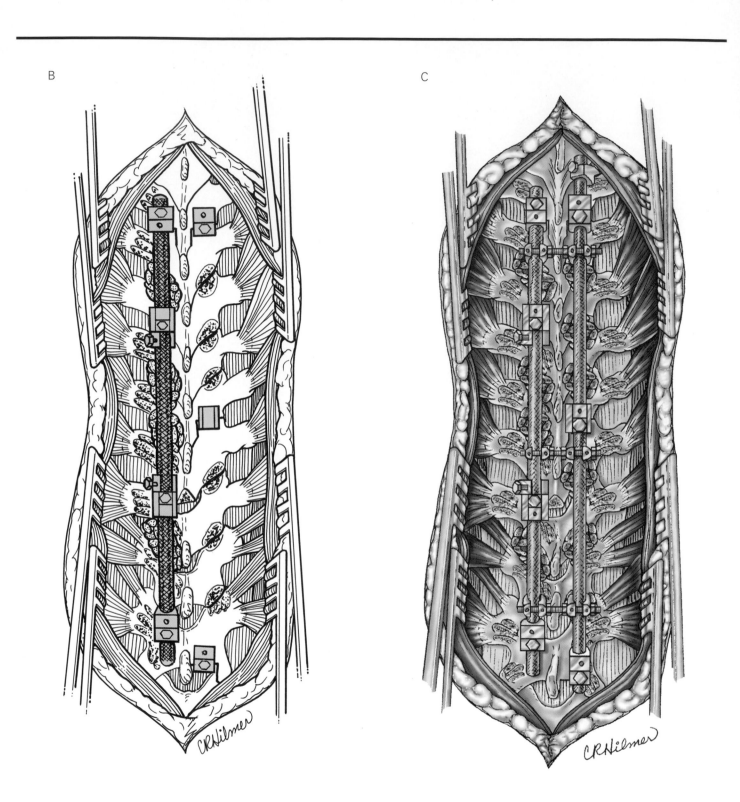

Figure 10.10 *(contd)*

B
Hooks are reseated after the rotation maneuver and facet excision and decortication are performed on the convex side prior to rod placement.

C
Final tightening and transverse connector placement.

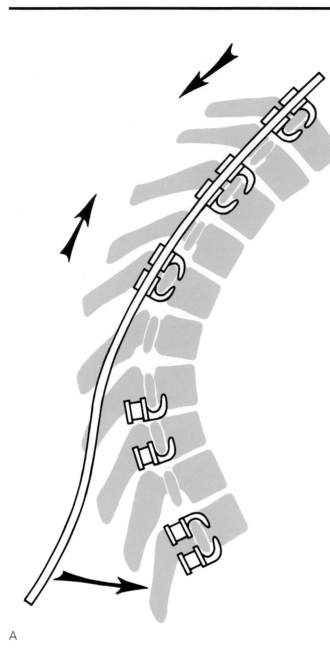

A

Figure 10.11

Posterior instrumentation for thoracic kyphosis.

A
The proximal portion is cantilevered to the distal portion of the kyphus, shortening the posterior column

B
The posterior instrumentation acts as a tension band.

Posterior instrumentation for Scheuermann's kyphosis

Several key concepts in the treatment of Scheuermann's kyphosis need to be followed for a successful outcome. All levels involved in the deformity should be instrumented. The instrumentation should be symmetric and extend caudally to at least the first neutral disc on standing lateral radiographs. Hooks should not be placed near the apex of the deformity to avoid canal penetration and iatrogenic spinal cord injury. Adjacent motion segments should not be injured to prevent junctional kyphosis.

Three pedicle–transverse process claws are placed above the apex of kyphus. The area below the kyphus is instrumented with symmetrically placed upgoing hooks and a distal claw. Two rods are then contoured to the desired final sagittal contour. Facet fusion is then performed. The rods are inserted into the upper thoracic portion of the deformity first. The most cranial claw is seated and tightened. A rod holder is then placed below the next lowest pedicle hook. Distraction between the rod holder and the pedicle hook causes compression between the upper claw and the pedicle hook. Once adequate compression is achieved, the lower claw is tightened and the process repeated for the next lowest claw. This sequence creates a tension band across the instrumented upper segments which evenly distributes forces across them (Fig. 10.11A).

The rods are then grasped and cantilevered into the lower open hooks and compressed in a cranial-to-caudal direction. This completes the creation of a tension band across the entire instrumented segment (Fig. 10.11B).

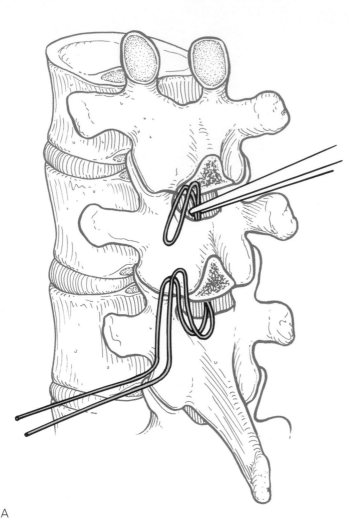

A

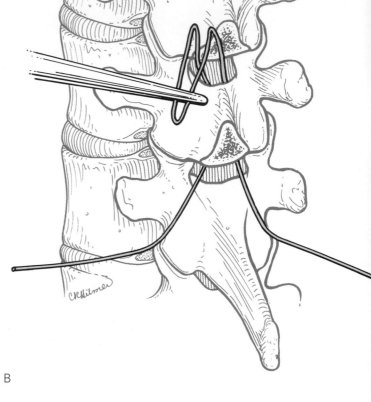

B

Figure 10.12

Sublaminar wire fixation technique.

A
Sublaminar wires are passed in a caudal-to-cranial direction.

B
The wire is advanced with even tension applied to both ends so that it always hugs the under surface of the lamina.

Sublaminar wire passage technique

Sublaminar wiring is an effective method of acquiring secure fixation to the spine. This technique requires attention to detail in the fashioning of the laminotomy sites and practice in wire bending and wire passage. An adequate laminotomy must be made to facilitate wire passage, but the size should be limited so that the mechanical strength of the lamina is not unduly compromised. The wire bend must be of sufficient length and shape to minimize wire penetration into the canal, and varies with the osteology of the particular level.

A double-action rongeur is used to remove the base of the spinous process. A Kerrison rongeur is then used to excise the ligamentum flavum and perform the laminotomy. The laminotomy often needs to extend into the medial aspect of the superior articular facet. Wires of No. 16 gauge are then bent for passage underneath the lamina. It is useful to bend the wire over the handle of a Cobb elevator and to place a compensatory bend

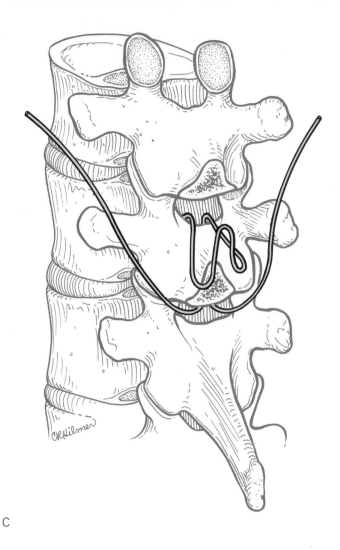

C

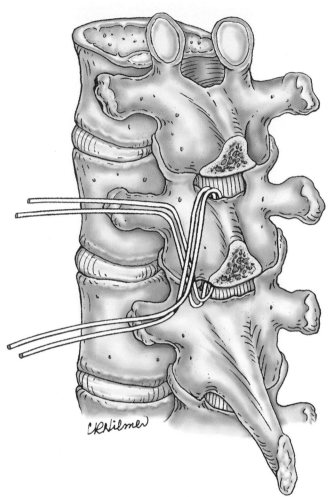

D

in the wire to facilitate passage. The primary bend can then be adjusted so that it passes beneath the lamina with minimal intrusion into the canal. Wider laminae require a longer radius of curvature than narrow laminae, where the wire bend will be C-shaped.

The wire is then passed by hand in a controlled fashion in a caudal-to-cranial direction. Wires should be passed in the midline where there is the maximum anterior-to-posterior canal space. The wire should be passed so that it hugs the under surface of the lamina and the tip grasped with a large needle holder when it presents in the cranial interlaminar space (Fig. 10.12A). The wire is then advanced with even tension on both ends pulling at all times away from the canal until sufficient wire has been passed (Fig. 10.12B). The wire is then folded over the lamina while still applying upward tension to prevent wire intrusion into the canal. The doubled wire is split and the separate arms are bent to either side for single wire constructs (Fig. 10.12C). In doubled wire constructs the bent wire is brought to the side to be instrumented first and folded over the lamina (Fig. 10.12D).

C
The wire is split and bent over the lamina for single wire constructs.

D
The wire is brought to the side to be instrumented first and bent over for double wire constructs.

Scoliosis correction using Luque instrumentation

The convex and concave methods are common techniques used in the correction of scoliosis with Luque instrumentation. In general, in lordoscoliosis the concave side should be done first. For lumbar curves, the convex side should be done first. This is similar to the approach taken with multiple hook-rod systems.

The Luque rod is inserted on the convex side first in the convex technique. The short arm of the L rod is placed above the spinous process and securely attached to the most proximal lamina involved in the fusion (Fig. 10.13A). The four next caudal levels are sequentially tightened to the rod. The opposite rod is inserted on the concave side of the curve with the short arm of the L rod above the spinous process to be fused. The remaining sublaminar wires are tightened and the rods levered in a parallel fashion to obtain correction (Fig. 10.13B). Wires should be tightened until a secondary twist appears and then trimmed and bent toward the midline (Fig. 10.13C).

Figure 10.13

Luque rod fixation technique.

A

The L rod is attached proximally to the convex side first and secured to the adjacent four segments. The concave rod is then attached distally.

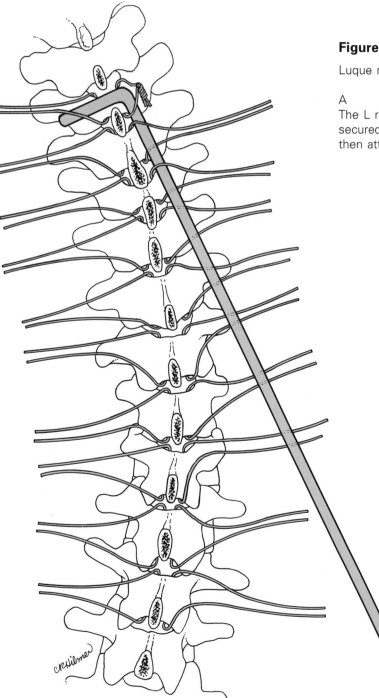

A

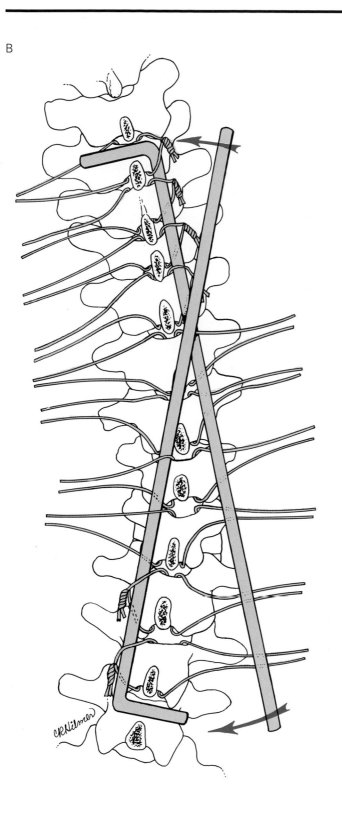

B

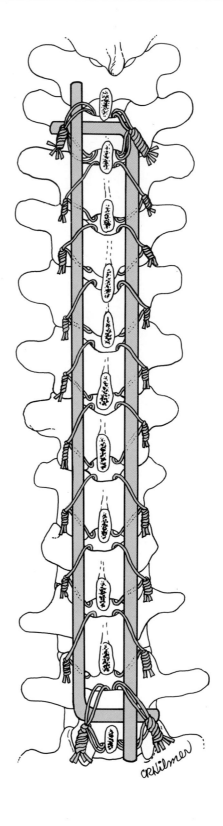

C

B
The proximal and distal rods are levered down to effect a correction.

C
Wires are tightened down alternately and correction is achieved. Double wires are recommended at the ends of the construct.

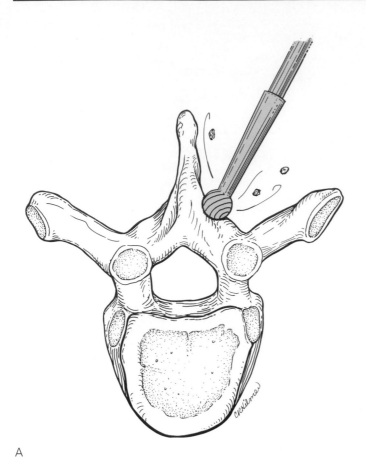

A

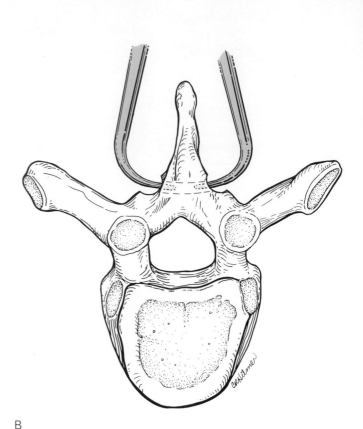

B

Figure 10.14

Drummond (Wisconsin) technique.

A
A high speed burr is used to mark the starting point in the midpoint of the base of the spinous process.

B
A large towel clip, Lewan clamp or curved awl is used to tunnel just above the internal cortex of the spinal canal.

C
Paired button–wire implants are passed at each level, except for the end vertebrae, which have unpaired implants passed from the concave to the convex side.

D
Final construct for a single thoracic curve.

Drummond (Wisconsin) technique

This technique provides secure wire fixation without wire penetration of the spinal canal. It is not indicated in patients with severe osteoporosis. This technique uses a Harrington distraction rod in the concavity of the curve and a Luque rod in the convexity. The advantage of the Wisconsin procedure is that it combines the benefits of the correction provided by a Harrington distraction rod with the segmental fixation of a wire-rod construct while avoiding wire penetration into the spinal canal. Although this technique provides excellent lateral correction it does not provide good correction in the sagittal plane, and is therefore less effective than segmental hook-rod constructs of the Cotrel-Dubousset type for correction of deformity.

A high speed burr is used to penetrate the outer cortex at the base of the spinous process (Fig. 10.14A). A large towel clip or curved awl is then used to make a hole in the base of the spinous process just

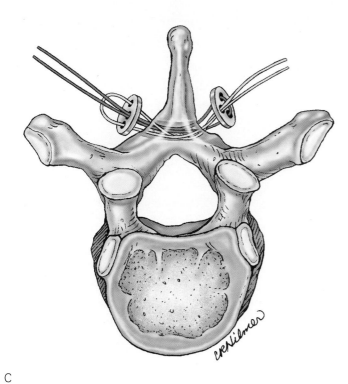

C

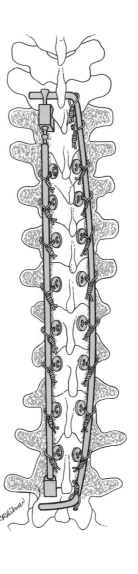

D

above the internal cortex of the spinal canal (Fig. 10.14B). Two Drummond button–wire implants are passed at each level from opposite sides. The beaded wire of the opposite paired implant is passed through the button on the opposite side so that forces are distributed over the base of the spinous process (Fig. 10.14C).

Hook sites for a Harrington distraction rod are prepared in the convexity of the curve. A pedicle hook is used in the upper level and an André anatomical hook is used in the lower level. Paired button–wire implants are then inserted in the levels to be instrumented using the technique described earlier. At both ends of the instrumentation, a single button–wire implant is placed from the concave to the convex side of the curve. Facet removal and decortication are performed over the concavity and the looped wires are opened to accept a Moe modified Harrington distraction rod with normal physiologic contour. The rod should be preloaded with two TSRH I-bolts, and these prepositioned near the ends of the construct. The rod is then distracted to correct the deformity.

A Luque rod with an 'L' at both ends is then contoured with the desired sagittal contour and undercontoured relative to the remaining deformity and loaded with two I-bolts. Convex facet excision and bone grafting and decortication are performed. The modified Luque rod is inserted on the convex side. The upper end of the Luque rod should lie beneath the ratchet portion of the Harrington rod and the lower portion just distal to the lower hook. Further correction is achieved by wire tightening, beginning in the center and working toward the ends, alternating between the convex and concave sides. Correction should primarily be achieved by pushing the rod toward the spine with a rod pusher and then tightening down the wires, rather than relying solely on wire twisting, which can lead to wire breakage. Additional Harrington rod distraction can also be used for further correction. After final correction and wire tightening and bone grafting, cross links are applied at opposite ends (Fig. 10.14D).

Bibliography

Cotrel Y, Dubousset J, Guillaument M (1988) New universal instrumentation in spinal surgery. *Clin Orthop* **227**:10

Denis F (1988) Cotrel–Dubousset instrumentation in the treatment of idiopathic scoliosis. *Orthop Clin North Am* **19**:291

Drummond DS (1992) Segmental spinal instrumentation with spinous process wires. In HS An and JM Cotler (eds), *Spinal Instrumentation*. Baltimore: Williams and Wilkins

Drummond DS, Guadagni J, Keene JS et al (1984) Interspinous process segmental spinal instrumentation. *J Pediatr Orthop* **4**:397

Goll S, Balderston R, Stambaugh J et al (1988) Depth of intraspinal wire penetration during passage of sublaminar wires. *Spine* **13**:503

Harrington PR (1960) Surgical instrumentation for management of scoliosis. *J Bone Joint Surg* **42A**:1448

Harrington PR (1988) The history and development of Harrington instrumentation. *Clin Orthop* **227**:3

Luque E (1982a) Segmental spinal instrumentation for correction of scoliosis. *Clin Orthop Rel Res* **163**:192

Luque E (1982b) The anatomic basis and development of segmental spinal instrumentation. *Spine* **7**:256

Shufflebarger HL, Clark CE (1988) Cotrel–Dubousset instrumentation. *Orthopaedics* **11**:1435

Shufflebarger HL, Clark CE (1990) Fusion levels and hook patterns in thoracic scoliosis with Cotrel–Dubousset instrumentation. *Spine* **15**:916

11

Lumbar decompressive procedures

Howard S An
Frederick A Simeone

Introduction

Patients with lumbar disc disease or spinal stenosis usually present with radicular leg pain with or without neurological deficits. The surgical outcome in patients with a herniated disc depends mostly on the proper indications and patient selection. An appropriate course of conservative treatment should be given for at least 2-3 months before considering surgery. The surgical patient should have dermatomal pain distribution, a positive tension sign or a focal neurological deficit and a correlating positive imaging study. The cauda equina syndrome and profound weakness should be managed more aggressively.

The great majority of spinal stenosis cases are as the result of degenerative changes in the intervertebral disc and facet joints, with resultant constriction of the spinal canal and neural foramina. Many patients with spinal stenosis may have concurrent herniated discs, and preoperative imaging studies should identify these lesions. Again the goal of surgery is to relieve neurogenic claudication, radicular pain, or neurologic deficits. It is crucial to identify sites of neural compression with neuroimaging studies, and the nerve roots to be decompressed should be clinically correlated. The techniques of surgery should include adequate decompression of symptomatic nerve roots while minimizing destabilization effects of laminectomy and facetectomy.

Anatomy

It is important to consider anatomical variations, which may affect the surgical approach, dissection, and ultimate completion of the procedure. Anatomic considerations include bony or neural anomalies as well as the anatomic location of disc ruptures. Correct localization of the appropriate level for surgery depends on careful preoperative examination of both the plain radiographs and neuroimaging studies. The intercrestal line crossing the top of the iliac crest usually passes through the L4-5 disc space, but variations exist among individuals. If the surgeon places his or her fingertips over the top of the iliac crest when the patient is in a kneeling position, he or she will be about 1-2 cm higher than the radiographic intercrestal line and must compensate for this accordingly. Also, 'lumbarization' or 'sacralization' of the last vertebral segments may confuse the surgeon in localizing the appropriate level. By comparing neuroimaging studies to the plain radiographs, the surgeon should be able to localize the appropriate level. Further identification of the correct level is aided intraoperatively by palpation of the sacrum, checking for mobile and immobile segments, and identification of the posterior elements and interlaminar space. However, the only foolproof method is an intraoperative localizing radiograph. Intraoperative radiographs should be obtained in those cases where variations in lumbosacral segmentation exist or any case where the surgeon is unsure of the correct level.

Bony variations or anomalies may also relate to posterior element deficiency. Spina bifida occulta is common. Also, the L5-S1 interlaminar space may be unusually wide in some cases. Careful review of the preoperative radiographs will reveal these anomalies. To prevent inadvertent dural tear or neural injury, one must palpate the bony structures with a finger before using a periosteal elevator. Although herniated lumbar discs typically occur in the posterolateral location, they may rupture laterally into the foramen, centrally or axially, or migrate as free fragments.

Precise preoperative localization of the disc pathology will aid the surgeon in making the proper surgical approach and avoiding neural injury. Unlike a posterolateral herniated disc, the foraminal herniated disc affects the nerve root numbered one above the ruptured disc. A foraminal herniated disc may be approached either by a medial facetectomy or a paraspinal muscle splitting approach, depending on the size and location of the disc fragment. If the herniated disc is mostly within the intervertebral foramen, the paraspinal splitting approach is preferred, to avoid complete resection of the facet joint. On the other hand, if the herniated disc is broad, occupying both the intracanal and foraminal regions, medial facetectomy is recommended. A central disc rupture causing bilateral leg pain should be approached by a bilateral hemilaminectomy or laminectomy, so that the disc can be removed from both sides. A massive central disc rupture presenting as a cauda equina syndrome requires emergency decompression by a midline laminectomy. Axillary disc ruptures are a consequence of disc migration into the axilla of the nerve root. A portion of the axillary herniated disc should be removed first in order to retract the nerve root safely for standard discectomy. Free or sequestered fragments are common. The surgical approach should be modified to extend either cephalad or caudad to remove the free fragment.

Finally, anatomic anomalies and variation may occur in the nerve roots. Preoperative imaging studies may reveal the majority of the anatomic variations and anomalies. Preoperatively, one should suspect these anomalies if multiple roots are involved or when radiographic and clinical findings do not correlate in a classical manner. Surgical management should respect the principle of exposing the nerve root to its lateral edge before manipulation. Often, more extensive bone removal is necessary to complete exposure and ensure safe decompression in these cases.

Indications

1. Laminotomy and discectomy for a herniated disc
2. Laminectomy for spinal stenosis
3. Paraspinal approach for foraminatomy or a foraminal herniated disc
4. A combination of partial or complete laminectomy, facetectomy, and discectomy for various nerve root compressive disorders.

Surgical techniques

Standard laminotomy and discectomy

The patient is placed in a kneeling position to decompress the abdomen. The use of a 3.5 magnified loupe and fiberoptic headlight is recommended. A midline incision rarely extends more than 4 cm (Fig. 11.1A). The location of the skin incision is estimated by palpating the iliac crest as the reference point. In doubtful cases, radiographic localization is recommended. Unilateral exposure of the spinous process, lamina, and facet capsule is made by subperiosteal dissection (Fig. 11.1B). A Taylor or self retaining retractor is positioned at the lateral aspect of the facet joint. The correct level is confirmed either by palpating the sacrum or radiographically. Access to epidural space is achieved by removal of the ligamentum flavum and the inferior margin of the proximal lamina on one

Figure 11.1

Lumbar laminotomy and discectomy .

A
The midline incision between the spinous processes is about 4 cm.

B
Unilateral exposure of the spinous process, lamina, and facet capsule. A Taylor retractor is positioned at the lateral aspect of the facet joint.

1 L5
2 Deep muscles of back
3 Spinous process
4 Facet joint
5 Psoas m.
6 Common iliac a.
7 Common iliac v.

Contd

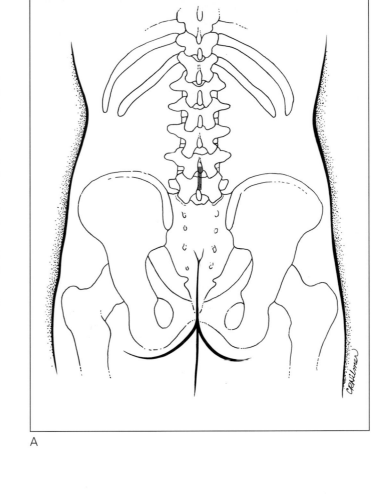

A

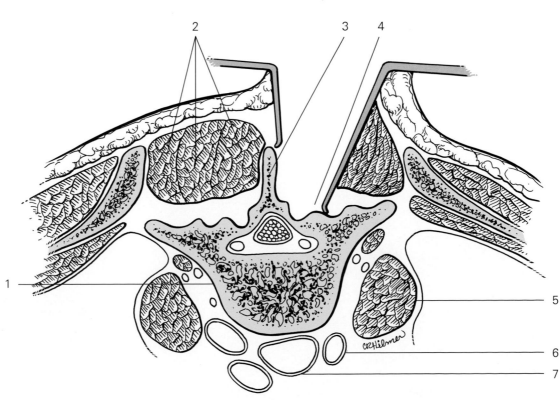

B

side. Using a curet, the ligamentum flavum is separated from the inferior lamina (Fig. 11.1C). The inferior aspect of the lamina is removed using a Kerrison rongeur (Fig. 11.1D). The lamina is removed proximally to the point where the ligamentum flavum is detached. At this time, an angled curet or probe is placed between the ligamentum flavum and the underlying dura, and the ligamentum flavum is separated from the dura. Packing cottonoid material

2

1

C

Figure 11.1 *contd*

C
A curet is used to separate the ligamentum flavum from the inferior lamina.

1 Ligamentum flavum
2 Lamina

D
The inferior aspect of the lamina is removed using a Kerrison rongeur.

D

between the dura and the ligamentum flavum may prevent dural tears. The ligamentum flavum is then excised using a knife or Kerrison rongeur (Fig. 11.1E). A different technique of epidural exposure may be performed at a larger L5–S1 interspace with less bony resection. The ligamentum flavum may be separated from the superior margin of the sacrum using a curet (Fig. 11.1F). A knife or Kerrison rongeur is then used to remove the ligamentum flavum. Using the Kerrison

E

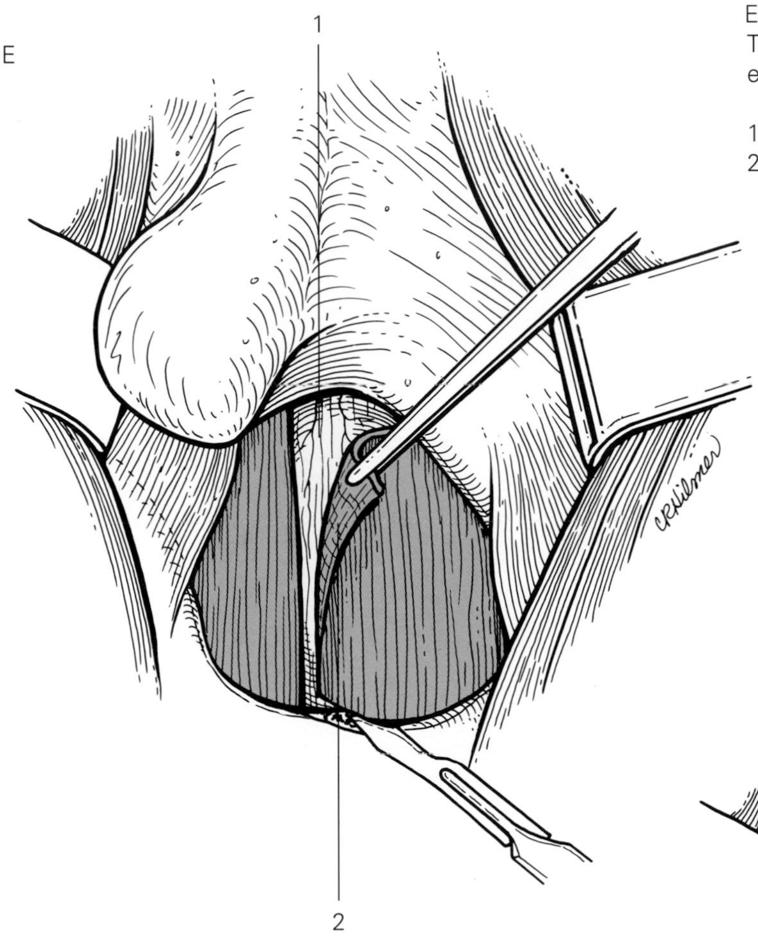

E
The ligamentum flavum is separated from the dura and excised using a knife or Kerrison rongeur.

1 Dura
2 Ligamentum flavum

F

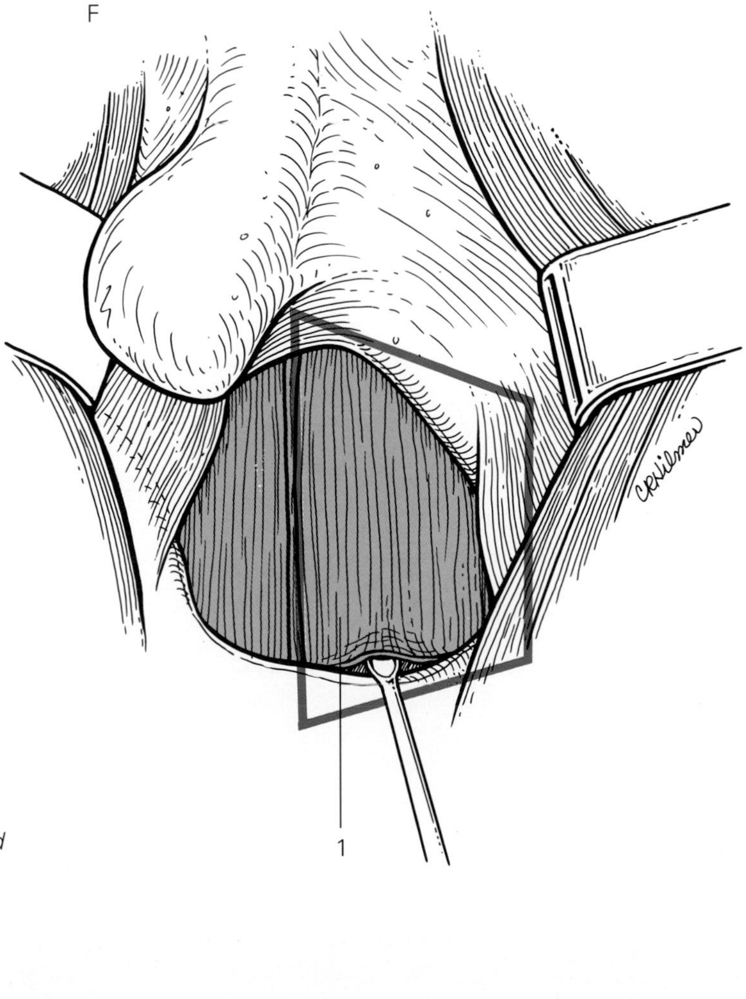

F
The ligamentum flavum is usually separated from the superior margin of the sacrum using a curet.

1 Ligamentum flavum

Contd

rongeur, exposure is carried out laterally, so that the lateral edge of the nerve root is visualized before it is retracted (Fig. 11.1G). Manipulation of the nerve root before adequate exposure invites neural injury. The surgeon may also need to undercut the medial aspect of the superior facet in patients with concomitant lateral recess stenosis pathology. By undercutting the superior articular process, the facet joint is largely undisturbed and mechanical stability is maintained.

The nerve root is then gently mobilized and retracted using a Penfield dissector. A cottonoid may be placed superiorly and inferiorly to medialize the nerve root. The nerve root is further medialized with a nerve root retractor, and the extruded or sequestered disc fragment is removed using a pituitary rongeur (Fig. 11.1H). If the herniated disc is contained by the posterior longitudinal ligament, a large rectangular window of annulus is opened for disc excision. The depth and

G

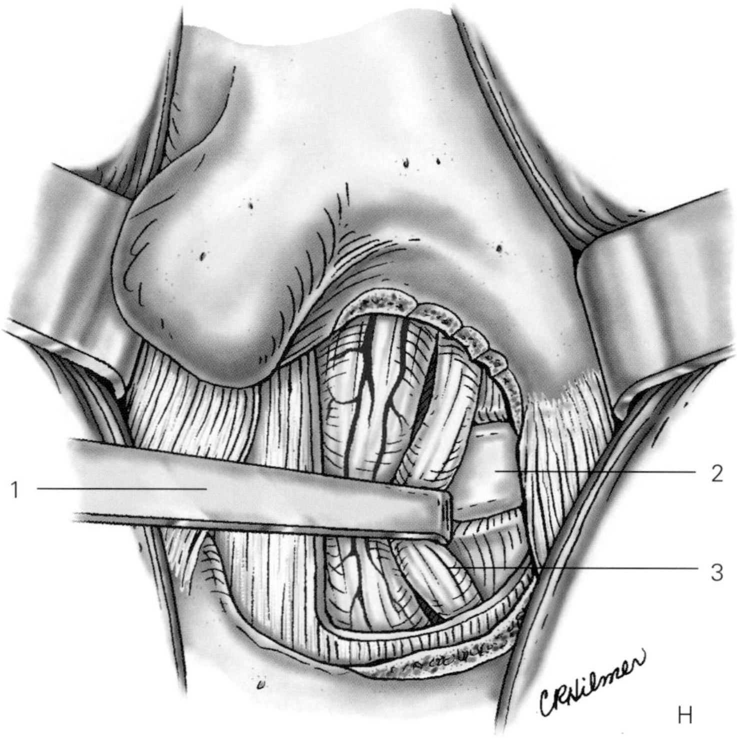

Figure 11.1 *(contd)*

G
The lateral edge of the nerve root is exposed and retracted.

1 Nerve root retractor
2 Intervertebral disc
3 Spinal n.

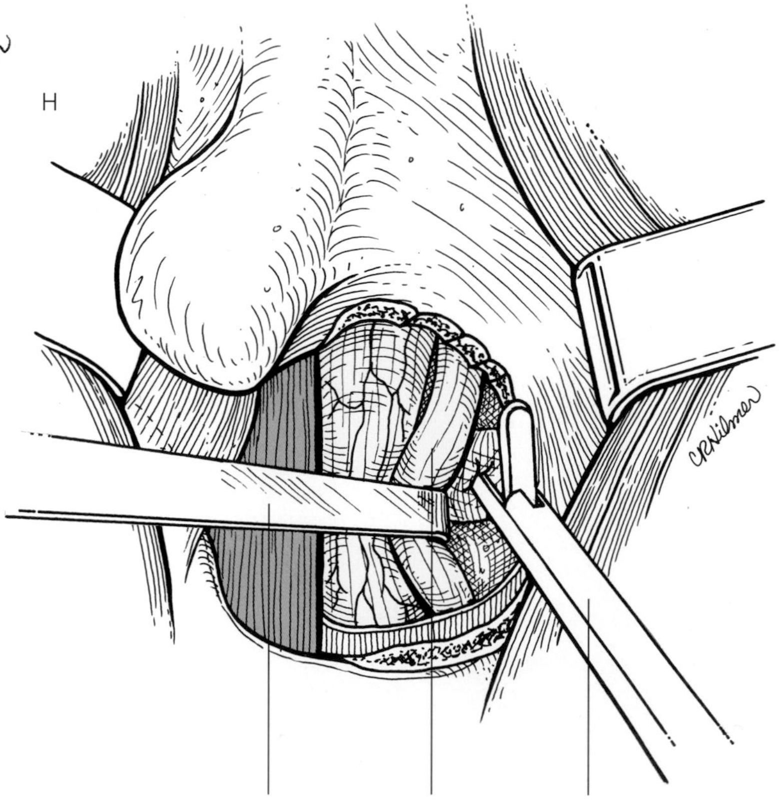

H
The nerve root is medialized with a nerve root retractor, and the extruded or sequestered disc fragment is removed using a pituitary rongeur.

1 Nerve root retractor
2 Spinal n.
3 Pituitary rongeur

width of penetration by the pituitary rongeur should be carefully monitored to avoid disastrous vascular injury (Fig. 11.1I). The pituitary rongeur may be marked at 2 cm from the tip to gauge the depth of the instrument during disc evacuation. The discectomy in the disc space should be done to remove loose fragments only. It is not recommended to remove the entire nucleus pulposus vigorously, as scarring and instability may result.

Finally, the excursion and course of the nerve root into the foramen is also palpated with a Fraser elevator (Fig. 11.1J). A tight nerve following discectomy may have further compression in the foramen. Thorough irrigation is done, followed by meticulous hemostasis. Hemostasis is aided by placing a thrombin-soaked gelfoam over the nerve root for 1–2 minutes. The author recommends removal of the gelfoam and placement of a thin fat graft to minimize epidural fibrosis.

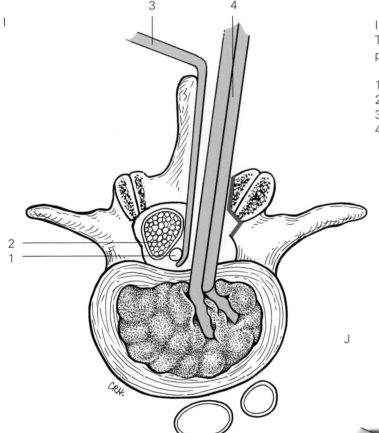

I

I

The cross-section of the intervertebral disc, showing the pituitary rongeur removing the nucleus pulposus.

1 Spinal n.
2 Dura
3 Nerve root retractor
4 Pituitary rongeur

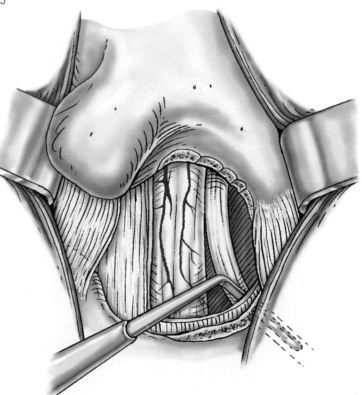

J

J

The course of the nerve root into the foramen is checked with a Fraser or dental probe.

Laminectomy

The key to successful completion of spinal stenosis surgery is thorough understanding of the patho-anatomy of the affected nerve root. The central stenosis is usually secondary to a combination of disc bulging, facet enlargement, and ligamentum flavum thickening. The techniques of laminectomy and removal of ligamentum flavum are straightforward. However, lateral stenosis may be confusing, as more than one mechanism may be responsible for the compression of the nerve root. A particular nerve root may be initially compressed by a herniated disc as it emerges from the dural sac. The next area of nerve root compression is within the lateral recess, as a result of hypertrophy of the superior facet. This is known as the lateral recess syndrome, and accounts for the majority of lateral spinal stenosis. Undercutting this lateral recess accomplishes decompression of the nerve root in most cases. Next, the nerve root exits just inferomedial to the pedicle, and 'pedicle kinking' may be responsible for compression of the nerve root. This phenomenon is more common in patients with scoliosis or spondylolisthesis. Partial or complete excision of the involved pedicle may be necessary to relieve this condition. Lastly, the neural foramen is frequently the area of nerve root compression. Within the foramen, the nerve root may be impinged between the subluxated superior facet and bony structures such as the foramen, pedicle, or vertebral body. Another common foraminal compression is secondary to a laterally bulging or herniated disc or annulus, which elevates the nerve root against the pedicle. On occasion, the L5 nerve root may be impinged by the L5 transverse process against the ala of the sacrum in L5 spondylolisthesis cases. All these areas of potential nerve root compression should be checked unless the medial–lateral excursion of the involved nerve root is at least 1 cm.

The kneeling position is again recommended, to reduce the intra-abdominal pressure and to minimize operative bleeding.

The midline skin incision is followed by a careful subperiosteal dissection of the paraspinous muscle (Fig. 11.2A). The exposure should be limited laterally to the pars interarticularis and facet joints, taking great care to preserve the facet capsule (Fig 11.2B). The spinous processes are initially removed using an

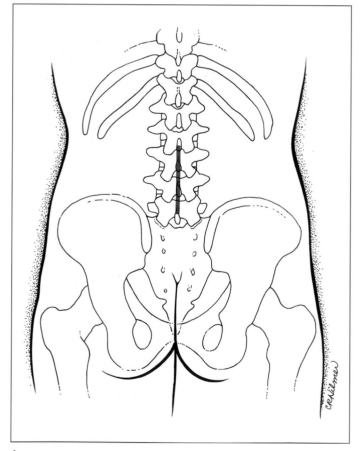

A

Figure 11.2

Lumbar laminectomy.

A

The midline skin incision is over the spinous processes of the involved vertebrae.

angled bone cutter (Fig. 11.2C). Before opening the canal itself, the operating physician should identify the location of the pedicle, which is the key to the subsequent dissection. The nerve root courses under the pedicle to exit into the foramen. The location of the pedicle and corresponding nerve root to be decompressed should be firmly established by the surgeon before proceeding with further dissection. After the ligamentum flavum has been cleanly exposed, a small curet is used to dissect the insertion of the ligament

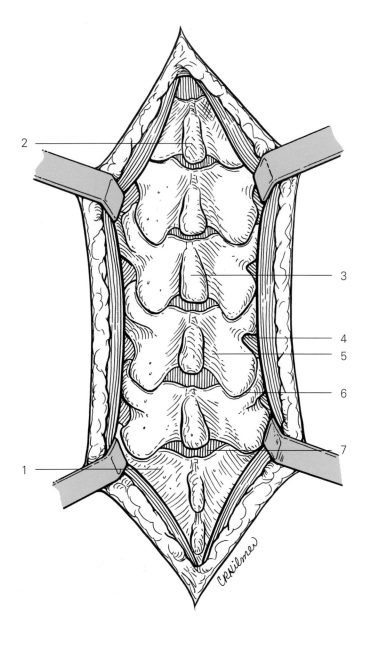

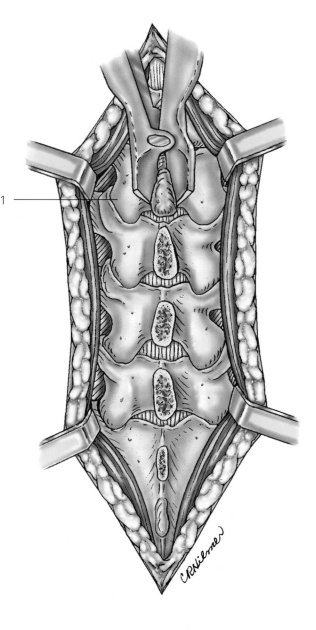

B
The exposure of the spinous processes, lamina, pars interarticularis and facet capsules is done.

1 Sacrum
2 L1
3 Spinous process
4 Pars interarticularis
5 Lamina
6 Facet joint
7 Ligamentum flavum

C
The spinous processes are then removed using an angled bone cutter.

1 L2 lamina

Contd

gently from the undersurface of the inferior lamina (Fig. 11.2D). When the inferior edge of the lamina has been exposed, a Kerrison punch or Lexcel rongeur is used to remove the bone of the lamina itself. This step is started in the midline, where the canal is most spacious, and then carried to the lateral sides of the spinal canal. When using the Kerrison punch, pressure should be directed dorsally, and it should not be rocked from side to side, to safeguard the dura underneath from damage (Fig. 11.2E). The cottonoid material can also be placed to displace the dural sac from the posterior elements. It is important to free adhesions between the anterior surface of the lamina and the dura as the dissection is carried out

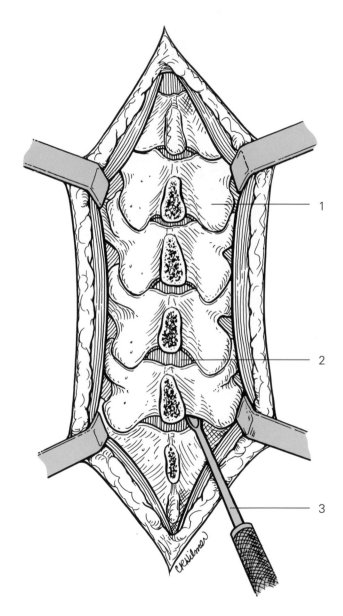
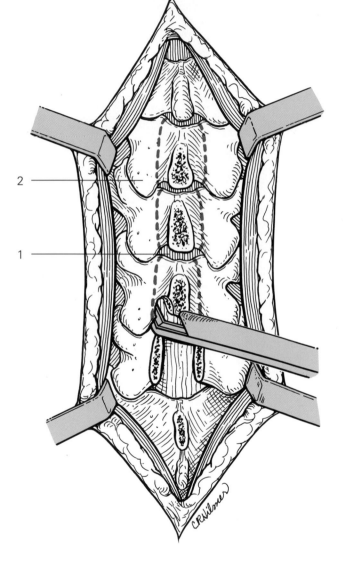

Figure 11.2 *contd*

D
After the ligamentum flavum has been cleanly exposed, a small curet is used to separate the ligamentum flavum from the undersurface of the inferior lamina.

1 L2
2 Ligamentum flavum
3 Curet

E
Laminectomy is done with a Kerrison rongeur from the caudal to cephalad direction.

1 Ligamentum flavum
2 L2

proximally. Any epidural bleeding should be controlled with bipolar cautery. This dissection is carried out to make a central trough extending in a distal–proximal direction over the symptomatic levels to be decompressed and extending laterally to the medial edge of the facet joint (Fig. 11.2F). At the level of the pars interarticularis, bony resection should not extend too laterally, to avoid postlaminectomy fractures of the pars interarticularis.

In patients with a central spinal stenosis secondary to congenitally short pedicles, midline dissection alone is adequate.

In the majority of patients, the area of stenosis extends to the lateral recess or foramen, and further

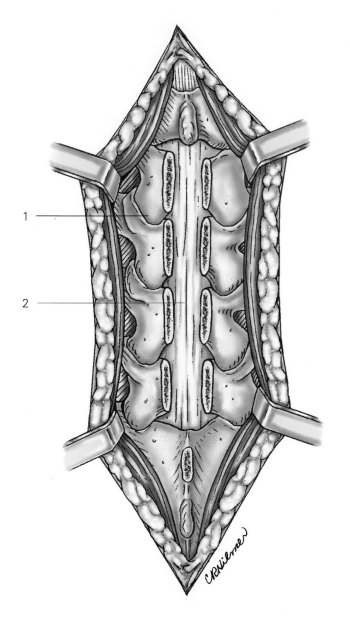

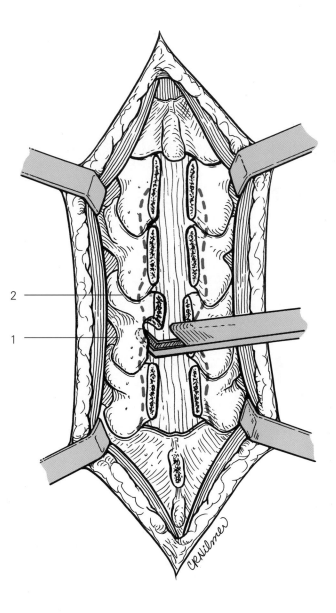

F
The midline laminectomy should extend to the lateral edge of the dura.

1 | 2
2 Dura

G
Decompression of the lateral recess or foramen is done by extending the laminectomy laterally and undercutting the superior facet with a 45° Kerrison rongeur.

1 Pars interarticularis
2 Facet joint

Contd

dissection is necessary. A 45° Kerrison rongeur is used to undercut portions of the superior facet, thus freeing the lateral recess. This maneuver is best accomplished from the opposite side (Figs. 11.2G, H). Dissecting instruments should always be parallel to the nerve root, minimizing the chances of grasping or transecting the nerve roots. Undercutting the facet allows decompression of the lateral recess without jeopardizing spinal stability (Fig. 11.2I). At this juncture, the nerve root should move at least 1 cm from a medial to a lateral direction. The intervertebral discs should be examined to rule out concurrent herniated discs. Further foraminal or extraforaminal decompression should be performed if the nerve is

H

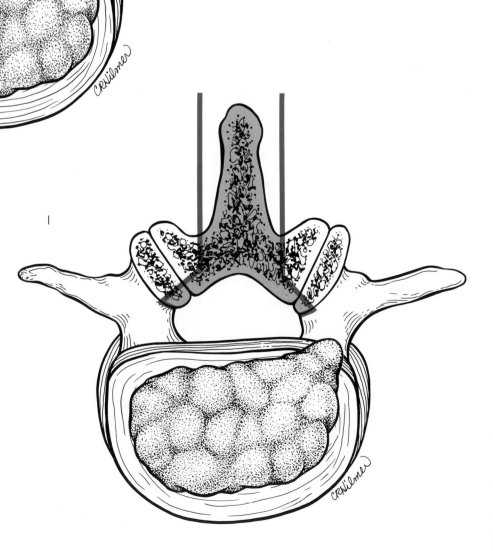

Figure 11.2 *(contd)*

H
Cross-sectional diagram showing the Kerrison rongeur undercutting the facet joint from the opposite side.

I
Laminectomy and partial facetectomy enlarges the central canal and the lateral recess without significant resection of the facet joint.

still tight at this time (Fig. 11.2J). The facet joint should be removed more laterally to look for the entrapment of the spinal nerve between the superior facet of the vertebra below and the posterolateral aspect of the vertebral body or pedicle of the vertebra above. The nerve can be decompressed by excising the tip of the superior facet or the entire facet joint. Another common place for nerve root entrapment is between the laterally bulging annulus or herniated disc and the pedicle of the supra-adjacent vertebra. In this case, decompression of the nerve root is performed by excising the lateral annulus. The nerve root is frequently seen exiting in a perpendicular direction instead of a normal oblique course, because the laterally bulging disc pushes the nerve root in a cephalad direction against the pedicle. If the nerve is still tight following annulus excision and foraminotomy, the inferomedial aspect of the vertebral pedicle may be resected for complete decompression of the nerve root.

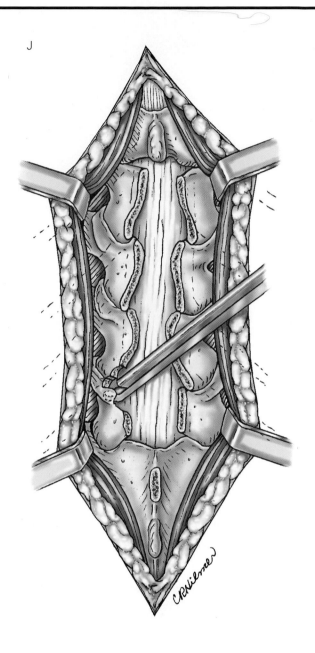

J

J
Foraminotomy is performed by following the nerve root into the foramen with a foraminotomy Kerrison rongeur.

The paraspinal muscle splitting approach

This approach is useful for cases that require exposure of the transverse processes and the intervertebral foramen without the need for central laminectomy. A far lateral herniated disc or a foraminal herniated disc is a typical case for utilizing this approach.

The patient is placed in the kneeling position. For bilateral exposures, either two paraspinal incisions or a longer midline incision can be made (Fig. 11.3A). The author prefers the paraspinal incision for unilateral exposure and the midline incision for bilateral exposure. The lateral incision is about two fingers' breadths or 1¾ inches (4.5 cm) from the midline. This incision should be over the junction between the multifidus and longissimus muscles. These muscles are well identified on the CT or MRI axial views, and the

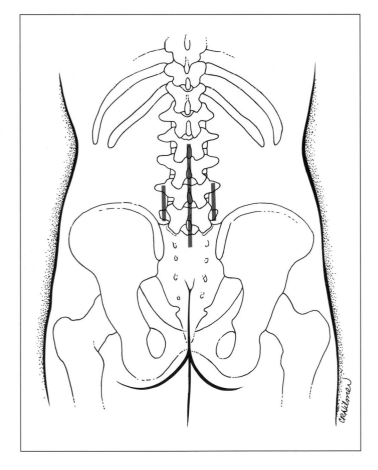

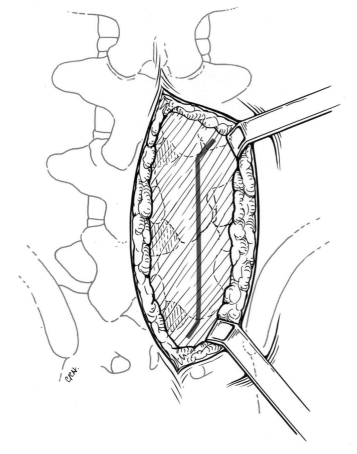

Figure 11.3

The paraspinal muscle splitting approach.

A
The skin incision may be in the midline or over the paraspinal muscles. The lateral incision is about two fingers' breadths or 1¾ inches (4.5 cm) from the midline.

B
The distal end of the fascial incision is curved toward the midline and the proximal end of the incision is curved laterally, so that retraction of the muscles becomes easier.

exact distance from the midline may be calculated preoperatively. Following mobilization of the skin and subcutaneous tissue, a fascial incision is made over the junction between the multifidus and longissimus muscles. The distal end of the fascial incision is curved toward the midline and the proximal end of the incision is curved laterally, so that retraction of the muscles becomes easier (Fig. 11.3B). The index finger is used to dissect between the longissimus and multifidus toward the edge of the facet capsule and trans-

verse processes (Fig. 11.3C). A periosteal Cobb elevator is used to expose the transverse processes or the ala of the sacrum, and the two Gelpi retractors or other self retaining retractors are placed (Fig. 11.3D). Procedures such as foraminotomy, discectomy, partial pedicle resection, or intertransverse fusion can be performed thought this approach. For the foraminotomy procedure, the lateral aspect of the superior facet, the pars interarticularis, the inferior part of superior transverse process, and the superior part of

C

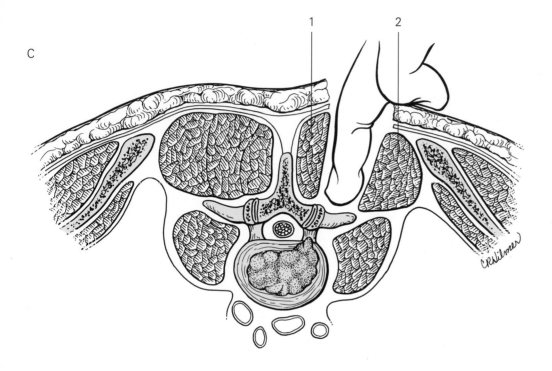

C
The index finger is used to dissect between the longissimus and the multifidus toward the edge of the facet capsule and the transverse processes.

1 Multifidus m.
2 Longissimus m.

D

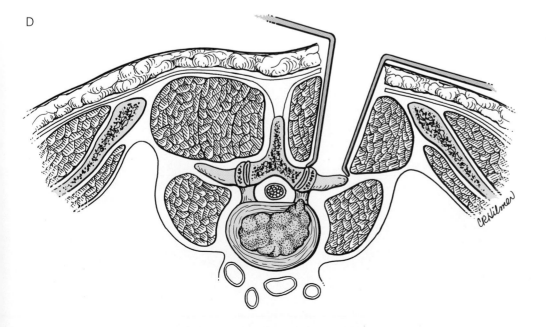

D
The exposure of the transverse processes or the ala of the sacrum is facilitated by Gelpi retractors or other self retaining retractors.

Contd

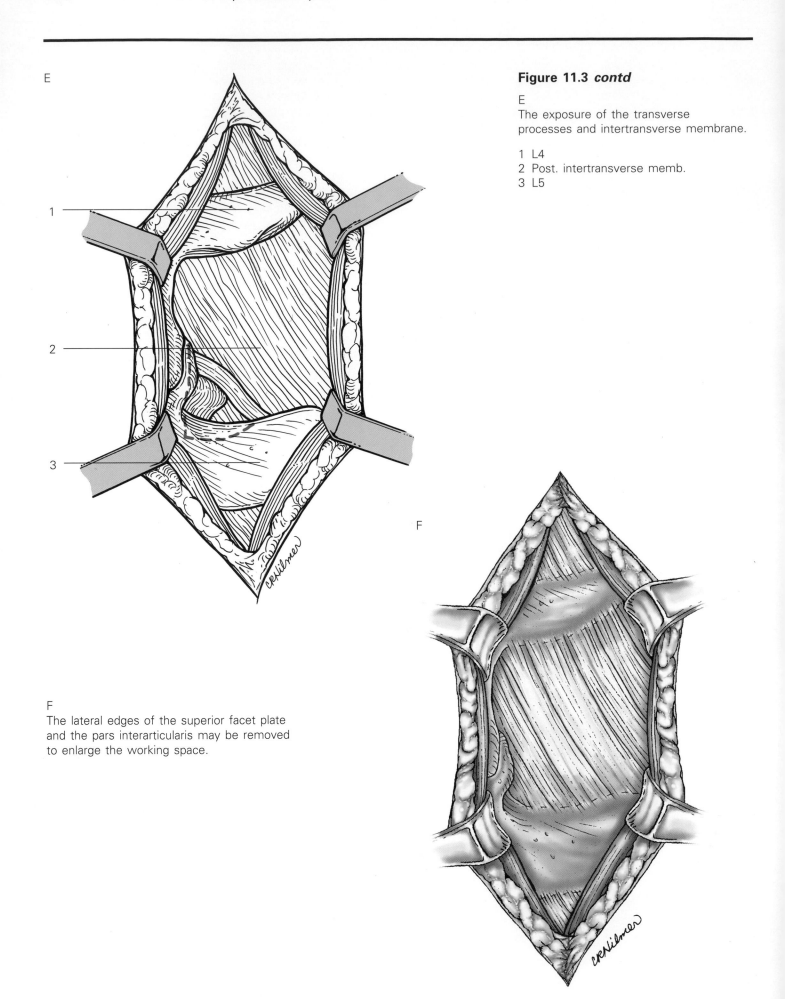

E

Figure 11.3 *contd*

E
The exposure of the transverse
processes and intertransverse membrane.

1 L4
2 Post. intertransverse memb.
3 L5

F

F
The lateral edges of the superior facet plate
and the pars interarticularis may be removed
to enlarge the working space.

G

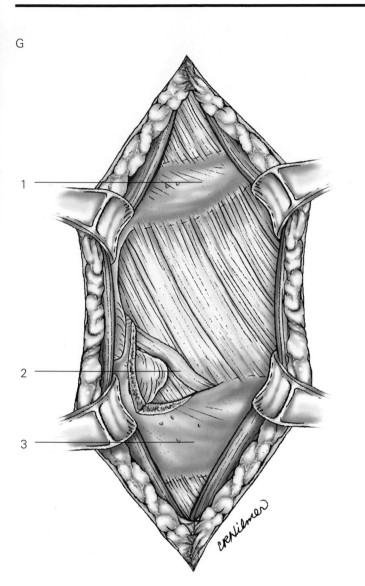

the inferior transverse process are exposed by using a curet to detach the muscle fibers (Fig. 11.3E). Any bleeding is controlled using bipolar coagulation to protect the nerve root. The lateral edges of the superior facet plate and the pars interarticularis may be removed using a Kerrison rongeur to enlarge the working space and to initiate the detachment of the intertransverse ligament (Fig. 11.3F). The intertransverse ligament is carefully detached from the lateral aspect of the pars interarticularis, the facet, and the inferior aspect of the transverse process. The nerve root and the disc herniation will be immediately identified. The nerve root is usually retracted toward the pedicle, and the disc fragment is removed. Following removal of the free fragment, the disc space may be entered, and the rest of the disc herniation can be removed in the usual fashion. It must be remembered that the depth of the disc space is smaller at the lateral corner, and the pituitary rongeur should not penetrate too deeply to avoid vascular injury. Occasionally, the nerve root may be retracted distally to remove a far lateral disc fragment. Great caution should be taken to minimize traction to the nerve root throughout the procedure. At the completion of the procedure, the nerve root should be mobile and should exit obliquely (Fig. 11.3G).

G
The intertransverse membrane is detached from the bony insertions to expose the nerve root.

1 L4
2 L4 n.
3 L5

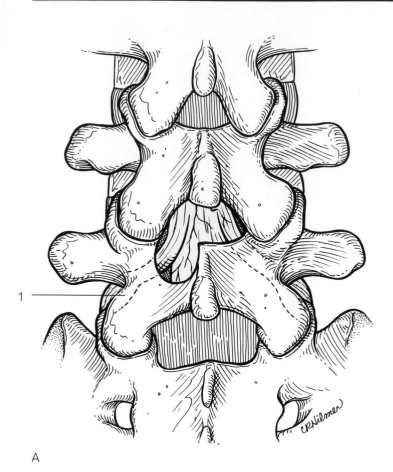

A

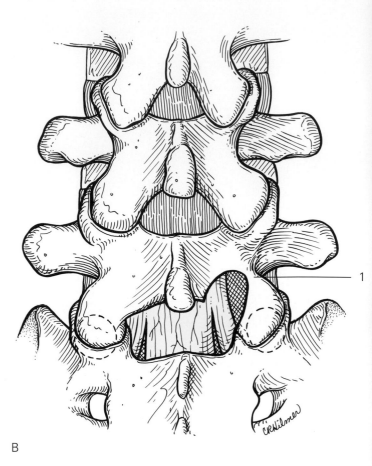

B

Figure 11.4

Modifications of laminotomy and foraminotomy.

A
Foraminotomy may be done by tracing the nerve root distally. The Kerrison rongeur is used to remove the bone overlying the nerve root into the foramen.

1 Involved foramen

B
Foraminotomy may be done by extending decompression superiorly and laterally toward the pars interarticularis and the intervertebral foramen above.

1 Involved foramen

C
The intervertebral foramen may be approached from the lateral aspect of the pars interarticularis.

D
Unilateral hemilaminectomy and partial facetectomy.

E
Bilateral hemilaminotomy or fenestration.

Modifications of laminotomy and partial facetectomy

Depending on the location of a herniated disc or osteophyte, the decompressive procedure should be modified to complete the decompression of the involved nerve root. Following a routine laminotomy and discectomy, the nerve root may still be impinged by the hypertrophic superior facet in the lateral recess. In this situation, the nerve root can usually be decompressed by extending the laminotomy both laterally and distally. The Kerrison rongeur is used to remove the bone overlying the nerve root into the foramen (Fig. 11.4A). On the other hand, if the nerve root compression is at the pars interarticularis level or the herniated disc fragment is located laterally and superiorly, bony decompression should be extended superiorly and laterally toward the pars interarticularis (Fig. 11.4B). Occasionally, the entire inferior facet must be removed to access the intervertebral foramen for nerve root decompression. The intervertebral foramen may be approached from the lateral aspect of the pars interarticularis, as discussed under the paraspinal muscle splitting approach (Fig. 11.4C).

Frequently, the nerve root compression is localized at multiple levels on one side owing to hypertrophic facets without significant central stenosis. In this

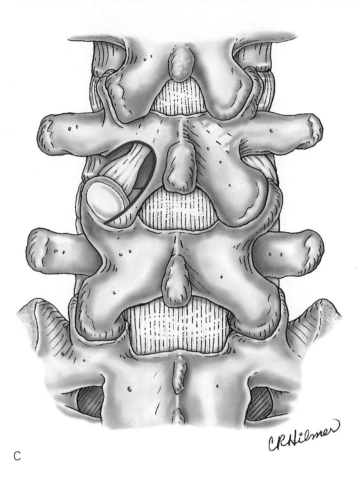

C

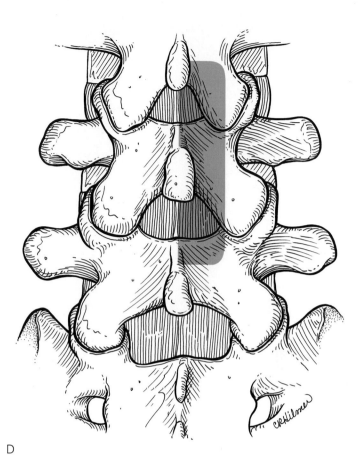

D

situation, unilateral hemilaminectomy and partial facetectomy may be performed (Fig. 11.4D). Special curved foraminotomy Kerrison rongeurs are helpful in performing adequate decompression of the lateral recess. Finally, some surgeons prefer to perform central canal decompression with preservation of the midline spinous processes and interspinous ligaments. This procedure is not recommended for severe stenosis cases. The area of stenosis is at the level of the disc and the facet joint, and adequate decompression may be achieved by bilateral hemilaminotomy or fenestration procedure (Fig. 11.4E). The preservation of the interspinous ligament and the spinous process may reduce the incidence of postlaminectomy instability.

Complications

Perforations of the dura may occur with or without nerve root damage, and may lead to pseudomeningocele formation, cerebrospinal fluid fistula, meningitis or wound healing problems. Dural tears may occur during excision of the ligamentum flavum, but more commonly during manipulation of the dural sac to free adhesions, particularly in a stenotic canal. Gentle handling of the dural sac largely avoids this complication. Dural tears

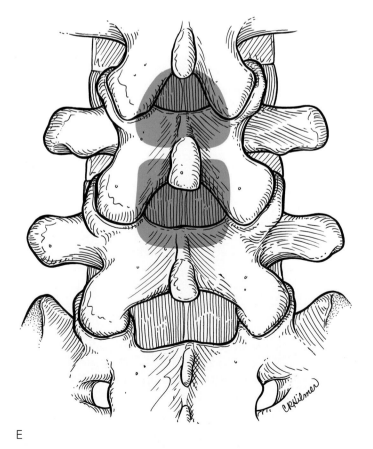

E

should be primarily closed using 6:0 or 7:0 nonabsorbable sutures in such a way as not to produce constriction of the cauda equina. A fascial or free fat graft may be used to augment the repair. The paraspinous muscle, overlying fascia, subcutaneous tissue and skin should be closed in multiple layers in a watertight manner. Drains should be avoided. Injuries to the nerve roots may result in sensory alteration, a motor deficit, or even sphinter dysfunction. Exposing the lateral aspect of the nerve root before manipulation is the key to prevention of nerve root damage. Excessive retraction with metallic instruments can be avoided by packing the nerve roots with cotton pledgets. Repeated manipulation and stretching of the nerve may result in the 'battered root syndrome'. Lacerations of the nerve root may occur if adequate visualization or identification of the nerve root is not achieved. A flattened nerve root over an extruded disc, excessive bleeding, and inadequate bony exposure may be the reasons for difficulty in identification of the nerve root. Also, failure to recognize nerve root anomalies may lead the unwary surgeon to injure the nerve root.

The abdominal structures anterior to the intervertebral disc are at risk of damage if the anterior annulus is violated during disc removal. The aorta bifurcates into the common iliac arteries at the L4–5 disc level. The right common iliac artery crosses the anterior surface of the L4–5 disc and fixes the left common iliac branch of the vena cava against the vertebral column. The structures lateral to the vessels are the ureters, and the terminal ileum lies anterior to the vessels. The injuries to the intra-abdominal structures may be catastrophic. In addition to reducing venous bleeding and giving better exposure of the disc space, the kneeling position allows the intra-abdominal contents to fall anteriorly, away from the vertebral column. One should avoid overzealous attempts to remove the entire nucleus. The surgeon should always be aware of the depth of the instrument in the disc space. By maintaining contact with the vertebral endplates, the surgeon has better depth perception. The pituitary rongeur with a depth marking is helpful in avoiding excessively deep penetration. Preoperative lateral lumbar spine radiographs should also be reviewed carefully to measure the depth of the intervertebral disc space.

Injuries to the great vessels, including the aorta, the inferior vena cava, and the iliac vessels, lead to shock and death unless prompt diagnosis and repair are performed. With partial injury to the vessel wall, delayed hemorrhage, false aneurysm, or arteriovenous fistula may result. The patients with arteriovenous fistula may present with increase in pulse pressure, tachycardia, dyspnea, and cardiac enlargement months or years after back surgery. Symptoms include high-output circulatory failure; and vascular repair is necessary in these patients.

Bowel injuries during lumbar disc surgery are uncommon. Injuries to the ileum and appendix are described in the literature. The patients may develop abdominal distention, rigidity, and peritonitis. Prompt diagnosis and treatment are important. Ureteral injuries are again mostly caused by the pituitary rongeur. Postoperative intervertebral disc space infection is uncommon. Persistent back pain several weeks after removal of the intervertebral disc is a sign of postoperative discitis. Elevated erythrocyte sedimentation rates are observed in most patients with discitis. Bone scans, tomograms, or magnetic resonance imaging are helpful in identifying changes associated with discitis earlier than plain radiography. The bacteria responsible for postoperative discitis are identified in less than 50 per cent of cases. The most common organisms cultured are *Staphylococcus* species. Early diagnosis and prompt treatment are important in the prevention of chronic infection. Occasionally, lumbar epidural abscesses may develop and frank paresis or paralysis may occur. Under these circumstances, immediate decompressive laminectomy is indicated.

The incidence of lumbar instability after decompression laminectomy varies depending on the patient's preoperative pathology and the extent of bony resection during surgery. The patients with degenerative spondylolisthesis frequently slip further, and fusion is recommended in the majority of cases. The extent of bony resection is probably the most important factor in the development of postoperative instability. Concomitant operation on the disc at the time of laminectomy may contribute to additional instability. Total laminectomy and bilateral facetectomy will make the spine unstable. The pars interarticularis should be preserved as much as possible. Postlaminectomy fractures of the pars interarticularis may cause progressive slippage. For the majority of routine spinal stenosis cases, at least half of the facet joint can be preserved by undercutting the superior facet and thus postoperative spondylolithesis can be prevented.

Conclusions

In summary, the success of lumbar decompressive procedures is primarily dependent on proper patient selection. With meticulous surgical techniques, the involved nerve roots should be adequately decompressed, but not excessively, to prevent postoperative instability. The surgeon should recognize the cases that require fusion in addition to decompression procedures.

Bibliography

An HS, Booth RE, Rothman RH (1991) Complications in lumbar disc disease surgery. In RA Balderston, HS An (eds) *Complications in Spine Surgery*, pp. 61–78. Philadelphia: W.B. Saunders

An HS, Glover JM (1994) Spinal stenosis: Historical perspectives, classifications, and pathoanatomy. *Sem Spin Surg* **6**:69–77

An HS, Haughton V (1993) Imaging considerations of lumbar spinal stenosis. *Sem CT, Ultras, and MRI* **14**:414–24

Booth RE (1986) Spinal stenosis. In LD Anderson (ed) *The American Academy of Orthopaedic Surgeons: Instructional Course Lectures*, pp. 420–35. St Louis: C.V. Mosby

Eismont FJ, Wiesel SW, Rothman RH (1981) The treatment of dural tears associated with spinal surgery. *J Bone Joint Surg* **63A**:1132

Johnsson KE, Willner S, Johnsson K (1986) Postoperative instability after decompression for lumbar spinal stenosis. *Spine* **11**:107–10

Kadish L, Simmons EH (1984) Anomalies of the lumbosacral nerve roots and anatomical investigation and myelographic study. *J Bone Joint Surg* **66B**:411

Kahanovitz N, Viola K, McCulloch JA (1989) Limited surgical discectomy and microdiscectomy. A clinical comparison. *Spine* **14**:79–81

Rothman RH, Simeone FA (1992) *The Spine*, 3rd edn. Philadelphia: W.B. Saunders

Stambough JL (1989) Surgical techniques for lumbar discectomy. *Sem Spine Surg* **1**:47–53

12

Microsurgery for lumbar disc disease

John A McCulloch

Introduction

Lumbar procedures are frequently performed without any magnification or with loupes. The advantage of loupes and fiberoptic illumination is principally improved visualization. For many reasons the operating microscope is superior to loupes. The most important of the reasons is maintenance of stereopsis or 3-dimensional viewing in the depths of a spinal wound. For surface surgery loupes are fine. For surgery deep in a lumbar spine, the only way 3-D vision can be maintained deep in a wound is with a wound long enough to accommodate one's fixed interpupillary distance, which is approximately 65 mm. To shorten that distance so one's incision is 'not much longer than the microsurgeon's' is to give up 3-D visualization. Every surgeon wants to see 'more and better', and for this reason those spinal surgeons who wish to see infinite depth in a small spinal wound and maintain 3-D vision have adopted the microscope. Additional reasons for using a microscope for spine surgery include:

(1) a parallel rather than an offset light source,
(2) the ability to achieve high magnification up to 10× for fine work,
(3) the ability to teach residents and others in the room, and
(4) the fixed focus of the microscope,

so that the surgeon can move around the room without having to refocus on the surgical field and to obtain relief from the fixed neck position necessary to use loupes.

There are biological advantages associated with minimally invasive spine surgery. Surgical wounds heal by either primary or secondary intention. A long midline spinal incision that is followed by elevation of paraspinal muscle over many segments has a greater potential for hematoma formation than a short single-segment muscle elevation. A large paraspinal hematoma has to be reabsorbed by granulation tissue formation or healing by secondary intention. A single-segment muscle elevation and retraction leaves behind limited dead space and less hematoma, and reduces healing by secondary intention. Finally, the benefits of ambulating a patient the day of surgery or even discharging the microdiscectomy patient on the day of surgery are too obvious to state. Such a patient has a major postoperative advantage over the patient with a more painful wound that results in longer bed rest and hospitalization.

While supporting the microscope for lumbar spine surgery, one should still point out that the microscope will not do the surgery for you. In fact, there are some disadvantages in using the microscope. Most importantly, the technical advance of using the microscope may not improve your surgical outcomes at all. Only 10 per cent of surgical success depends on technique, while 90 per cent of successful surgical outcomes still depend on good clinical judgment leading one to operate on the correct patient.

The biggest problem with the microscope is reduced peripheral vision. Within the 5 cm diameter field of vision of the microscope, excellent visualization of tissues is achieved; but outside that field, the visualization is lost. If the surgical procedure takes the operative area to the edge of the microscope field, the scope should be moved so that the center of the microscope field is adjusted. Another problem with the learning curve of the microscope is that many tissues, such as empty severed epidural veins, residual strands of ligamentum flavum, strands of annulus, and some strands of proteoglycan-filled nucleus, may resemble 'strands of nerve rootlets'. This point may be advantageous, in that it makes the surgeon much more cautious, and may reduce the complication rate of dural tears and root damage. A small amount of bleeding into a limited operative field interferes with visualization and the completion of the surgical exercise. The difference between 25 ml of blood loss and 100 ml of blood loss under the microscope is significant. Every effort in preoperative preparation (i.e., stopping anti-inflammatory medication), in assuring proper patient positioning on the operating room table with the abdomen free of pressure, and in intraoperative control of hemorrhage has to be made to avoid this disadvantage. Wilson and associates (1981) reported an increased rate of disc space infection after microsurgery. This is most likely to be because of the presence of the microscope directly over the wound. Although the microscope is sterilely draped, there are parts of the microscope that are exposed (eyepieces) that have the potential to contaminate the wound.

And the limited operating space between the microscope and the wound introduces another element of potential break in proper surgical technique that can result in wound contamination.

Indications

1. Laminotomy and discectomy for a herniated disc
2. Laminectomy for spinal stenosis
3. A paraspinal approach for foraminatomy or a foraminal herniated disc.

Surgical techniques

Lumbar laminotomy and discectomy

The operation can be done under general anesthesia, spinal anesthesia, or local anesthesia. This author prefers general anesthesia. Most surgeons use a variation of the kneeling frame that relieves pressure on the abdominal cavity and reduces back flow through Batson's plexus, in turn reducing epidural bleeding. Some surgeons prefer the Wilson frame to reduce lumbar lordosis further; but more intraoperative bleeding is expected with the Wilson frame. This author uses the Andrews frame. Another important point in positioning is the correct identification of the level of intervention.

The author's preferred method is to use an image intensifier to mark the level of intervention before prepping and draping.

A 1-inch (2.5 cm) skin incision is made straddling the interspinous marking line (Fig. 12.1A, B). Moving the incision just lateral to the midline facilitates the fascial flap (Fig 12.2A). Making a midline fascial incision not only destroys the integrity of the supraspinous ligament; it removes a good buttress for the medial post of the frame retractor. The short rotators insert at the inferior portion of the spinous process (Fig. 12.2B). Trying to dissect subperiosteally in this region will result in deflection of the Cobb elevator by the tendon into paraspinal muscles, resulting in excessive bleeding. Rather, dissect down the spinous process inferior to the interlaminar space to be exposed. Slip the Cobb elevator over the facet joint, retract the muscle and detach multifidus muscle (Fig. 12.2C). With the Cobb elevator in position, insert the muscle blade of the self retaining frame retractor (Fig. 12.3A). Next position the hook in the inter-

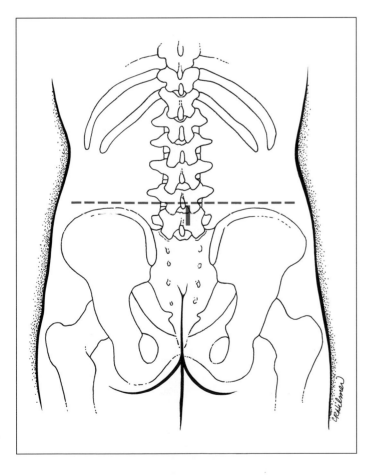

Figure 12.1

Skin incision for microscopic laminotomy and discectomy.

A
A 1-inch (2.5 cm) skin incision is made straddling the interspinous marking line.

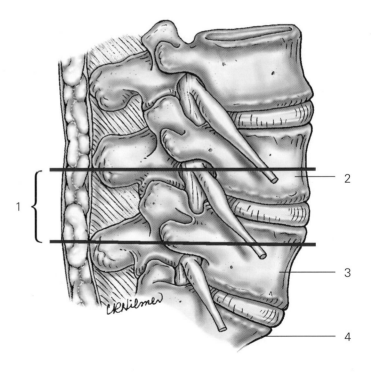

B
The skin incision is from the middle of the spinous process to the next spinous process, centered over the intervertebral disc.

1 Incision
2 L4
3 L5
4 Sacrum

A

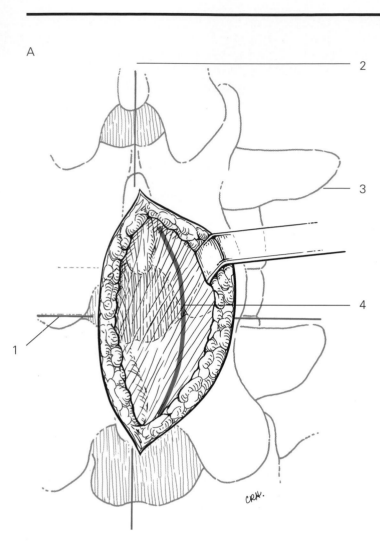

B

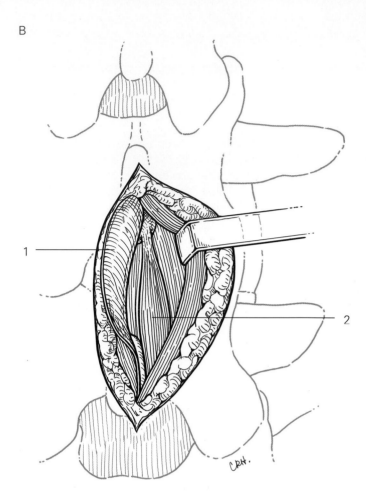

Figure 12.2

Deeper dissection for microscopic laminotomy and discectomy.

A
The fascia is divided just lateral to the midline to facilitate the fascial flap.

1 Marking line, inf. edge of disc space
2 Midline marking line
3 L4
4 Fascial incision

B
The short rotator muscles are detached from the inferior portion of the spinous process and retracted laterally.

1 Fascial flap
2 Multifidus m.

C
Dissection of the muscles is done laterally to expose the spinous processes, lamina, and facet capsule.

C

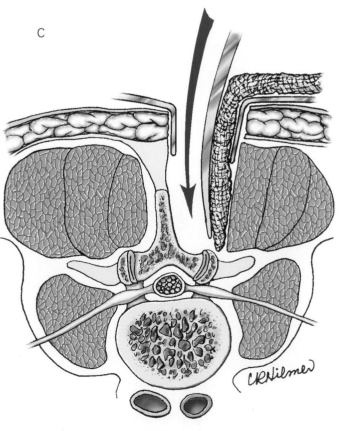

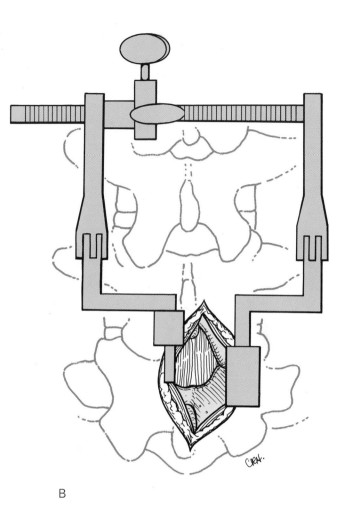

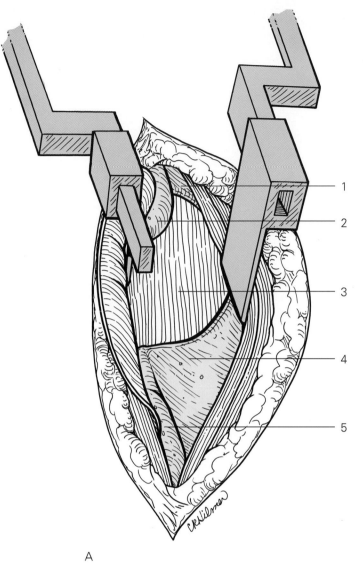

A

B

Figure 12.3

Exposure for microscopic laminotomy and discectomy.

A

Dissection of muscles should expose the superior and inferior lamina and the ligamentum flavum.

1 Lamina
2 Spinous process
3 Ligamentum flavum
4 Lamina
5 Spinous process

B

A self retaining retractor is positioned so that the smaller blade is in the midline and the larger blade retracts the muscles laterally.

spinous notch so that it does not stand proud and overhang the operative field (Fig. 12.3B). By choosing various combinations of blades and hooks, the retractors can be rotated or tilted. For a simple discectomy, choose the shortest midline post with the longest lateral muscle blade to keep the retractor flat.

Some surgeons use the microscope from the skin incision forward. This author prefers to make the incision with no aids, and to secure the retractor in perfect position before moving the microscope over the field. (Obviously the microscope is draped in a sterile fashion before this stage.) Under the microscope, the initial procedure is the fashioning the ligamentum flavum flap. Identify the 'safety net'. This immediately identifies the inferior tip of the inferior facet and serves as the starting point for the ligamentum flavum flap. There are three steps in fashioning the flap (Fig. 12.4A). First, separate the ligamentum flavum origin from the anterior aspect of the superior lamina. This is best done with an angled curet. Next,

A

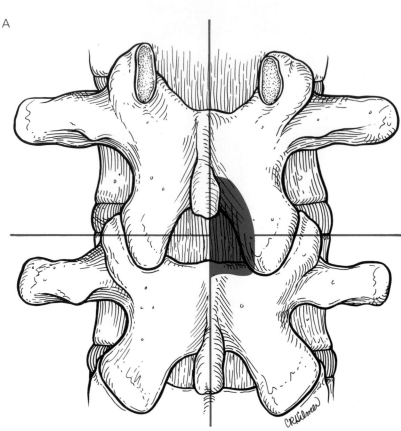

Figure 12.4

Laminotomy and resection of ligamentum flavum procedure.

A

The areas of dissection include bony resection of the laminae and ligamentum flavum.

B
Following resection of the inferior part of the superior lamina, the ligamentum flavum is freed from the superior part of the inferior lamina and the capsular insertion.

1 Ligamentum flavum

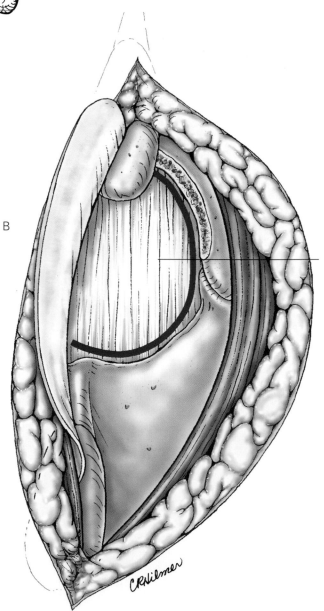

B

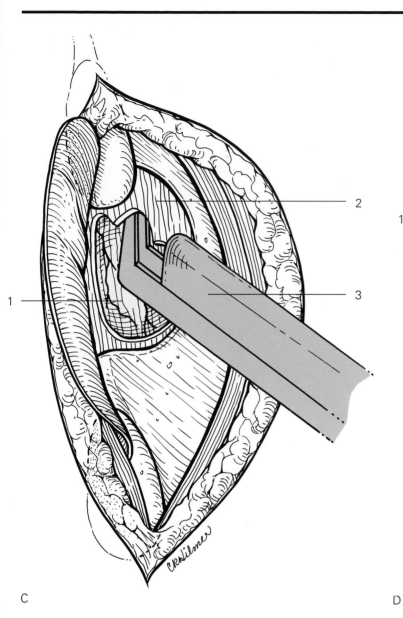

C

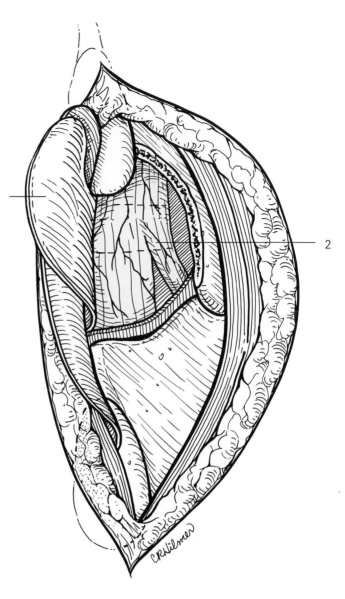

D

C
The ligamentum flavum may be excised and widened superiorly and laterally.

1 Dura
2 Ligamentum flavum
3 Kerrison rongeur

D
The ligamentum flavum may be elevated as a flap.

1 Ligamentum flavum flap
2 Nerve root

detach the ligamentum flavum insertion from the inferior lamina (Fig. 12.4B). Finally, separate the ligamentum flavum and the fat pad from its capsular insertion (Fig. 12.4C). Then elevate the flap just enough to see the lateral edge of the nerve root, and then tuck the flap under the root, retract the root medially and identify the disc space (Fig. 12.4D). The ligamentum flavum may be excised if the interlaminar space is small or if better exposure is needed. The nerve root is further medialized with a nerve root retractor, and the extruded or sequestered disc fragment is removed using a pituitary rongeur.

In the upper lumbar spine there is more lamina overhang with each succeeding disc space. In addition, the interpedicular distance narrows, the neurological contents of the spinal canal increase and exposure of the disc space becomes more difficult. The entry in to higher levels becomes more difficult

A

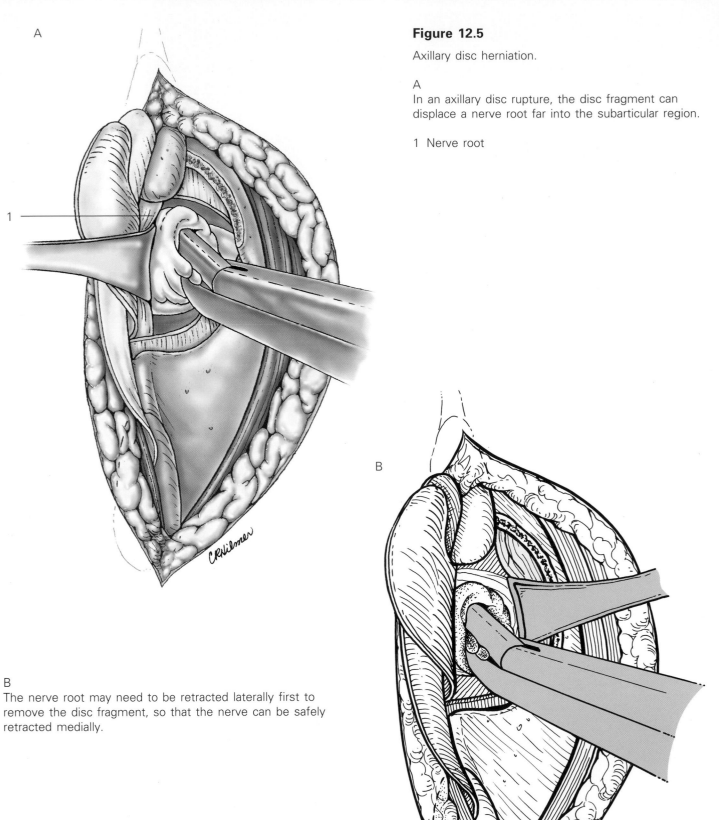

1

Figure 12.5

Axillary disc herniation.

A

In an axillary disc rupture, the disc fragment can displace a nerve root far into the subarticular region.

1 Nerve root

B

B

The nerve root may need to be retracted laterally first to remove the disc fragment, so that the nerve can be safely retracted medially.

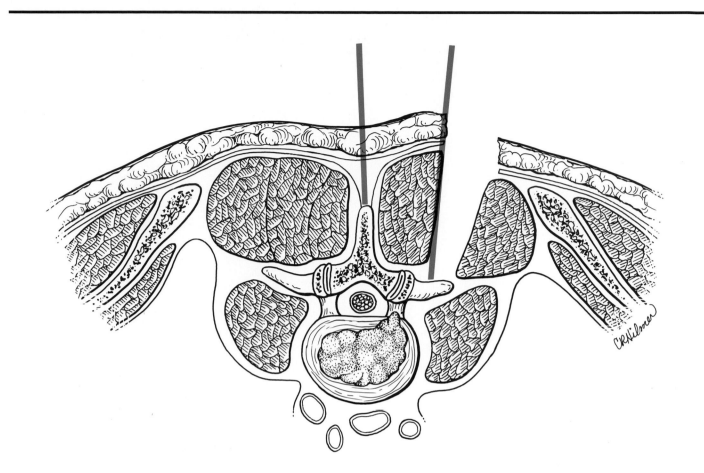

Figure 12.6

A foraminal herniated disc may be approached through
Wiltse's muscle splitting paraspinal approach.

in a short obese patient with narrow disc space and retrospondylolisthesis. A wider bony resection is required to overcome these difficulties. Disc herniations may be protruding, extruded, or sequestered. Extruded and sequestered discs may migrate. To prevent retained pathology and continuing symptoms it is essential to know where migrated discal fragments or bony pathology may be, relative to the surgical anatomy of a lumbar segment. In completing the decompressive procedure, remove all bony encroachment and all ruptured discal material interfering with nerve root function. Once the root is free and mobile, one must decide what to do with intradiscal material that has the potential to become a recurrent disc rupture. For a contained disc herniation, it is best to be conservative by dilating the annular fibers with an elevator without making a square or cruciate incision. For noncontained or transannular disc herniation, loose fragments in the disc space should be removed through the annular rent. It is not recommended to remove the entire

nucleus pulposus vigorously, as the purpose of the surgery is to decompress the nerve root rather than removing the disc. Disc herniations usually occur in the posterolateral quadrant of the disc space; but they can migrate as extruded and sequestered fragments. In an axillary L5–S1 disc rupture, the disc fragment can displace a nerve root far into the subarticular region and out of direct view, where it can be damaged by the unwary surgeon (Fig. 12.5). A foraminal disc herniation is more common at the L4–5 and L3–4 levels, and it should be approached through Wiltse's muscle splitting paraspinal approach (Fig. 12.6). Nerve root anomalies causing double root involvement are not rare, and being aware of these situations will prevent complications. Allowing that the MRI scan was properly interpreted and all pathology seen on MRI was dealt with at surgery, the nerve root should be free and mobile at completion. For the closure of the laminectomy defect the ligamentum flavum flap is used instead of fat graft. Drains are not routinely necessary.

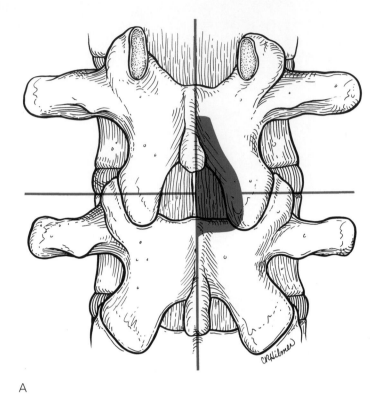

A

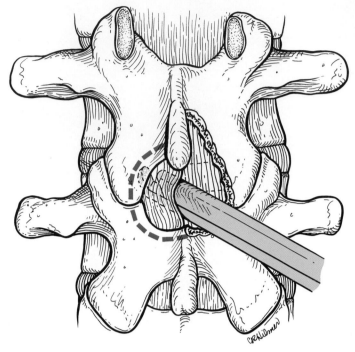

B

Figure 12.7

Microscopic laminectomy.

A
The cephalad lamina is removed proximally until the origin of the ligamentum flavum fibers is seen, the medial edge of the facet joint is resected, and the superior edge of the caudad lamina is removed.

B
Using the midline cleft of the ligamentum flavum, the medial portion of the ligamentum flavum is removed, moving cephalad to caudad. By retracting and saving the interspinous ligament, the contralateral side of the spinal canal can be undercut.

C
A bilateral decompression of spinal stenosis through a unilateral interlaminar window is possible.

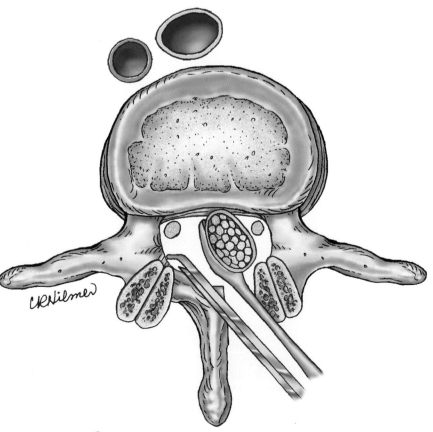

C

Microsurgery for spinal canal stenosis

Spinal stenosis can be divided into central canal stenosis and lateral zone stenosis. Central canal stenosis is a true circumferential encroachment on cauda equina territory, with annular bulging anteriorly with or without a spondylolisthesis, facet joint hypertrophy laterally, and ligamentum flavum infolding posteriorly. Note that the predominant location of the lesion in acquired spinal canal stenosis is largely in the central canal; but lateral zone stenosis should not be overlooked. Using the knowledge of the attachment of the ligamentum flavum, it is possible to decompress the lesion in spinal canal stenosis with a limited microsurgical exposure. The cephalad lamina is removed proximally until the origin of the ligamentum flavum fibers is seen (Fig. 12.7A). Next, remove the medial edge of the facet joint. Finally, complete the interlaminar decompression by removing the superior edge of the caudad lamina, which removes the insertion of the ligamentum flavum. Another useful anatomical fact during this decompression is the cleft that usually separates the right and left leaves of the ligamentum flavum. Using this natural division, it is easy to remove the medial portion of the ligamentum flavum, moving cephalad to caudad. By retracting and saving the interspinous ligament and rotating the patient away from the ipsilateral side, it is possible to use the magnification and illumination of the microscope to see the contralateral side of the spinal canal (Figs. 12.7B,C). With careful preparation it is possible to do a bilateral decompression of spinal stenosis through a unilateral interlaminar window

Complications

1. A short 1-inch incision and force into deeper structures may result in damage to the cauda equina, the vascular tree, and even the bowel or the genito-urinary system.
2. Dural tears and root injury are usually due to technical factors, such as poor exposure, excessive force, or manipulation. Use the proper instrumentation with precision. In an inadvertent durotomy, repair with a watertight seal is mandatory. One may ignore an anterior dural tear, as it will tamponade itself.
3. The incidence of recurrent disc ruptures following a routine microdiscectomy is about 2–5 per cent. The microscope is especially valuable for dealing with this problem.

Conclusion

The magnification and illumination offered by the microscope is a useful addition to a spinal surgeon's armamentarium. Remembering the weaknesses, traps, and special complications of least invasive spine surgery makes the microscope an indispensable addition to most spine surgical practices.

Bibliography

Goald HJ (1986) A new microsurgical reoperation for failed lumbar disc surgery. *J Microsurgery* **7**:63–6

Kahanovitz N, Viola K, McCulloch JA (1989) Limited surgical discectomy and microdiscectomy. A clinical comparison. *Spine* **14**:79–81

Scoville WB, Corkilig G (1973) Lumbar disc surgery: Technique of radical removal and early mobilization. *J Neurosurgery* **39**:265–9

Spengler DM (1982) Results with limited excision and selective foraminotomy. *Spine* **7**:604–7

Tullberg T, Isacson J, Weidenhielm L (1993) Does microscopic removal of lumbar disc herniation lead to better results than the standard procedure? *Spine* **18**:24–7

Williams RW (1978) Microlumbar discectomy: A conservative surgical approach to the virgin herniated lumbar disc. *Spine* **3**:175–82.

Wilson DH, Harbaugh R (1981) Microsurgical and standard removal of the protruded lumbar disc: A comparative study. *Neurosurgery* **8**:422–7

Wiltse LL (1984) Alar transverse process impingement of the L5 spinal nerve: The far-out syndrome. *Spine* **9**:31–8

13

Posterior lumbar fusion procedures

Howard S An

Introduction

Interlaminar fusion of the lumbar spine was originally described by Hibbs and Albee in 1911 for tuberculosis, and it was subsequently extended to include a variety of pathological conditions of the spine. Several authors, such as Watkins (1959), Stauffer (Stauffer and Coventry 1972), and Wiltse (Wiltse and Bateman 1965), have reported their experiences with transverse process fusion of the lumbar spine. It has become the standard fusion technique for the past several decades. Posterior lumbar interbody fusion (PLIF) following lumbar disc removal was reported by Jaslow (1946), and PLIF has been reported by several authors, including Cloward (1953), Crock (1983), Lin (1977), and Simmons (1985). In this chapter, indications for lumbar fusion and techniques of posterolateral fusion and PLIF will be discussed.

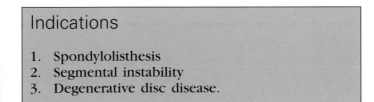

Indications

1. Spondylolisthesis
2. Segmental instability
3. Degenerative disc disease.

Surgical techniques

Intertransverse posterolateral fusion

A kneeling position using an Andrews-type frame lessens blood loss by reducing the intra-abdominal venous pressure. Alternatively, a four-poster frame may be used to extend the hips.

This position can help in maintaining better lumbar lordosis. A midline incision is made for routine cases. Bilateral lateral incisions, popularized by Wiltse, may be utilized in some cases, where midline decompression is not needed. In cases of previous infection or dural tear, the lateral incisions may be preferred. Following a midline skin incision, electrocautery is utilized to deepen the incision to the fascia. The exposure of the spinous processes should extend to an additional level. For example, the spinous processes from L3 to S2 should be exposed for a fusion from L4 to the sacrum. Using Cobb elevators, the dissection should stay subperiosteally, and the paraspinous muscles are retracted with the sponges. Each side is dissected alternately so that the self retaining retractors can gradually be placed more deeply. The exposure of the spinous processes is followed by exposure of the lamina and facet joints. The facet capsules of the cephalad facet joints not included in the fusion should be carefully preserved. The pars interarticularis and transverse processes are exposed using cautery and Cobb elevators. Great care must be taken not to break off the transverse process. The intertransverse membrane connects the transverse processes, and this membrane should not be penetrated. The blood vessels just lateral to the pars interarticularis should be cautiously approached and coagulated if bleeding is encountered.

The exposure of the ala of the sacrum is frequently compromised owing to its relative anatomic inaccessibility. The ala of the sacrum is best exposed by dissecting just lateral to the L5–S1 facet joint. The Cobb elevator can be used to retract and dissect muscles off the lateral gutter between the ala and the L5 transverse process. The exposure of the fusion bed in this area is critical for successful fusion. After exposing the transverse processes and the ala of the sacrum, the muscles and capsules should be cleaned so that the exposed bone continues from the transverse process, the pars interarticularis, and the lateral

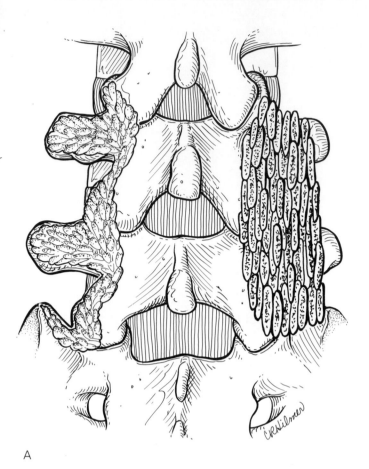

A

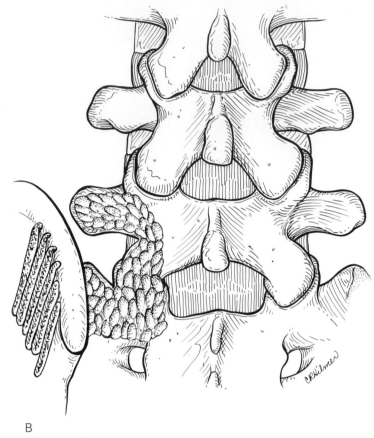

B

Figure 13.1

Intertransverse process fusion of the lumbar spine.

A
Exposed bone continues from the transverse process, the pars interarticularis, and the lateral aspect of the facet joint to the next transverse process, and bone grafts are packed over these decorticated surfaces of bone.

B
Corticocancellous graft, primarily cancellous graft, is harvested from the posterior iliac crest.

aspect of the facet joint to the next transverse process (Fig. 13.1A).

At this time, laminectomy and foraminotomy is performed if indicated. The facet surfaces are denuded of their articular cartilage using a narrow double-action rongeur. Corticocancellous graft, primarily cancellous graft, is harvested from the posterior iliac crest (Fig. 13.1B). This can usually be accomplished through the same midline incision by elevating the subcutaneous tissue off the lumbar dorsal fascia. Alternatively, the fascial splitting approach can be utilized, by splitting the lumbar dorsal fascia from the fascia overlying the paraspinal muscles. The fascial attachment over the posterior iliac crest is divided, and subperiosteal dissection will expose the outer iliac crest. In patients with a wide pelvis, the exposure of the iliac crest through the midline skin incision may be difficult. The preoperative pelvic radiograph will help in determining whether a separate incision over the iliac crest is to be preferred. The iliac crest from the non-painful side should be harvested, to differentiate the postoperative donor site pain from the residual preoperative radicular pain. Large

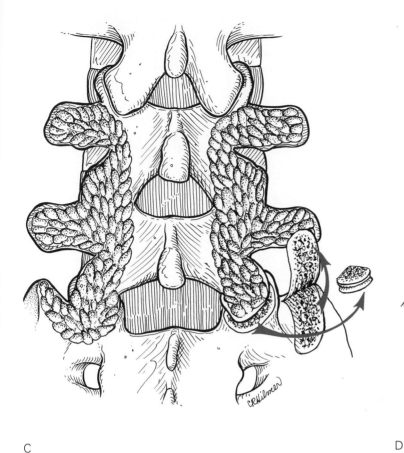

C

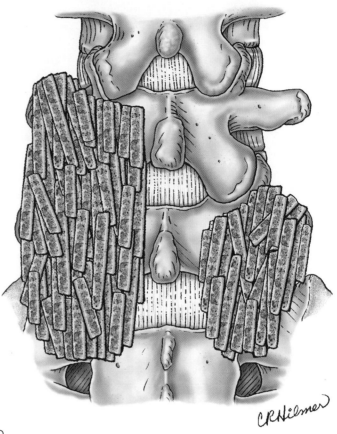

D

amounts of corticocancellous graft can be harvested in the shape of long strips (Fig. 13.1A).

Decortication of the transverse process, the lateral gutter, and the sacral ala are performed carefully (Fig. 13.1A). The decortication may be done using the rat-tooth Leksell double action rongeur or power burr. The graft is carefully tamped within the denuded facets and placed in the lateral gutters which have been created lateral to the facet joint (Fig. 13.1A). Using a curved osteotome, a flap of bone may be created on the ala of the sacrum. This flap of bone is flipped over so that it contacts the transverse process of L5 (Fig. 13.1C). In addition to the inter-transverse fusion, interlaminar fusion may be augmented if laminectomy has not been performed. The lamina is carefully decorticated, and long strips of bone graft are placed to bridge from one lamina to the next lamina (Fig. 13.1D). A plug of bone wax or thrombin-soaked gelfoam may be used to control bleeding from the iliac crest. Careful hemostasis is important in the prevention of hematoma formation. Separate drains in the midline line wound and donor site are placed.

C

A flap of bone may be created on the ala of the sacrum and flipped over, so that it contacts the transverse process of L5.

D

In addition to the intertransverse fusion, interlaminar fusion is done if laminectomy has not been performed. The lamina is carefully decorticated, and long strips of bone graft are placed to bridge from one lamina to the next lamina.

Posterior lumbar interbody fusion

PLIF is a technique that involves insertion of the bone grafts into the disc space by retracting the nerve roots. Great care must be taken to avoid damage to the nerve roots. Other possible complications associated with PLIF may be anterior vessel damage through penetrating the anterior annulus, posterior bone graft migration, perineural fibrosis, and pseudarthrosis.

The technique of PLIF is exacting, and the complications can be avoided with meticulous preparation of the interbody space and careful insertion of the grafts. There are many variations of the PLIF. The author prefers the technique of filling the disc space with bone blocks or cages to restore the disc height and stability. PLIF requires midline laminectomy and partial facetectomy to expose the nerve roots. The medial border of the lateral facets should be removed out to the pedicle. The nerve roots should be completely decompressed out to the foramen so that they are free and mobile. By using a lamina spreader, the disc space is distracted (Fig. 13.2A). Alternatively, pedicle screws may be used to distract the motion segment if pedicle screw instrumentation is to be used for the stabilization procedure. Discectomy is performed bilaterally while retracting the nerve roots. An osteotome is then used to remove the endplates (Fig. 13.2B). Curets and pituitary rongeurs are used to clean out the intervertebral disc space (Fig. 13.2C). The disc is removed to the lateral and anterior edges of the annulus (Fig. 13.2D). Alternatively, specialized instruments may be used to

A

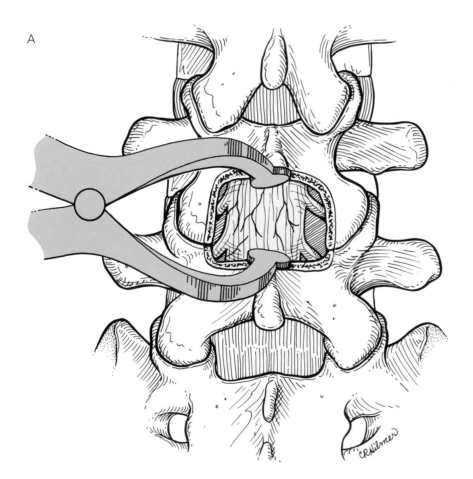

Figure 13.2

Posterior interbody fusion of the lumbar spine.

A

Midline laminectomy and partial facetectomy expose the nerve roots out to the foramen so that they are free and mobile. By using a lamina spreader, the disc space is distracted. Alternatively, pedicle screws may be used to distract the motion segment if pedicle screw instrumentation is used for the stabilization procedure.

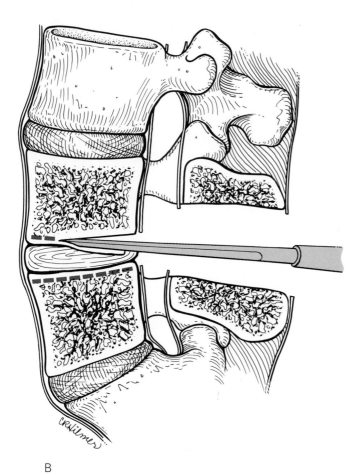

B

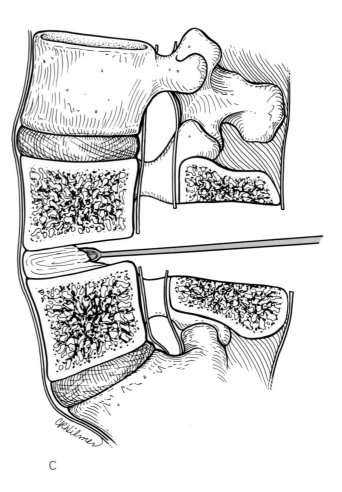

C

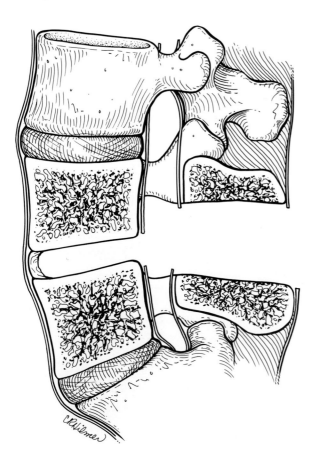

D

B
An osteotome is used to remove the endplates, followed by thorough removal of the intervertebral disc.

C
Curets and pituitary rongeurs are used to clean out the intervertebral disc space.

D
The disc is removed to the lateral and anterior edges of the annulus.

Contd

remove the disc and endplates en bloc (Fig. 13.2E). A cannulated rectangular osteotome or chisel is used to cut a precise rectangular space on the pathologic interspace to be fused (Fig. 13.2F).

The insertion of bone grafts or cages is carried out next. Using a lamina spreader the disc space is distracted. Morselized bone grafts are inserted, first into the anterior aspect of the space. A spacer of appropriate size is placed on one side (Fig. 13.2G). An

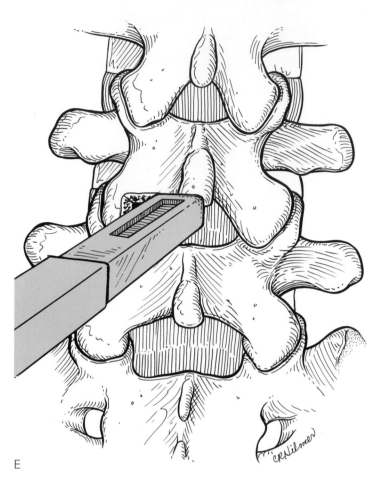

E

Figure 13.2 *(contd)*

E

A specialized instrument may be used to remove the disc and endplates *en bloc*.

F

A cannulated rectangular osteotome or chisel is used to cut a precise rectangular space on the pathologic interspace to be fused.

G

A spacer of appropriate size is placed on one side.

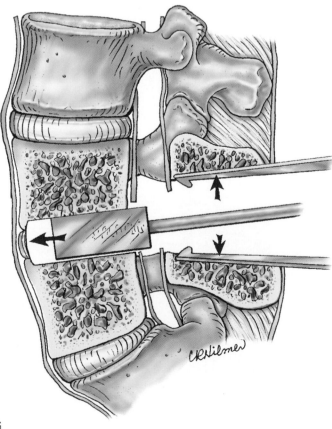

F

G

appropriate-size bone graft is then placed on the opposite side (Fig. 13.2H). Either an autograft or an allograft bone plug can be used, but the autograft bone is expected to achieve a better rate of union. Another bone block may be inserted by moving the bone block medially (Fig. 13.2I). The spacer is then removed, and additional bone blocks can be inserted on the opposite side. Three or four bone blocks can be inserted in the space. The grafts should be 3–4 mm

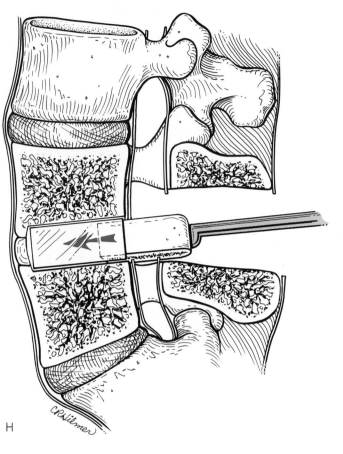

H
An appropriate-size bone graft is placed on the opposite side.

I
Three to four bone blocks may be inserted by moving the bone blocks medially.

Contd

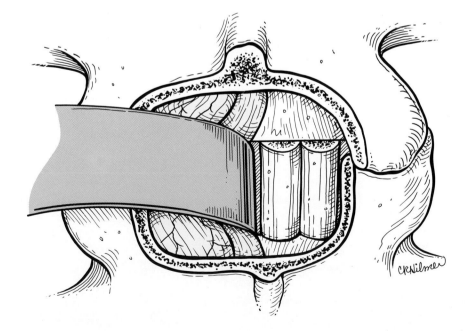

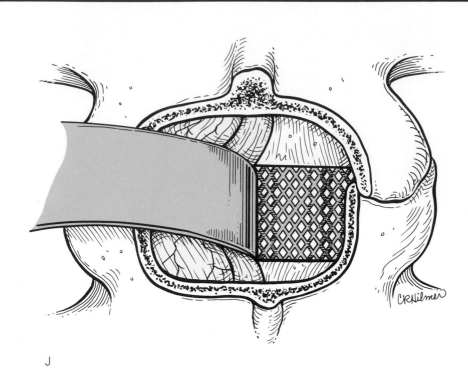

J

Figure 13.2 *(contd)*

J
Cages filled with chips of autograft may be inserted instead of bone blocks.

K
Morselized autogenous bone grafts should be placed into the anterior aspect of the space, and the cage should be inserted in the posterior aspect of the vertebral body.

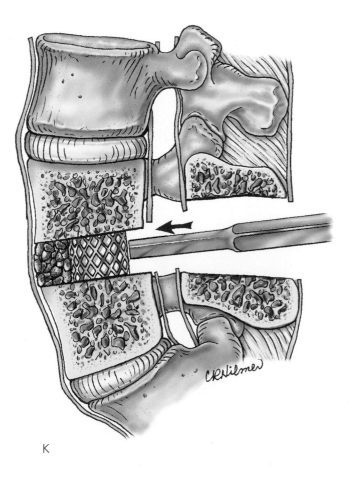

countersunk from the posterior margin of the vertebral body. The grafts should be under compression loading and quite stable. Alternatively, cages instead of bone blocks may be used to enhance stability (Fig. 13.2J). Again morselized autogenous bone grafts should be placed into the anterior aspect of the space (Fig. 13.2K). The cages should be filled with morselized bone and placed into both sides of the interbody space. The cages should be placed in the posterior two-thirds of the vertebral body, about 3 mm anterior to the posterior vertebral margin.

A fat graft is placed anteriorly between the dura and the grafts, as well as posteriorly over the dura. Following PLIF, posterolateral fusion or instrumentation may be augmented to enhance fusion rates. If instrumentation is to be performed, compression loading should be applied to enhance the stability of the graft or cage and to maintain lumbar lordosis.

K

Bibliography

Cloward RB (1953) The treatment of ruptured lumbar intervertebral discs by vertebral body fusion: Indications, operative technique, after care. *J Neurosurg* **10**:154–68

Crock HV (1983) *Practice of Spinal Surgery.* New York: Springer-Verlag

James A, Nisbet NW (1953) Posterior intervertebral fusion of the lumbar spine. Preliminary report of a new operation. *J Bone Joint Surg* **35**:181–7

Jaslow IA (1946) Intercorporal bone graft in spinal fusion after disc removal. *Surg Gyn Obstet* **82**:215–18

Lin PM (1977) A technical modification of Cloward's posterior lumbar interbody fusion. *Neurosurg* **1**:118–24

Ma GW (1985) Posterior lumbar interbody fusion with specialized instruments. *Clin Orthop* **193**:57–63

Simmons JW (1985) Posterior lumbar interbody fusion with posterior elements as chip grafts. *Clin Orthop* **193**:85–9

Stauffer RN, Coventry MB (1972) Posterolateral fusion of the lumbar and lumbosacral spine. *J Bone Joint Surg* **54A**:1195–204

Watkins MB (1959) Posterolateral bone grafting for fusion of the lumbar and lumbosacral spine. *J Bone Joint Surg* **41A**:388–95

Wiltse LL, Bateman JG (1965) Experience with transverse process fusion of the lumbar spine. *J Bone Joint Surg* **47A**:848–9

14

Posterior lumbar instrumentation procedures

Howard S An

Introduction

Posterolateral fusion is a well-established procedure. However, the rate of pseudarthrosis is relatively high without spinal fixation. In addition, if the spine is unstable or deformed, an instrumentation system must be used to stabilize the spine. The spinal implants may also be used to improve the rate of fusion. There are numerous techniques of spinal instrumentation for the lumbar spine. Translaminar facet joint fixation, pedicle screw instrumentation, and sacral fixation techniques will be described in this chapter. The other techniques, such as Harrington rods, Luque rods, Knodt rods, etc., require multiple level fusion of the lumbar spine, and may produce a flat back deformity; and thus these procedures have fallen into disfavor. The pedicle screw instrumentation provides the best stability, and thus is the preferred method of posterior stabilization, particularly for trauma and deformity cases. The translaminar facet joint screw fixation may be utilized in the relatively stable spine or as an adjunct fixation.

Indications

1. Pedicle screw instrumentation for lumbar burst fractures
2. Pedicle screw instrumentation for spondylolisthesis or deformities
3. Pedicle screw instrumentation for degenerative disc disease
4. Translaminar facet joint fixation for degenerative disc disease
5. Intrasacral rod fixation for spondylolisthesis or deformities.

Surgical techniques

Translaminar facet joint screw fixation

Magerl developed the technique of translaminar facet joint screw fixation (Magerl 1984). A midline incision is made and subperiosteal dissection of the paraspinous muscles is performed, exposing the spinous processes, laminae, facet joints, pars interarticularis, and transverse processes (Fig. 14.1A). The facet joint capsule is excised and the joint cartilage is scraped. A guide is placed so that the screw is inserted from the base of the spinous process, through the lamina, across the facet, ending at the attachment of the transverse process to the pedicle (Fig. 14.1B). Because of the angle of insertion, the drill and screwdriver are usually inserted percutaneously. Drilling is done using a 3.2 mm AO drill bit.

An appropriate-size 4.5 mm AO cortical screw is then inserted (Fig. 14.1C). At the lumbosacral level, a longer screw can be inserted into the sacral ala. Another screw is inserted from the opposite side in the same manner (Fig. 14.1D). The starting points and directions must be chosen in such a way that the screws pass through the lamina perpendicular to the facet joint and to the junction between the pedicle and the transverse process (Fig. 14.1E). Posterolateral fusion is then performed in the routine manner (Fig. 14.1F).

A

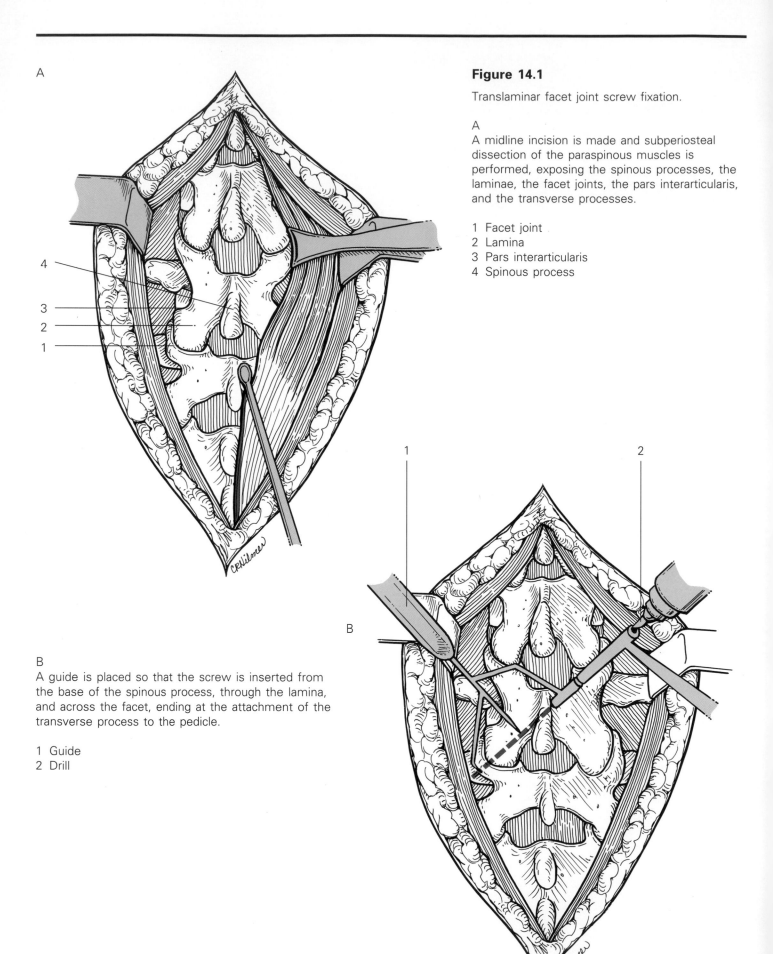

Figure 14.1

Translaminar facet joint screw fixation.

A

A midline incision is made and subperiosteal dissection of the paraspinous muscles is performed, exposing the spinous processes, the laminae, the facet joints, the pars interarticularis, and the transverse processes.

1 Facet joint
2 Lamina
3 Pars interarticularis
4 Spinous process

B

A guide is placed so that the screw is inserted from the base of the spinous process, through the lamina, and across the facet, ending at the attachment of the transverse process to the pedicle.

1 Guide
2 Drill

C

Contd

C
A cortical screw or some other type of screw is
then inserted through the drill hole.

D

D
Another screw is inserted from the opposite side in
the same manner.

E

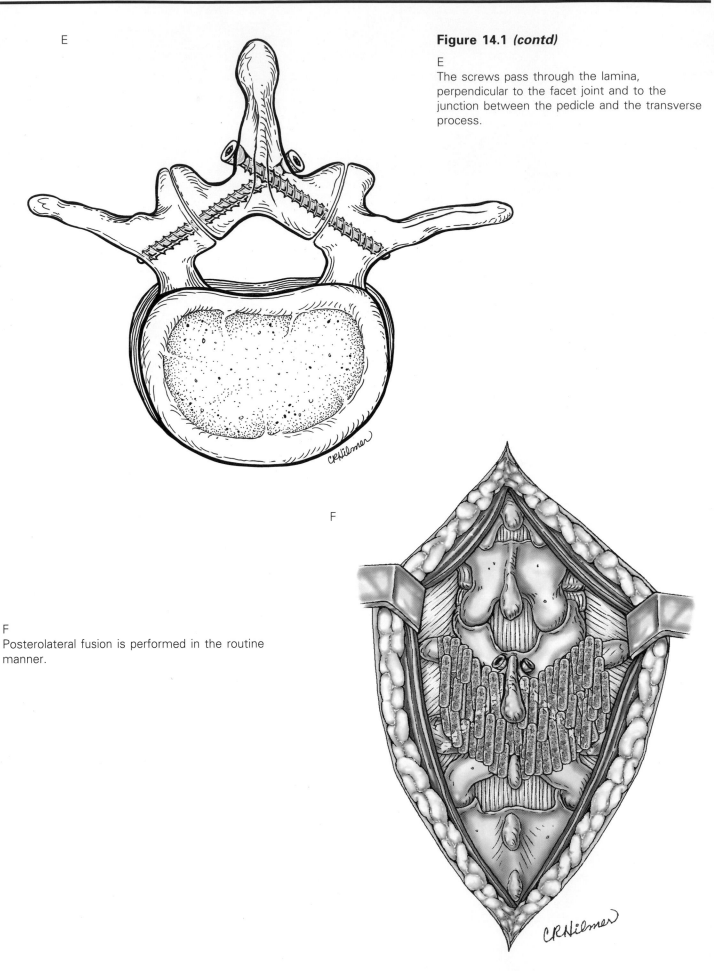

Figure 14.1 *(contd)*

E
The screws pass through the lamina, perpendicular to the facet joint and to the junction between the pedicle and the transverse process.

F

F
Posterolateral fusion is performed in the routine manner.

Pedicle screw instrumentation

In addition to pedicle screw fixation, the transpedicular approach may be utilized for biopsy, decompression, or eggshell procedure for kyphosis correction. The key to transpedicular procedures is the anatomic identification of the pedicle. Knowledge of pedicular anatomy in relation to neural structures is crucial to avoid complications. Preoperative assessment of the pedicle height, width, and angulation is important.

The exposure of posterior elements of the lumbar spine is routinely performed. It is important to expose the junction between the pars interarticularis and the transverse process, which are anatomic landmarks for the pedicle entrance point. The pedicle entrance point is situated at the crossing of two lines (Fig. 14.2A). The vertical line is the extension of the facet joint in line with the bony crest coming from the superior articular facet. This vertical line is about 2–3 mm lateral from the pars interarticularis, and slants slightly laterally, going from L4 to S1 (Fig. 14.2A). The horizontal line passes through the middle of the insertion of the transverse process, or 1–2 mm below the joint line. The sacral entrance point is at the lower point of the

L5-S1 articulation on the elevated ridge of bone. The entrance point of the pedicle is about 2 mm lateral from the center of the pedicle, so that the screw can be inserted without disturbing the facet joint above, and so as to medialize the screw for better fixation.

The nerve root is situated just medial and inferior to the pedicle as it exits into the intervertebral foramen. Therefore one must avoid the area medial and inferior to the pedicle, to prevent damage to the nerve root. A small rongeur or burr is used to decorticate the pedicle entrance (Fig. 14.2B). A Steinmann pin or pedicle marker is placed about 1 cm deep, and radiographs should confirm the proper entrance point and path of the pedicle. A blunt instrument is advanced carefully through the pedicle into the vertebral body (Figs. 14.2C, D). The amount of medial angulation depends on both the level and the starting point. Preoperative axial CT or MRI cuts will guide the entrance point and medial angulation.

A thin probe is used to feel the walls of the pedicle (Fig. 14.2E). Tapping is done at all the pedicles, followed by insertion of the proximal screw of appropriate diameter and length (Fig. 14.2F). At this time, the transverse processes, the pars interarticularis, and

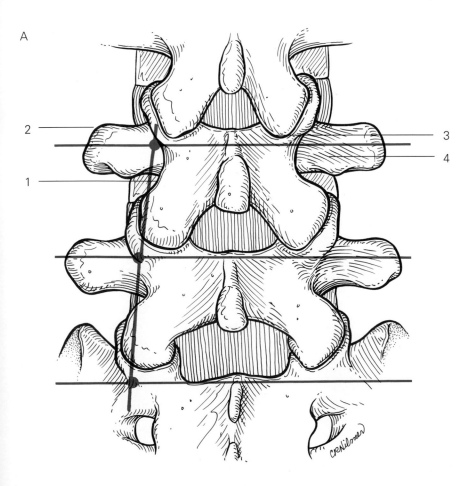

A

Figure 14.2

Pedicle screw instrumentation.

A
The pedicle entrance point is crossed by a vertical line that connects the lateral edges of bony crest, which is the extension of the pars interarticularis, and the horizontal line that bisects the middle of the transverse processes.

1 Pars interarticularis
2 Transverse process
3 Inf. edge of facet joint
4 Lat. edge of inf. articular crest

Contd

Figure 14.2 *(contd)*

B

A small rongeur or burr is used to decorticate the pedicle entrance.

B

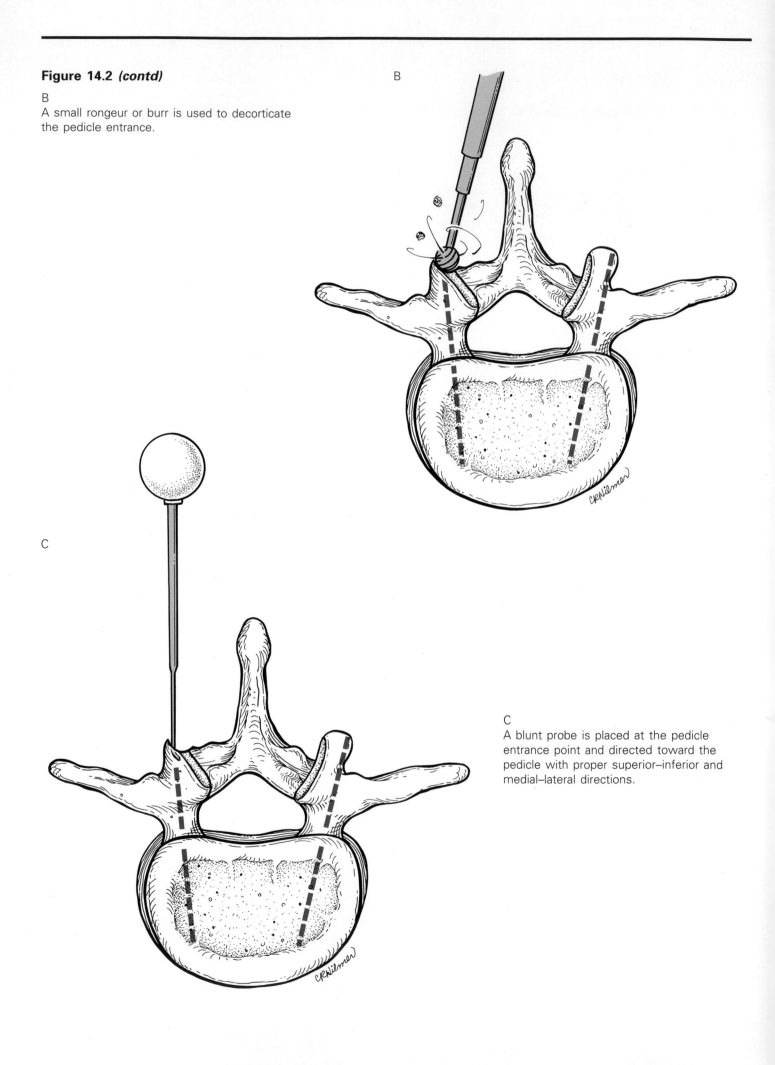

C

A blunt probe is placed at the pedicle entrance point and directed toward the pedicle with proper superior–inferior and medial–lateral directions.

D

D
The blunt instrument is advanced through the
pedicle into the vertebral body.

E

E
A thin probe or depth gauge is used to feel
the walls of the pedicle and measure the
depth of the pedicle.

Contd

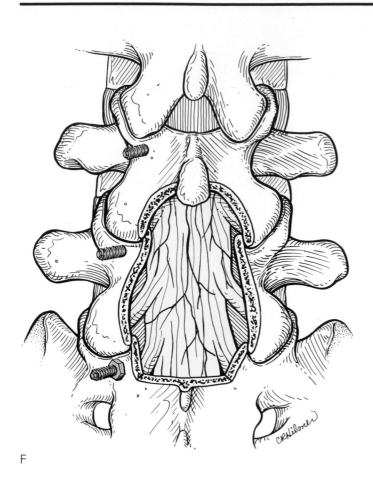

F

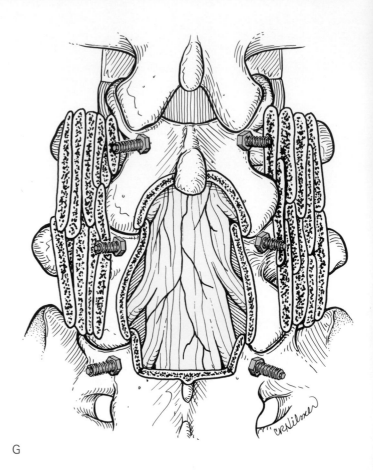

G

Figure 14.2 *(contd)*

F
Pedicle screws are inserted after tapping.

G
After decortication, bone grafts are placed between transverse processes and into the facet joints.

the lateral wall of the facet joint should be meticulously decorticated, and bone grafts are laid (Fig. 14.2G). The rest of the screws are then inserted into the pedicles. It is recommended that the decortication and grafting should be done prior to insertion of the rest of the screws, so that the screws are not in the way of the grafting procedure. The pedicle screw should be directed medially and inserted close to the anterior cortex of the vertebral body, but not penetrating the cortex (Fig 14.2H). The screws should be parallel to the endplates or slightly angled upward to engage the more dense bone adjacent to the endplate (Fig. 14.2I).

Following the insertion of all the screws, either plates or rods are connected to the screws. The plates or rods must be contoured to conform to the lordotic lumbar spine. The rods may be prebent or bent after connecting to the screws with in situ bending devices. Depending on the pathology, the rods can also be used to distract or compress the motion segment. With any techniques, the preservation of lumbar lordosis is important.

H

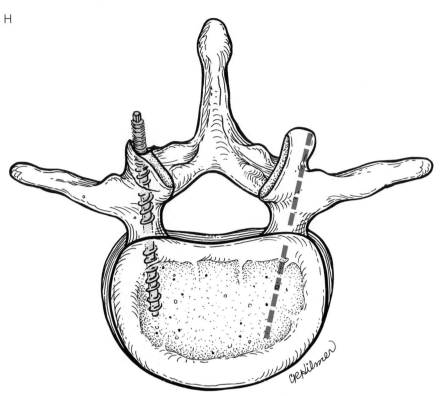

The pedicle screw should be directed medially, and inserted close to the anterior cortex of the vertebral body, but not penetrating the cortex.

I

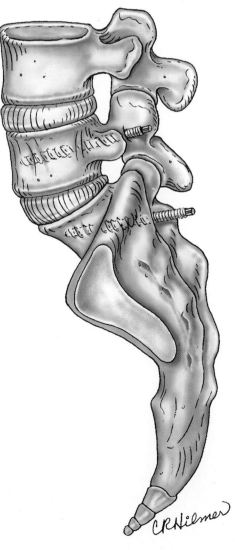

I

The pedicle screws should be parallel to the endplates or slightly angled upward to engage the more dense bone adjacent to the endplate.

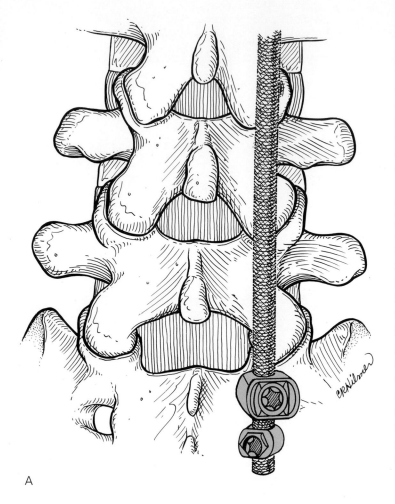

A

Sacral fixation

Posterior exposure of the sacrum is done through a vertical midline incision. One must be careful to avoid dural tear in the midline, particularly in patients with occult spina bifida. Posterior sacral foramina are richly surrounded by venous structures, and can be sources of significant bleeding. The sacrum is most commonly exposed for extension of instrumentation and fusion down to the sacrum.

The most common method of fixation to the sacrum is the S1 screw or ala screw. The entrance point of the sacral screw is at the lower point of the L5–S1 articulation on the elevated ridge of bone. The screw is directed medially about 20° and 10° superiorly toward the sacral promontory. This sacral screw may purchase on the anterior cortex to enhance the fixation. Alternatively, lateral ala screw insertion technique may be utilized. A 2 mm drill bit is inserted into the dimple of S1 and directed 35° laterally and parallel to the sacral endplate. The drill bit will usually rest on the caudal tip of the L5 spinous process. The drill is pushed anteriorly until it abuts the anterior cortex. The drill hole is enlarged with larger drill bits or curets and the sacral screw is inserted without tapping. Purchase on the anterior cortex can be achieved with this screw as well. The 2 mm hole is enlarged to 3.5 mm and the drill bit is advanced just

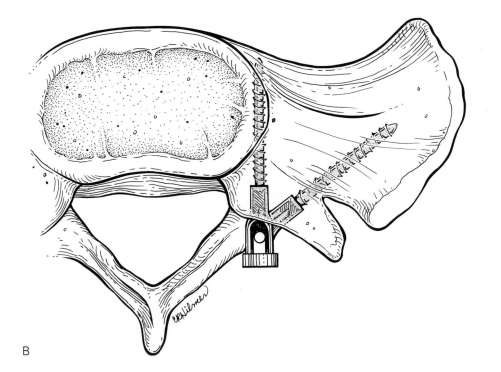

B

Figure 14.3

Sacral screw techniques.

A
The entrance point of the S1 screw is just at the lower point of the L5–S1 articulation on the elevated ridge of bone, and the screw is directly medially toward the sacral promontory. Alternatively, a lateral ala screw can be inserted, starting slightly lower at the dimple of S1, and directed laterally toward the ala. Both medial and lateral screws may be utilized.

B
The S1 medial screw is directed medially about 20° and 10° superiorly toward the sacral promontory, and the lateral ala screw is directed 35° laterally and parallel to the sacral endplate.

through the anterior cortex of the lateral sacral ala. Use a depth gauge to select the correct-length screw; the screw should not project more than 2 mm beyond the anterior cortex of the sacrum. This lateral screw may be inserted slightly inferiorly so that both the medial and the lateral screws may be inserted into the sacrum (Figs. 14.3A, B). Additionally, an S2 screw may be inserted. The S1 and S2 foramina are exposed. Find the point that is two-thirds distal to the inferior edge of the S1 foramina and two-thirds the distance from the true midline to a line that bisects the mid-portion of the S1–S2 foramina. The posterior cortex is opened with a burr, and the screw is directed 40–45° laterally. This screw is pointed toward the anterolateral corner of the S1–S2 ala (Figs. 14.3C, D). The instrumentation system used will also determine the specific technique of sacral screw fixation.

Sacral fixation may be inadequate despite the use of screws, particularly in cases which require longer constructs. Jackson's intrasacral fixation may enhance the stability of sacral fixation by transpedicular endplate screw fixation and intrasacral rod insertion to provide sacroiliac buttressing effect. Additionally, more anterior and distal insertion of the rods reduces the momentum acting on the rods and screws. In situ contouring of the rods is easier because of the greater distance between the L5 and S1 screw heads. Following exposure of the sacrum, a guide pin is

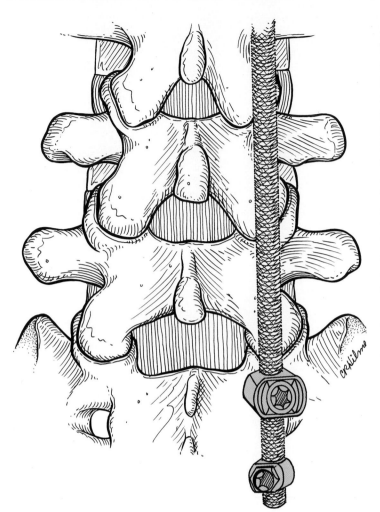

C

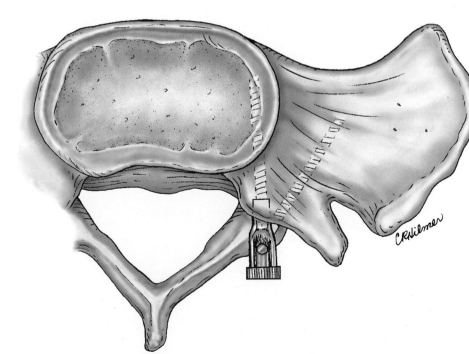

D

C
The entrance point of the S2 screw, about two-thirds distal to the inferior edge of the S1 foramina and directed 40–45° laterally.

D
The S1 screw is directed medially about 20° and the S2 screw is directed 40° toward the anterolateral corner of the S1–S2 ala.

inserted at a point just proximal to the posterior S1 neuroforamen (Fig. 14.4A). It is directed 10° medially and cephalad, so that it penetrates the sacral endplate anteriorly (Figs. 14.4B, C). The screw is inserted so that the screwhead is buried in bone. The bone and part of the L5–S1 facet joint is removed, so that an angled sacral curet can be introduced into the sacrum (Fig. 14.4D). The curet is passed through the oblique canal of the screwhead and directed laterally and distally into the lateral sacral mass, but not across the sacro-iliac joint (Fig. 14.4E). A rod is bent and cut to length and inserted into the lateral sacral mass using a rod gripper (Figs. 14.4F, G). The rods can be further contoured using in situ benders and connected to the lumbar pedicle screws (Fig. 14.4H).

There are other types of sacropelvic fixation, such as iliosacral screws, iliac screws, and Galveston pelvic fixation, and the individual techniques each offer certain advantages and disadvantages. The techniques of sacropelvic fixation are still evolving, and continued research is needed to develop a technique that is biomechanically sound, safe, and easy for the surgeon.

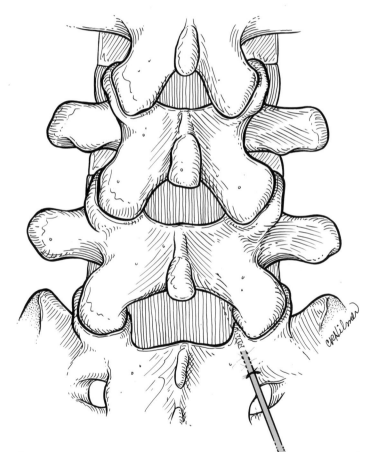

A

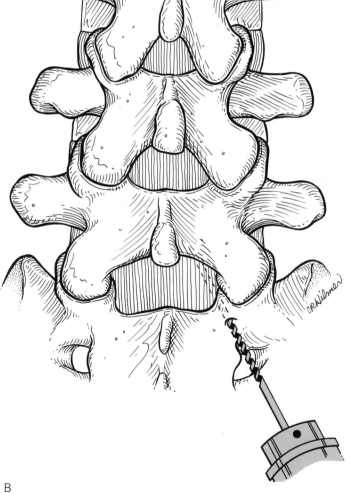

B

Figure 14.4

Jackson's intrasacral rod technique.

A
A guide pin is inserted at a point just proximal to the posterior S1 neuroforamen.

B
The drill is passed with radiographic confirmation.

C

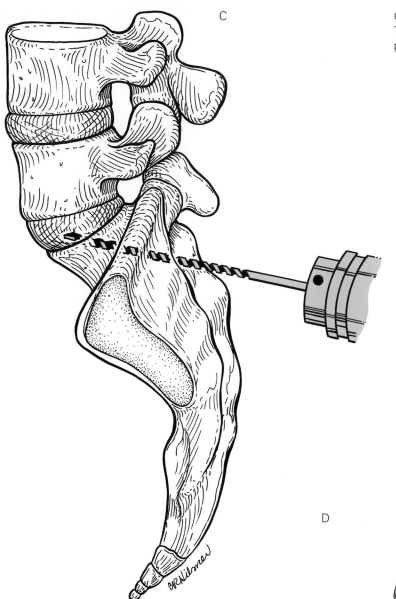

C
The drill is directed 10° medially and cephalad, so that it penetrates the sacral endplate anteriorly.

D

D
The bone and part of the L5–S1 facet joint is removed, so that an angled sacral curet can be introduced into the sacrum.

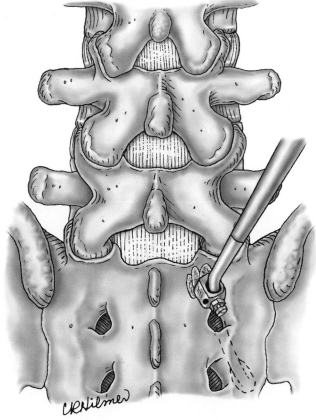

Contd

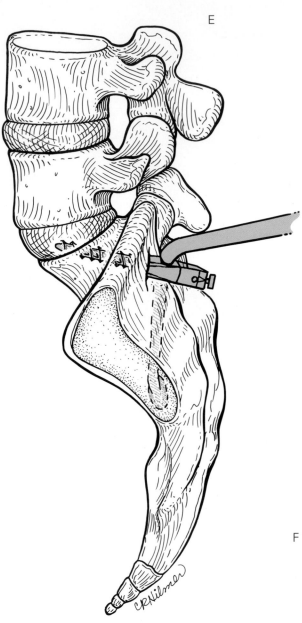

E

Figure 14.4 *(contd)*

E
The curet is passed through the oblique canal of the screwhead and directed laterally and distally into the lateral sacral mass, but not across the sacroiliac joint.

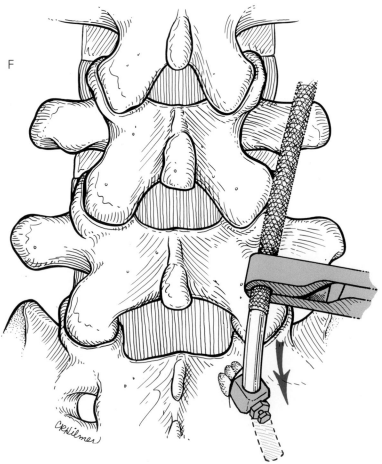

F

F
A rod is bent and cut to length and inserted into the lateral sacral mass using a rod gripper.

G

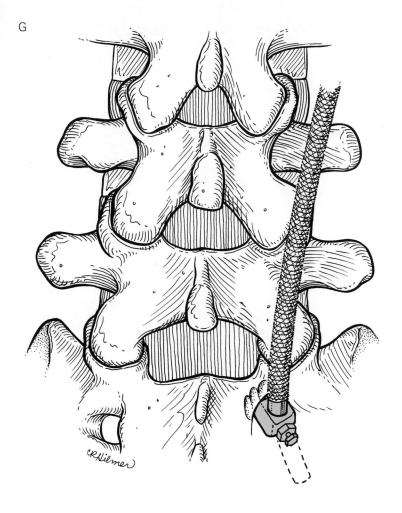

G

The smooth end of the rod is advanced into the sacrum.

H

In situ bending devices may be used to bend the rod into lumbar lordosis.

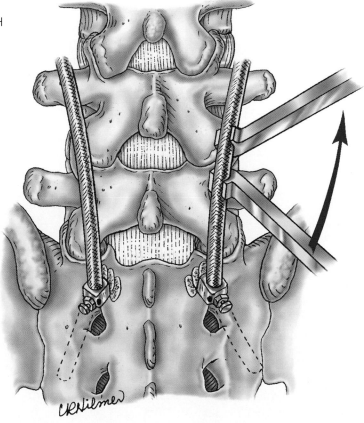

Complications

Nerve root or cauda equina injury is rare during lumbosacral fusion procedures unless laminectomy and foraminotomy are performed at the same time. On the other hand, reduction of spondylolisthesis is associated with a high incidence of neurologic deficits, particularly L5 nerve root injury. Dural tears and cauda equina syndrome are other potential complications. Reduction of spondylolithesis is rarely necessary. Results of in situ fusion for a mild to moderate degree of slippage are satisfactory. Even in patients with a severe degree of slippage, bilateral lateral in situ fusions can be successful if the slip angle is relatively normal. Reduction and stabilization of a severe kyphotic lumbosacral junction is one the most difficult procedures. One should reduce the lumbosacral kyphosis, but resist the temptation to reduce anterior translation completely.

Nerve root injuries may be associated with pedicle screw instrumentation. It is important to identify the pedicle entrance point accurately to avoid neural injury. Plain radiographic confirmation of the pedicle is helpful. Avoid drilling into the pedicle. A blunt probe should be used, so that the dense cortex of the pedicle will prevent penetration outside the pedicle. Use of pedicle screws of the correct diameter and length prevents the contact of the screw with the neural structures. Compression across the instrumented segments should be avoided, as the intervertebral foramen may become smaller and may cause iatrogenic foraminal stenosis. To circumvent this problem, the disc space may be distracted first with a graft or cage, and then a compression force may be applied with the pedicle screw instrumentation. Sacral screws may be inserted without penetrating the anterior cortex in most cases. The lumbosacral plexus and vascular structures are at risk when the anterior cortex of the sacrum is perforated, particularly if the screw is too long.

The incidence of pseudarthrosis has become less with the use of rigid instrumentation such as pedicle screw instrumentation. However, there are many other factors associated with the development of pseudarthrosis. Patients who smoke cigarettes are at increased risk for the development of pseudarthrosis. Patients with previous failed fusion, grade III or IV spondylolisthesis, or multiple-level involvement may have poor outcomes. The key to prevention of pseudarthrosis is meticulous surgical technique and bone grafting.

Anterior interbody fusion should also be considered in cases where posterolateral bone grafting alone may not be adequate. Those with a high grade slip angle and translation should be considered for anterior interbody fusion or posterior lumbar interbody fusion. Loss of correction and instrument problems may be related to the development of pseudarthrosis, but may also occur independently. There seems to be a high incidence of hook dislodgement and instrument failure when a distraction instrumentation is used in the lumbosacral junction. The pedicle screw instrumentation is more rigid, and provides a greater stability. However, screw breakage and loss of correction are also reported even after pedicle screw instrumentation.

Conclusions

In summary, posterior lumbar instrumentation systems are invaluable in providing reduction and stabilization for deformity and trauma cases. The instrumentations may also be used to enhance fusion rates in selected cases. The choice of instrumentation depends on the patient's pathology and the surgeon's experience. The techniques of various instrumentations are important to master, but the basic techniques of fusion and bone grafting should not be compromised.

Bibliography

An HS (1992) Surgical exposure and fusion techniques of the spine. In HS An, JM Cotler (eds), *Spinal Instrumentation*. Baltimore: Williams & Wilkins

An HS, Balderston RA (1991) Complications of scoliosis, kyphosis and spondylolisthesis surgery. In RA Balderston, HS An (eds), *Complications in Spine Surgery*. Philadelphia: W.B. Saunders

An HS, Lynch K, Toth J (1995) Comparison between allograft and autograft in adult posterolateral lumbar spine fusion. *J Spin Dis* **8**:131–5

Carlson GD, Abitbol JJ, Anderson DR et al (1992) Screw fixation in the human sacrum. *Spine* **17**:S196–203

Farcy JPC, Rawlings BA, Glasman SD (1992) Technique and results of fixation to the sacrum with iliosacral screws. *Spine* **17**:S190–5

Jackson RP (1994) Jackson intrasacral fixation and segmental corrections with adjustable contoured translating axes. *Spine: State Art Rev* **8**:307–41

Jacobs RR, Montesano PX, Jackson RP (1989) Enhancement of lumbar spine fusion by use of translaminar facet joint screw. *Spine* **14**:12–15

Magerl FP (1984) Stabilization of the lower thoracic and lumbar spine with external skeletal fixation. *Clin Orthop* **189**:125–41

Steffee AD, Brantigan JW (1993) The variable screw placement spinal fixation system. *Spine* **18**:1160–72

15

Anterior exposures and fusion techniques of the lumbar spine

Howard S An
Lee H Riley III

Introduction

Anterior approaches to the thoracolumbar junction and lumbar spine are well described in the literature. The thoracolumbar junction is best exposed by the extensile thoracoabdominal approach, and the lumbar spine is usually exposed by retroperitoneal approaches (Fig. 15.1). The thoracolumbar junction and the upper lumbar spine are typically approached from the left in the lateral decubitus position, and the lower lumbar spine and lumbosacral junction can be exposed either from the left in the lateral position or anteriorly in the supine position. The transperitoneal approach can also be utilized for the extensile exposure of the lumbo-sacral junction. There are a variety of anterior fusion techniques for the lumbar spine. Attention to details in the exposures and fusion techniques will prevent the majority of complications associated with anterior approaches of the thoracolumbar spine.

Indications for anterior approaches

1. Burst fractures with canal compromise and neurologic deficits
2. Anterior discectomy and fusion for deformities
3. Anterior discectomy and fusion for degenerative disc disease
4. Corpectomy for tumors and infections.

Thoracoabdominal approach to T10–L3

The patient is placed in a lateral decubitus position with the left side up. The left-sided approach is preferred to avoid the liver and vena cava on the right side. A skin incision is made over the 10th rib from the lateral border of the paraspinous musculature to the costal cartilage. The incision is curved anteriorly to the edge of the rectus sheath (Fig. 15.2A). The dissection is extended down to the muscle layers to the periosteum of the 10th rib (Fig. 15.2B). The key is to access the retroperitoneal space by splitting the costal cartilage after removal of the 10th rib (Fig. 15.2C). The removal of the rib is done by cutting the rib at the angle of the rib and at the junction of the rib and costal cartilage. The neurovascular bundle on the inferior surface of the rib should be protected. After removing the rib, the pleura is incised and the lung is retracted. The costal cartilage is then split along its length. Under the retracted split tips of costal cartilage, the retroperitoneal space is identified by the light areolar tissue. Blunt dissection is performed to mobilize the peritoneum from the undersurface of the diaphragm and abdominal wall. After the peritoneum is retracted, the external oblique, internal oblique, and transverse abdominis muscles of the abdomen are divided one layer at a time. The next step entails circumferential incision in the muscular portion of the diaphragm adjacent to the costal margin. The diaphragm is incised circumferentially 1 inch (2.5 cm) from its peripheral attachment to the chest wall (Fig. 15.2D). Marker stitches or clips are placed for resuturing the

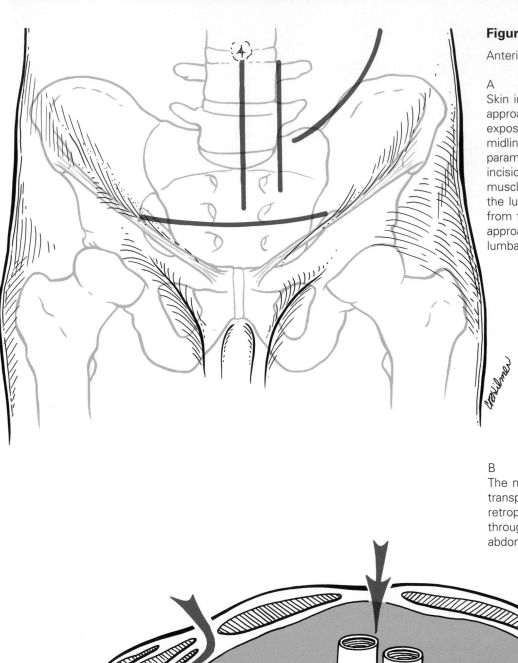

Figure 15.1

Anterior approaches to the lumbar spine.

A
Skin incisions for the lumbar spine approaches. The lumbar spine may be exposed through transperitoneal vertical midline or transverse incisions. The paramedian approach utilizes the skin incision along the rectus abdominis muscle and retroperitoneal dissection to the lumbar spine. The curvilinear incision from the left is for the retroperitoneal approaches to the lateral aspect of the lumbar spine.

B
The midline arrow indicates the transperitoneal approach, and the retroperitoneal approaches can be made through the paramedian or through the abdominal muscles.

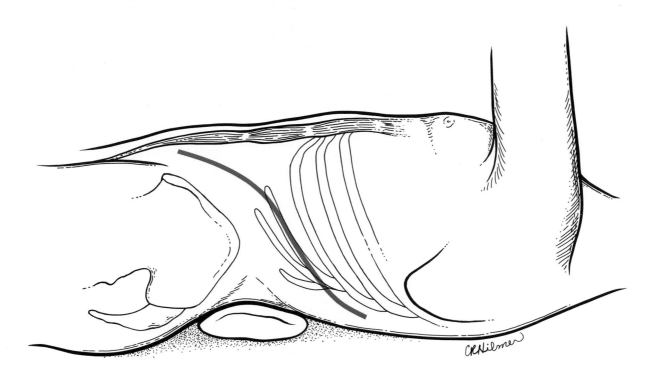

Figure 15.2

Thoracoabdominal approach to T10–L3.

A
A skin incision is made over the 10th rib from the lateral border of the paraspinous musculature to the costal cartilage. The incision is curved anteriorly to the edge of the rectus sheath.

B
The dissection is extended down to the muscle layers to the periosteum of the 10th rib.

1 Lattissimus dorsi m.
2 Serratus anterior m.
3 External oblique m.
4 Sheath of rectus abdominis m.
5 10th rib

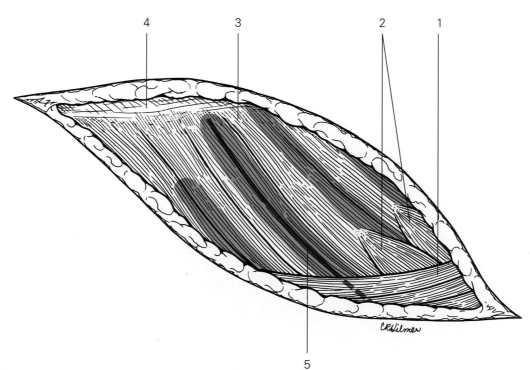

Contd

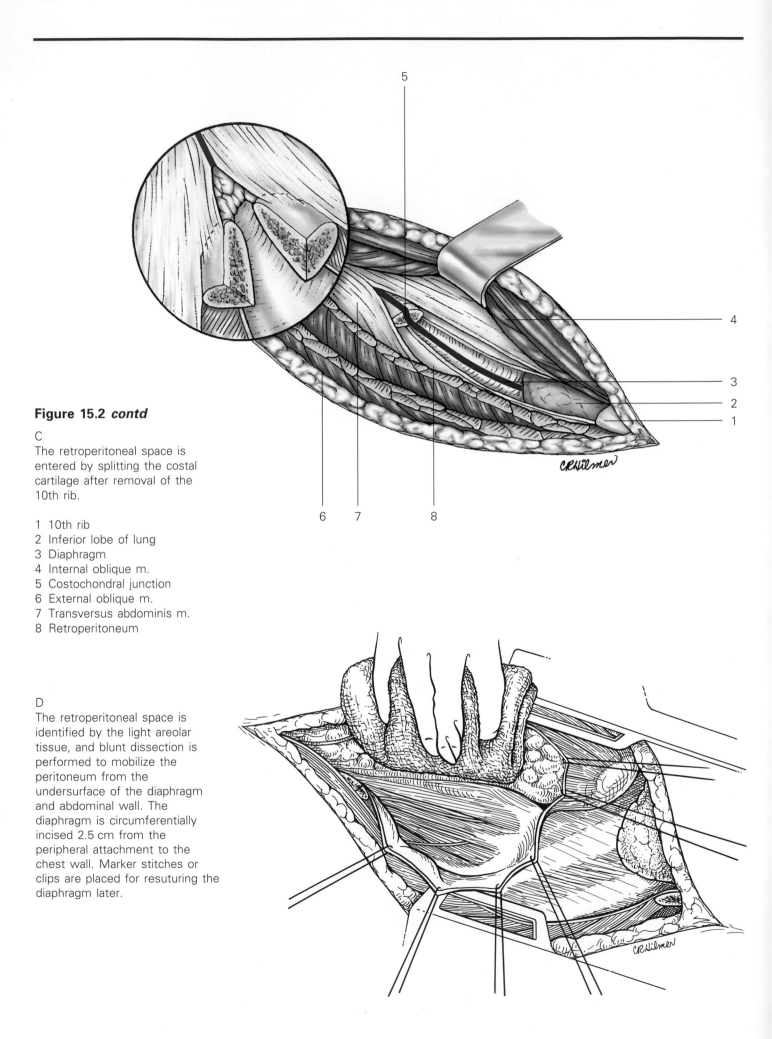

Figure 15.2 *contd*

C
The retroperitoneal space is entered by splitting the costal cartilage after removal of the 10th rib.

1 10th rib
2 Inferior lobe of lung
3 Diaphragm
4 Internal oblique m.
5 Costochondral junction
6 External oblique m.
7 Transversus abdominis m.
8 Retroperitoneum

D
The retroperitoneal space is identified by the light areolar tissue, and blunt dissection is performed to mobilize the peritoneum from the undersurface of the diaphragm and abdominal wall. The diaphragm is circumferentially incised 2.5 cm from the peripheral attachment to the chest wall. Marker stitches or clips are placed for resuturing the diaphragm later.

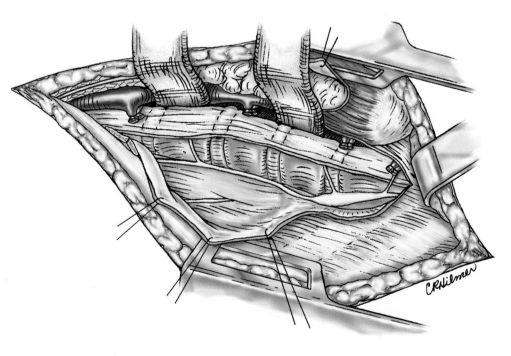

E
The aorta is mobilized by
ligating segmental vessels
as necessary.

1 Diaphragm
2 Ureter
3 Segmental vessels

F
The spine is exposed to the
opposite cortex by mobilizing
vessels and placing malleable
retractors.

diaphragm later. For the exposure of the T12–L1 region,
the crus of the diaphragm is cut and mobilized. The
segmental vessels are tied and ligated as necessary to
mobilize the aorta (Fig. 15.2E). Malleable retractors are
positioned to expose the thoracolumbar junction (Fig.
15.2F).

For the exposure of the thoracolumbar junction,
either an 11th rib or a 12th rib approach may be
utilized while remaining in the extrapleural and
retroperitoneal spaces. These exposures entail splitting
the tip of the costal cartilage, and the parietal pleura
is carefully mobilized from the undersurface of the rib
bed. The peritoneum is mobilized anteriorly, and the
retroperitoneal space is bluntly dissected toward the
spine. These approaches give less extensile exposure
of the thoracolumbar junction as compared with the
thoracoabdominal approach, but in them the dissection does not involve the pleural cavity.

Retroperitoneal flank approaches to L2–L5

In the lower lumbar region, a standard retroperitoneal flank approach is used (Fig. 15.3A). The level of the incision varies according to the level of the spine approached. The patient is placed in the right lateral decubitus position with the left side up. The retroperitoneal exposure utilizes the division of the abdominal muscles and blunt dissection through the retroperitoneal space toward the psoas muscles and the spine. The skin incision extends from the midaxillary line to the edge of the rectus sheath (Fig. 15.3B). Dissection is through the external oblique, internal oblique, and transversus abdominis muscles (Fig. 15.3C–D). The retroperitoneal space is entered laterally by identifying the retroperitoneal fat, taking care to avoid penetration of the peritoneum just lateral to the rectus sheath. Blunt finger dissection anterior to the psoas muscle should lead to the spine. One should identify the genitofemoral nerve on the anterior surface of the psoas muscle, and the sympathetic chains medial to the muscle (Fig. 15.3E). Extreme caution must be used to avoid injuries to the ureter, which can be identified medially along the undersurface of the peritoneum, and the pulsating aorta, which is easily palpated (Fig. 15.3F). The aorta is mobilized and a retractor is positioned around the vertebral body (Fig. 15.3G). The segmental vessels are ligated to expose the valleys of the vertebral bodies. At the L4–L5 region, the iliolumbar vein should be identified and ligated to mobilize the great vessels. For the approach to L5–S1, the midline within the vascular bifurcation should be palpated by passing the finger over the left common iliac artery. The left common iliac vein is retracted to the left and cephalad, while the middle sacral vein and the superior hypogastric plexus are retracted to the right bluntly.

Figure 15.3

Retroperitoneal flank approach to L2–L5.

A

The level of the incision varies according to the level of the spine approached. The patient is placed in the right lateral decubitus position with the left side up.

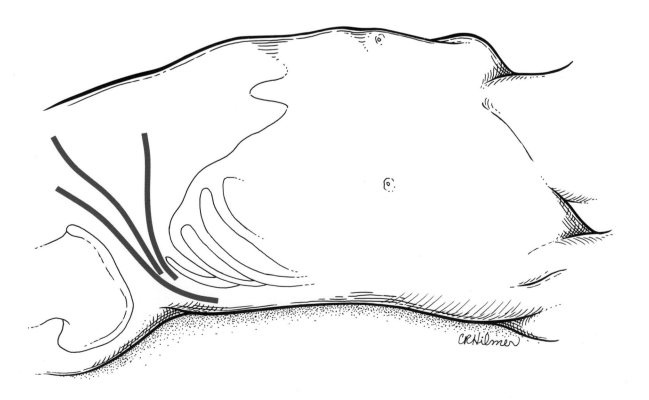

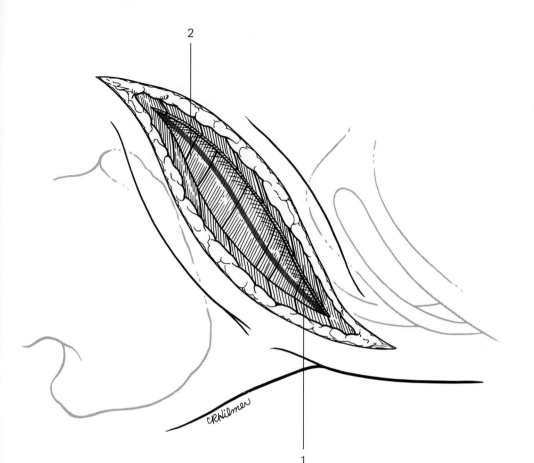

B
The skin incision extends from the midaxillary line to the edge of the rectus sheath. Dissection is through the external oblique, internal oblique and transversus abdominis muscles.

1 External oblique m.
2 Internal oblique m.

C
The transversus abdominis muscle fascia is thin and very close to the peritoneum.

1 Transversus abdominis m.
2 Transversalis fascia
3 Internal oblique m.
4 External oblique m.

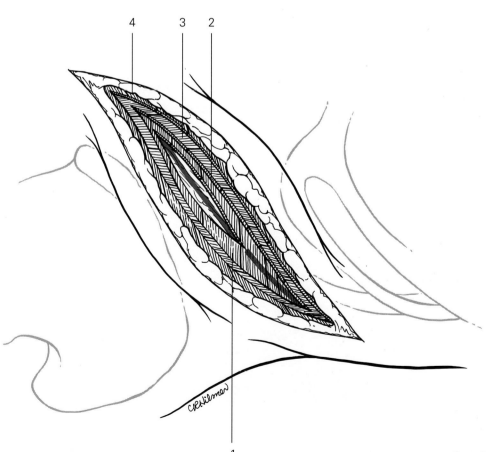

Contd

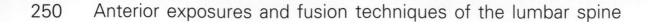

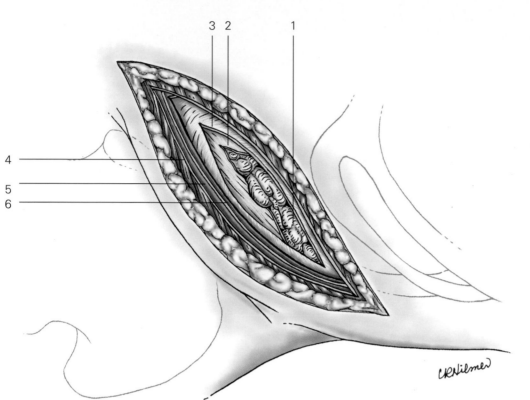

Figure 15.3 *contd*

D

The retroperitoneal space is entered laterally by identifying the retroperitoneal fat, taking care to avoid penetration of the peritoneum just lateral to the rectus sheath.

1 Retroperitoneal fat
2 Peritoneum
3 Transversalis fascia
4 External oblique m.
5 Internal oblique m.
6 Transversus abdominis m.

E
Blunt finger dissection anterior to the psoas muscle and reflection of the peritoneum anteriorly should expose the spine. One should identify the genitofemoral nerve on the anterior surface of the psoas muscle, and the ureter along the undersurface of the peritoneum.

1 Left ureter
2 Fascia over psoas major m.
3 Retroperitoneal fat
4 External oblique m.
5 Internal oblique m.
6 Transversus abdominis m.
7 Genitofemoral n.

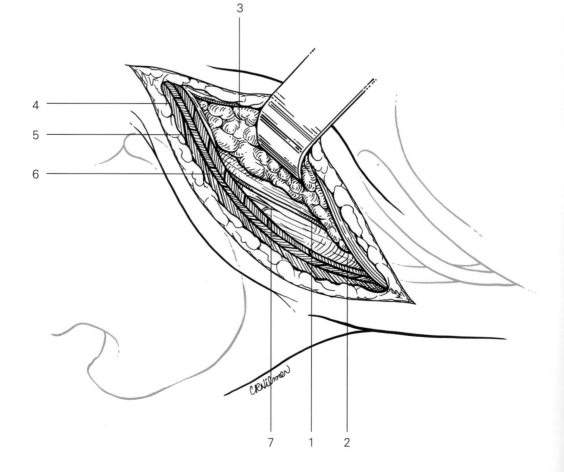

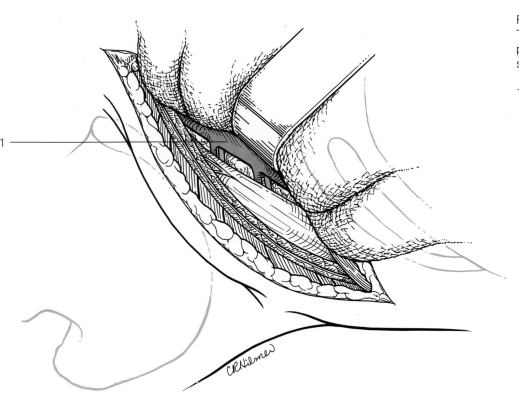

F
The pulsating aorta is easily palpated and mobilized by ligating segmental vessels.

1 Aorta

1

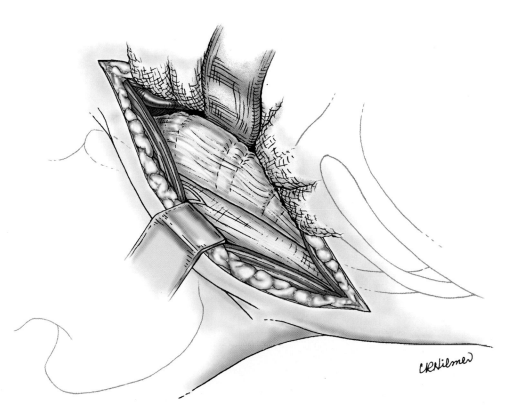

G
Malleable retractors are positioned around the vertebral body.

Paramedian retroperitoneal approach to L3–S1

This approach is made in the supine position. The anterior exposure of the lower lumbar vertebrae and the sacrum is better with this technique. The lateral edge of the rectus abdominis muscle is palpated, and a vertical incision is made (Fig. 15.4A). The length of the incision depends on the number of vertebrae that need to be exposed. The dissection is made to the level of abdominal fascia. The lateral border of the rectus abdominis muscle is palpated, and an incision is made in the anterior rectus sheath along the lateral edge of the muscle (Fig. 15.4B). The fibers of the rectus muscle are retracted medially to expose the posterior rectus sheath and the arcuate line (Fig. 15.4C). The inferior aspect of exposure should not go beyond to the level of inferior epigastric vessels (Fig. 15.4D). Great caution is taken to preserve these vessels and to preserve any innervation to the rectus abdominis muscle. The arcuate line divides the posterior rectus fascia proximally and the transversalis fascia distally. The preperitoneal space can then be entered and blunt dissection leads to the retroperitoneal space and the anterior aspect of the spine. The peritoneum is mobilized medially, and the dissection is carried down to the iliac vessels. Identify the psoas muscle, aorta, iliac artery and vein, genitofemoral nerve, ureter, and sympathetic chain and the superior hypogastric plexus (Fig. 15.4E). For the exposure of L3–L5, the psoas muscle is mobilized laterally off the vertebral bodies, and the left segmental vessels are identified and ligated, and the aorta and iliac vessels are mobilized medially (Fig. 15.4F–G). The iliolumbar vein should be ligated for the exposure of L4–L5. For the exposure of L5–S1, the aortic bifurcation at the L4–L5 is further dissected and the vessels are retracted laterally to enter the L5–S1 disc (Fig. 15.4H).

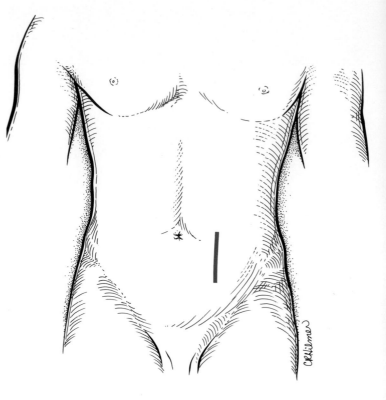

Figure 15.4

Paramedian retroperitoneal approach to L3–S1.

A

The lateral edge of the rectus abdominis muscle is palpated, and a vertical incision is made.

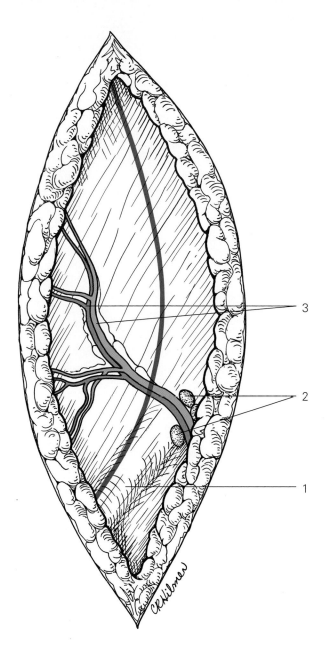

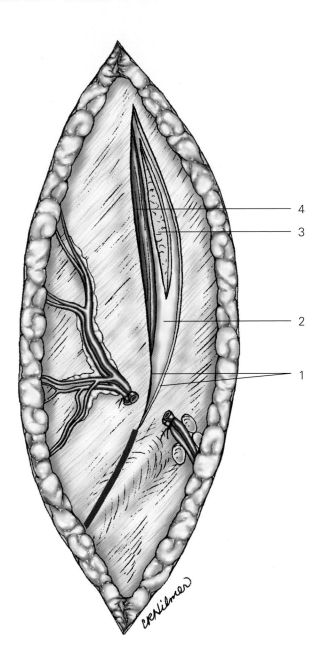

B
An incision is made in the anterior rectus sheath along the lateral edge of the muscle. Superficial epigastric vessels may be ligated as necessary.

1 External spermatic fascia
2 Superficial inguinal lymph nodes
3 Superficial epigastric vessels

C
The fibers of the rectus muscle are retracted medially to expose the posterior rectus sheath. The posterior rectus sheath is very close to the peritoneum.

1 Superficial rectus sheath
2 Deep rectus sheath
3 Peritoneum
4 Rectus abdominis m.   *Contd*

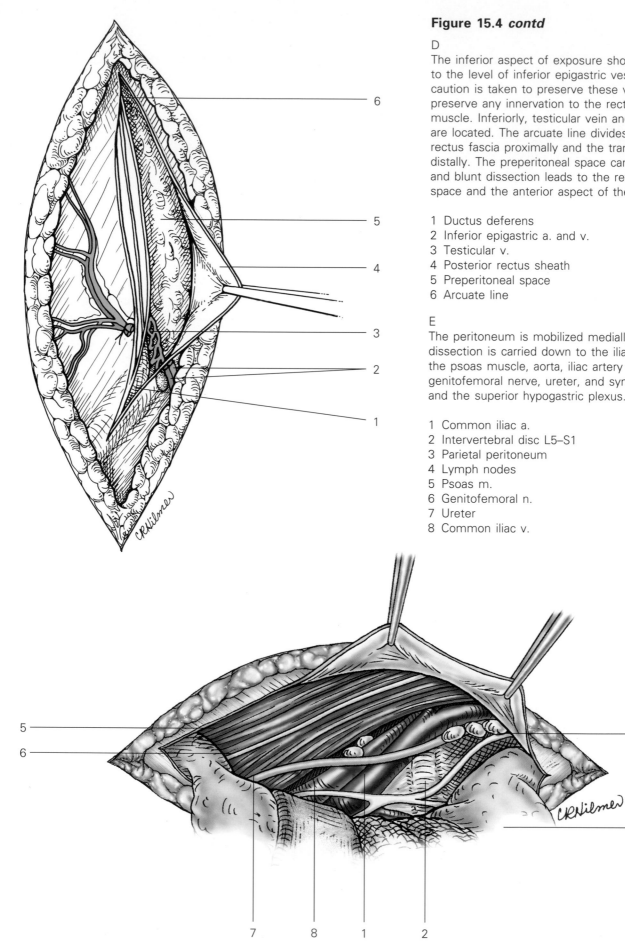

Figure 15.4 *contd*

D

The inferior aspect of exposure should not go beyond to the level of inferior epigastric vessels. Great caution is taken to preserve these vessels and to preserve any innervation to the rectus abdominis muscle. Inferiorly, testicular vein and ductus deferens are located. The arcuate line divides the posterior rectus fascia proximally and the transversalis fascia distally. The preperitoneal space can then be entered and blunt dissection leads to the retroperitoneal space and the anterior aspect of the spine.

1 Ductus deferens
2 Inferior epigastric a. and v.
3 Testicular v.
4 Posterior rectus sheath
5 Preperitoneal space
6 Arcuate line

E

The peritoneum is mobilized medially, and the dissection is carried down to the iliac vessels. Identify the psoas muscle, aorta, iliac artery and vein, genitofemoral nerve, ureter, and sympathetic chain and the superior hypogastric plexus.

1 Common iliac a.
2 Intervertebral disc L5–S1
3 Parietal peritoneum
4 Lymph nodes
5 Psoas m.
6 Genitofemoral n.
7 Ureter
8 Common iliac v.

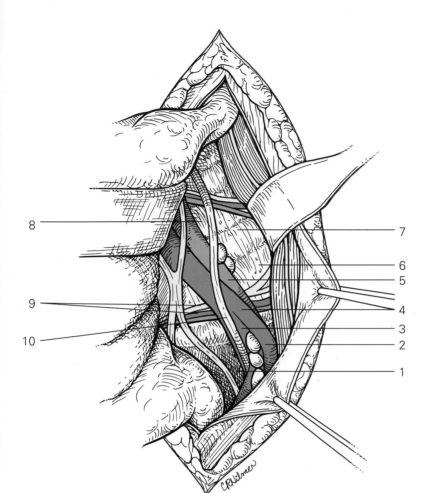

F–G
For the exposure of L3–L5, the psoas muscle is mobilized laterally off the vertebral bodies, and the left segmental vessels are identified and ligated, and the aorta and iliac vessels are mobilized medially.

F
1 Promontory
2 External iliac a.
3 Internal iliac a.
4 Left common iliac a.
5 Right common iliac v.
6 L5
7 L4, L5 disc
8 L4
9 Intercostal a. and v.
10 Ureter

G
1 Internal iliac a.
2 External iliac a.
3 Left common iliac a.
4 L5
5 L4
6 L4, L5 disc
7 Intercostal a. and v.
8 Ureter
9 Promontory of sacrum

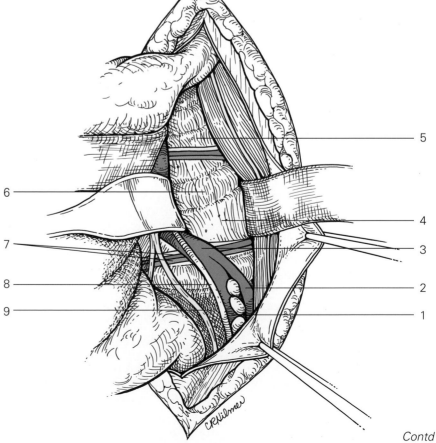

Contd

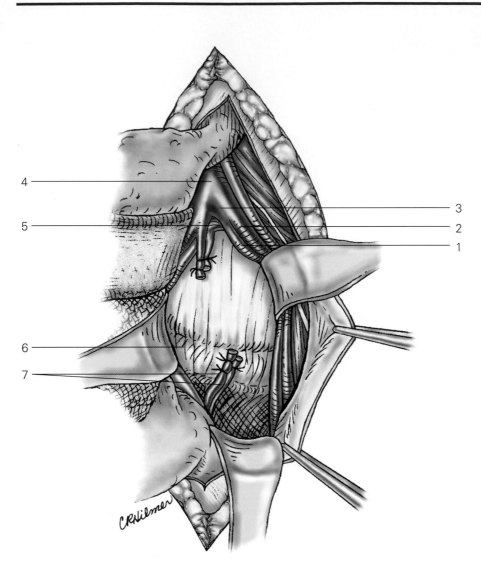

Figure 15.4 *contd*

H
For the exposure of L5–S1, the aortic bifurcation at L4–L5 is further dissected and the vessels are retracted laterally to enter the L5–S1 disc.

1 Internal iliac a.
2 External iliac a.
3 Left common iliac a.
4 Aorta
5 Right common iliac v.
6 L5–S1 disc
7 Middle sacral a. and v.

Transperitoneal approach to the lumbosacral spine

A transperitoneal approach through a vertical or transverse incision in the lower abdomen provides an excellent exposure to the lumbosacral junction (Fig. 15.5A). The patient is in the supine position with the lumbosacral spine hyperextended. The transverse incision requires transection of the rectus abdominis muscle, and the vertical incision splits the rectus abdominis muscle in the midline linea alba (Fig. 15.5B). Following division of the anterior rectus sheath, the conjoined fascia of the posterior rectus sheath and abdominal fascia is opened to the peritoneum (Fig. 15.5C). The perineum is carefully divided, and the bowel contents are mobilized away from the aorta and iliac vessels (Fig. 15.5D). The aortic bifurcation is palpated at the L4–L5 region (Fig. 15.5E). Saline infiltration of the tissue over the anterior surface of the sacral promontory may be done to elevate the posterior peritoneum off the vascular structures. The posterior peritoneum is opened and the L5–S1 disc identified. The sacral artery runs down along the anterior aspect of the sacrum and may be ligated for distal exposure. Great caution should be taken to protect the left iliac vein in the aortic bifurcation and to preserve the superior hypogastric plexus, which is important to sexual function. Electrocautery must be avoided to prevent damage to the hypogastric plexus. The left common iliac artery and left common iliac vein are retracted to the left, and the hypogastric plexus and right iliac vessels are retracted to the right. Retractors or Steinman pins can be used to expose the L5–S1 region (Fig. 15.5F). Exposure can be extended to the L4–L5 region by mobilizing the great vessels to the right after ligating the L4–5 vessels, including the iliolumbar vein. Take care not to injure the left ureter, which crosses the left common iliac vessels over the sacroiliac joint.

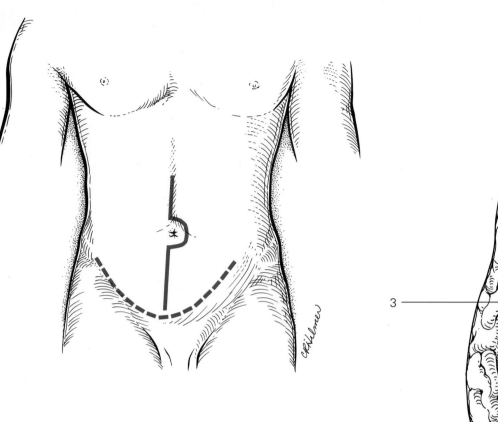

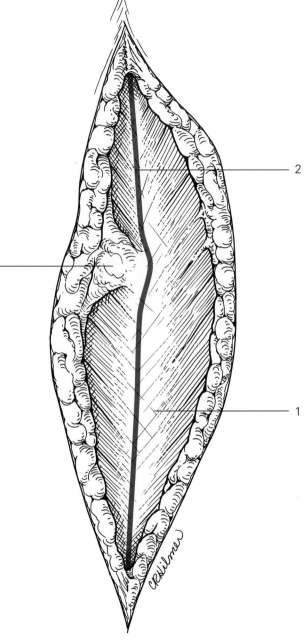

Figure 15.5

Transperitoneal approach to L4–S1.

A

A transperitoneal approach can be made through a vertical or transverse incision in the lower abdomen.

B
The vertical incision splits the rectus abdominis muscle in the midline linea alba.

1 Rectus abdominis m.
2 Linea alba
3 Umbilicus

Contd

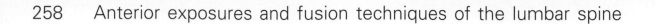

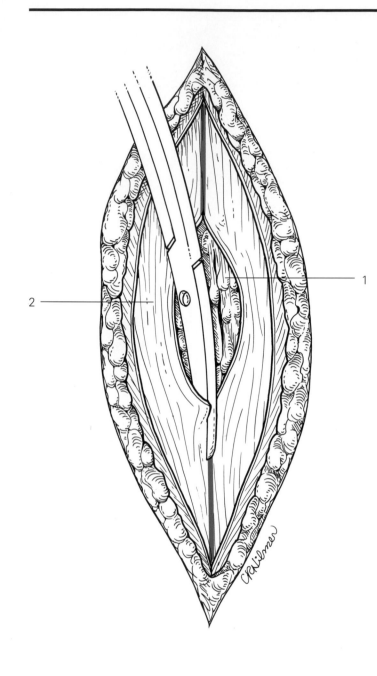

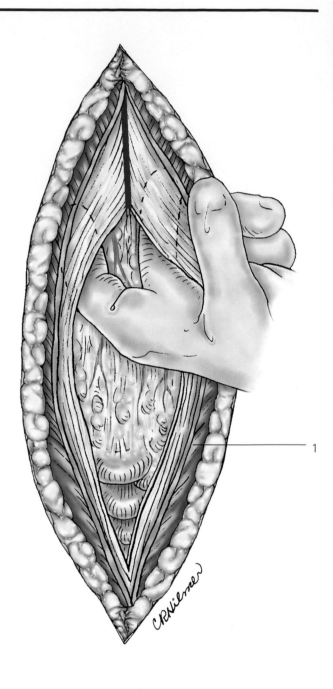

Figure 15.5 *contd*

C
Following division of the anterior rectus sheath, the conjoined fascia of the posterior rectus sheath and abdominal fascia is opened to the peritoneum.

1 Omentum
2 Parietal peritoneum

D
The perineum is carefully divided, and the bowel contents are mobilized away from the aorta and iliac vessels.

1 Rectus abdominis m.

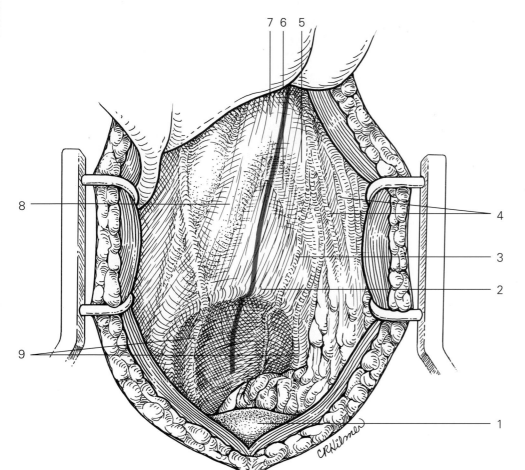

E
The aortic bifurcation is palpated at the L4–L5 region and the sacral promontory is easily palpated. The posterior peritoneum is opened and the L5–S1 disc identified.

1 Bladder
2 Sacral promontory
3 Superior rectal a.
4 Sigmoid a.
5 Left common iliac a.
6 Left common iliac v.
7 Aorta
8 Right common iliac a.
9 Ureter

F
The sacral artery runs down along the anterior aspect of the sacrum and may be ligated for distal exposure. The iliac vessels are mobilized and retracted for L5–S1 exposure.

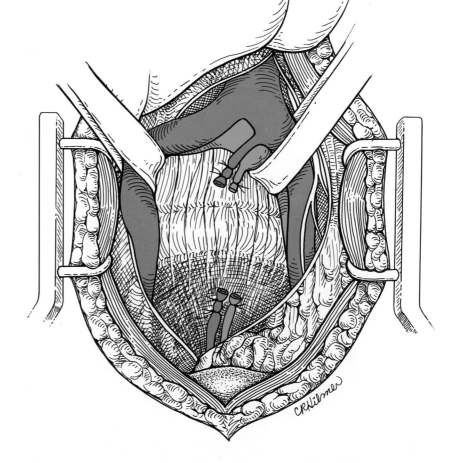

Lumbar fusion techniques

Following corpectomy, the vertebral body must be reconstructed with a tricortical iliac crest bone graft or other graft materials that provide good axial stability and bone healing. If the bone graft is used alone without a fixation device, it is recommended that the graft is well countersunk from the upper endplate above and lower endplate below (Fig. 15.6A–C). If a fixation device is used anteriorly, the graft should extend from the lower endplate above and upper endplate below, and screws are inserted into the vertebral bodies (Fig 15.6D). Prior to inserting the graft, the operating room table should be flexed at the level that corresponds to the corpectomy site. This technique provides more space for the graft to be inserted, and the table should be flexed back to the neutral position to lock the graft in the interspace.

The techniques of anterior interbody fusion in the lower lumbar spine vary widely among different authors. Nonetheless, the technique should consist of meticulous excision of the entire disc material, preparation of the endplates to provide stability and vascularity, and insertion of biomechanically sound bone graft or spacer (Fig. 15.6E). The graft or spacer should be biologically compatible to provide fusion of the construct.

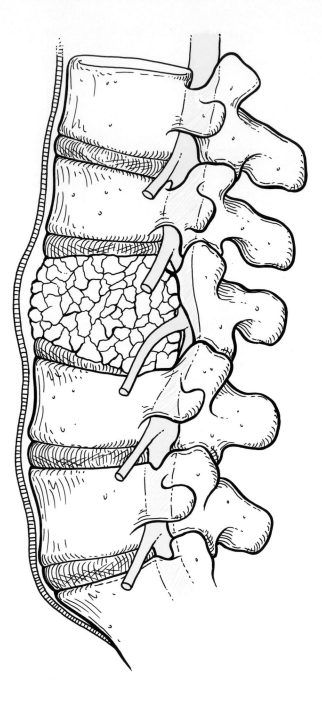

Figure 15.6

Anterior fusion techniques of the lumbar spine.

A
A schematic illustration of burst fracture of the lumbar spine with canal compromise.

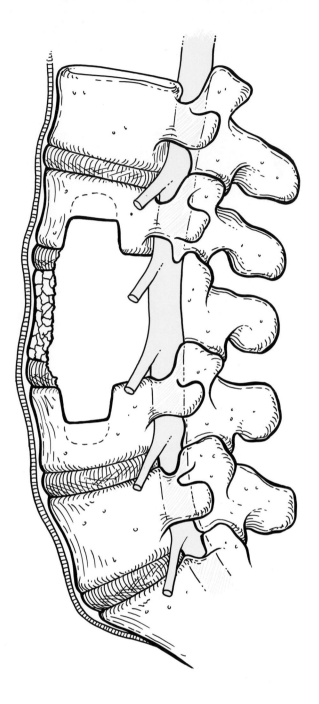

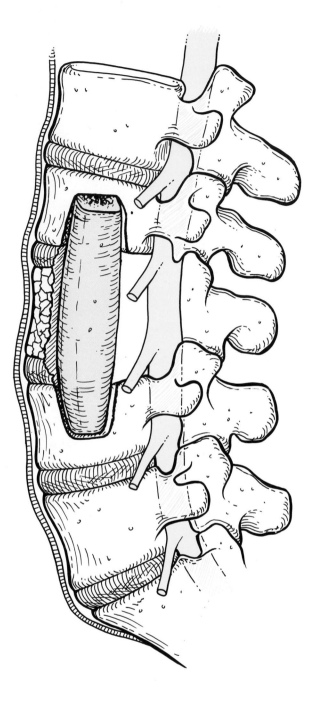

B
Corpectomy is performed to the level of the dura for adequate decompression of the thecal sac.

C
A tricortical iliac crest bone graft is utilized to provide structural support. The graft is well countersunk from the upper endplate above and lower endplate below.

Contd

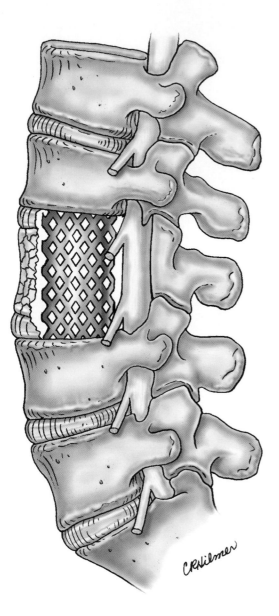

Figure 15.6 *contd*

D
Harm's cage is shown, which extends from the lower endplate above and upper endplate below, and screws are inserted into the vertebral bodies for plating or rodding.

E
Interbody fusion in the lower lumbar spine involves meticulous excision of the entire disc material, preparation of the endplates to provide stability and vascularity, and insertion of biomechanically sound bone graft. The graft should be biologically compatible to provide fusion of the construct. A femoral ring allograft with cancellous autograft in the middle of the ring can be used as shown.

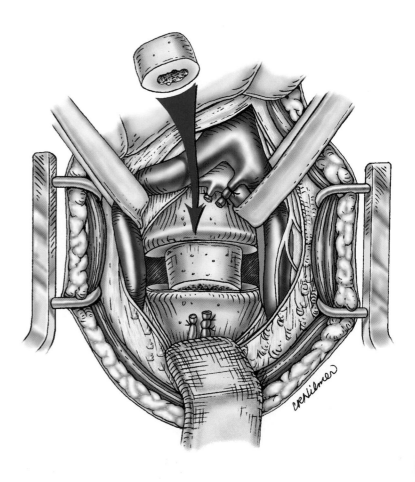

Complications

Potential complications during anterior dissection along the lower lumbar spine and sacrum include hemorrhage from great vessel injury, retrograde ejaculation and sterility from superior hypogastric sympathetic plexus injury, sympathectomy effect, ureteral injury, spleen injury, chylous leakage, and bowel injury. Injuries to the neural structure are possible during discectomy or corpectomy procedures. Bone graft collapse or pseudarthrosis is relatively common, and the techniques of fusion should be exacting to minimize these late complications. The closure of the abdominal muscles should be tight to prevent postoperative hernia or weakening of the abdominal wall. Excessive retraction or denervation of the rectus abdominis muscle may result in weakening or protuberance of the abdominal wall, particularly following the paramedian retroperitoneal approach.

Bibliography

Barber B (1987) Anterior lumbar interbody fusion: step-by-step procedures and pitfalls. In AH White, RH Rothman, CD Ray (eds) *Lumbar spine surgery*, pp. 368–82. St Louis: Mosby

Cotler HB, Cotler JM, Stoloff A, et al (1985) The use of autograft for vertebral body replacement of the thoracic and lumbar spine. *Spine*, **10**:748–56

Crock HV (1982) Anterior lumbar interbody fusion: indications for its use and notes on surgical technique. *Clin Orthop*, **165**:157

Freebody D, Bendall R, Taylor RD (1971) Anterior transperitoneal lumbar fusion. *J Bone Joint Surg*, **53B**:617–27

Harmon PH (1963) Anterior extraperitoneal lumbar disc excision and vertebral bone fusion. *Clin Orthop*, **16**:169–98

Hodgson AR, Stock FE (1957) Anterior spinal fusion. *Br J Surg*, **44**:266

Hodgson AR, Stock FE, Fang HSY, et al (1960) Anterior spinal fusion: the operative approach and pathologic findings in 412 patients with Pott's disease of the spine. *Br J Surg*, **48**:172–78

16

Anterior thoracolumbar instrumentations

Howard S An

Alexander J Ghanayem

Thomas A Zdeblick

Kiyoshi Kaneda

Introduction

Anterior instrumentation for the thoracolumbar and lumbar spine to reduce a scoliotic curve using vertebral body screws and a cable was pioneered by Dwyer (1969). This interest in anterior instrumentation devices for the correction and stabilization of scoliosis was further developed by the work of Hall and Zielke (Zielke 1982). At the present time, there are numerous anterior instrumentation systems available to correct scoliotic deformities, such as anterior TSRH (Danek Inc., Memphis, Tennessee), anterior ISOLA (Acromed, Inc., Cleveland, Ohio), anterior Moss–Miami (Depuy–Motech Inc., Warsaw, Indiana), Kaneda rods (Acromed Inc., Cleveland, Ohio), etc. Anterior instrumentations have also been utilized to decompress the spinal canal for trauma and tumor cases. In order to restore the stability of the spinal column, an anterior strut graft is placed anteriorly along with an anterior instrumentation system. Anterior instrumentation after anterior decompression has been advocated as a single-stage procedure to reduce the morbidity of a two-stage procedure. An anterior device designed by Dunn (1984) had excellent initial results in both the reduction and fixation of thoracolumbar burst fractures. Vascular complications, however, led to the discontinuation of the device. The Kostuik–Harrington device (Kostuik 1983) was then developed for anterior stabilization following decompression and strut grafting. Other devices included low-profile plate systems such as the Armstrong contoured anterior plate or Syracuse I-Plate. These devices did not provide sufficient rigidity of the construct, particularly in axial rotation. Modern instrumentations such as the Texas-Scottish-Rite Hospital (TSRH) screw and rod system (Danek Inc., Memphis, Tennessee), Kaneda rod system (Acromed Inc., Cleveland, Ohio), Z-Plate (Danek Inc., Memphis, Tennessee), Synthes Thoracolumbar Locking Plate anterior plate (Synthes Inc., Paoli, Pennsylvania) and University Plate (Acromed Inc., Cleveland, Ohio) give improved biomechanical characteristics and thus are more commonly used. Kaneda (Kaneda et al 1984) developed an anterior fixation device that employs vertebral body staples and screws connected by two threaded longitudinal rods that are crosslinked. Zdeblick (Zdeblick et al 1993) developed the Z-Plate, which is low profile and dynamic. An and McGuire developed the University plate, which can also distract the corpectomy site to insert the graft with ease and to compress the strut graft to enhance the stability of the construct. In-vitro biomechanical testing has also provided data in support of these anterior instrumentations of the thoracolumbar spine. The surgical techniques of the Zielke and TSRH rod systems for the correction of thoracolumbar or lumbar scoliotic deformities will be described. The surgical techniques of the Z-Plate, University Plate, and Kaneda rod will be described for fracture and tumor cases.

Indications

1. Zielke or solid rod instrumentation for isolated thoracolumbar or lumbar scoliosis. Contraindications include the presence of kyphotic deformity, compensatory thoracic curve > 30°, severe osteoporosis, and infection.
2. Z-Plate, University Plate, and Kaneda rod types of instrumentation for burst fractures, tumors, and kyphotic deformities. An anterior instrumentation may be utilized in conjunction with bone graft following thoracic disc excision. Contraindications include severe osteoporosis, infection, and fracture-dislocations.

Surgical techniques

The patient should be positioned in the true lateral position on an operating table so that the table can flex over the area of the spine. A vacuum deflatable bean bag supplemented by restraints is placed over the greater trochanter to maintain the patient's position. Care must be taken to protect the skin underneath these restraints over the shoulder and greater trochanter. Care must also be taken in padding the ulnar and peroneal nerves at the elbow and knee, respectively, and padding all bony prominences. An axillary roll should also be placed. It is imperative that the patient's coronal axis be perpendicular to the floor prior to the start of the procedure and that the surgeon is confident that the patient will not roll anteriorly or posteriorly from this position. Knowing and maintaining the patient in the true lateral position will enable the surgeon to allow proper insertion angles of fixation vertebral screws and installation of the plate or rod stabilizing devices in the proper axis. This technical point is useful regardless of which anterior instrumentation system is being used.

Zielke instrumentation

In 1976 Zielke introduced a modification of the Dwyer procedure that corrects both the coronal plane deformity and rotational deformity of scoliosis, also known as ventral derotation spondylodesis (VDS). This system utilizes vertebral body screws that are connected by a threaded rod, providing fine adjustment to the compression force. This system is primarily used for correcting isolated thoracolumbar or lumbar deformities, and the main advantage over posterior instrumentations is that fewer levels are required to fuse, allowing more mobile segments to remain distal to fusion. This system may also be applied to the anterior aspect of the thoracic spine, but the indications, advantages, and outcomes of anterior rod instrumentations are not well delineated at this time for thoracic scoliosis.

The surgical techniques for VDS are exacting. The exposure of the thoracolumbar spine is made over the convexity of the curve. The bed of the tenth rib is usually utilized for a thoracoabdominal approach.

The vertebral bodies are exposed, and segmental arteries and veins are isolated and ligated individually. The vertebral bodies are exposed circumferentially to the opposite side, and malleable retractors are positioned to protect the great vessels (Figure 16.1A). Radiographs are obtained to confirm the levels of dissection. First, meticulous removal of the intervertebral...

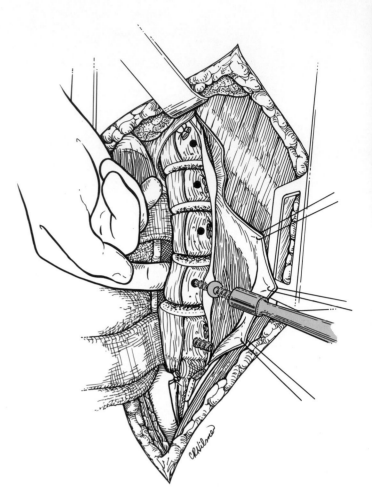

Figure 16.1

Zielke anterior instrumentation.

A
The vertebral bodies are exposed circumferentially to the opposite side, and malleable retractors are positioned to protect the great vessels. Removal of the intervertebral discs is done to the posterior longitudinal ligament, and the annulus on the concave side of the curve should be excised as well. Zielke screws are placed in the middle of each vertebra from the superior–inferior aspect and one-third posteriorly from the anterior–posterior aspect. The surgeon should palpate the opposite cortex and the tip of the screw to confirm the proper length of the screw.

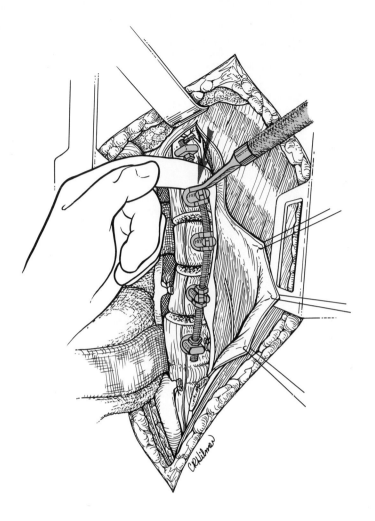

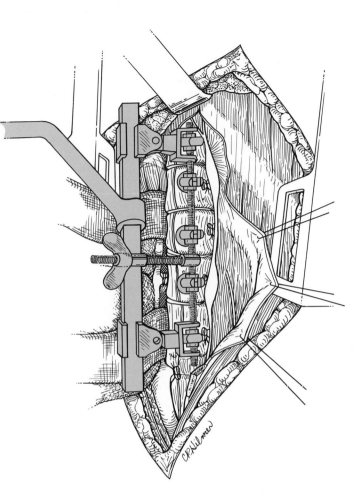

B
Zielke staples may be used as anchors at the proximal and distal ends of the instrumentation system, and plain washers used in the middle segments. The 3.2 mm threaded rod is placed over the screw heads.

C
The derotation and lordosing bridge is attached to the threaded rod that is anchored to each screw. When the spine is maneuvered into derotation and lordosis, the disc space should open up anteriorly. Morselized bone graft is placed in the disc space.

Contd

bral discs is performed. The disc material is removed to the posterior longitudinal ligament, and the annulus on the concave side of the curve should be excised as well. The endplates should be fish scaled to enhance the fusion rate. Zielke screws are placed in the middle of each vertebra from the superior–inferior aspect and posteriorly one-third from the anterior–posterior aspect. An awl is used to make the initial entry point, and an appropriate length screw is inserted to the opposite cortex. The surgeon should palpate the opposite cortex and the tip of the screw to confirm the proper length of the screw. Zielke

staples may be used as anchors at the proximal and distal ends of the instrumentation system, and plain washers used in the middle segments. The 3.2 mm threaded rod is placed over the screw heads (Figure 16.1B). The derotation and lordosing bridge is attached to the threaded rod that is anchored to each screw (Figure 16.1C). When the spine is maneuvered into derotation and lordosis, the disc space should open up anteriorly. Morselized bone graft is placed in the disc space. In order to enhance lordosis of the lumbar spine, a structural graft or cage may be placed anterior to the line of the compression rod.

Compression is applied in the corrected position, thus locking the spine in the lordotic and derotated position (Figure 16.1D). The excess rod is trimmed, and a chest tube insertion and closure are performed as usual. Postoperatively, a thoracolumbosacral orthosis (TLSO) is worn for 5–6 months.

Anterior TSRH instrumentation

The Zielke rod represents a flexible rod system that gives fine adjustment during instrumentation. The TSRH rod is a rigid system, which may give more powerful corrective force and more stable constructs. The indications for rigid rod systems for scoliosis are essentially the same for the Zielke rod. The TSRH system utilizes 4.8 mm or 6.4 mm diameter rods and 5.5 mm and 6.5 mm diameter screws. The screws may be standard or variable angle types.

After exposure, disc excision, and endplate preparation, the screws are placed in the posterior third of the vertebral bodies. The prongs of the staple should go into the endplate (Figure 16.2A). The rod is contoured for lordosis between L1 and L3 and relatively straight between T11 and L1. Eye bolts are then placed on the rod, and the rod is seated in each screw successively. The rod is seated from the caudal to the cephalad direction (Figure 16.2B). The rod is rotated 90° into lordosis using the hexagonal end wrench or rod gripper (Figure 16.2C). The disc spaces are packed with morselized bone grafts and the instrumentation is compressed and tightened (Figure 16.2D). Postoperatively, a TLSO is worn for 5–6 months.

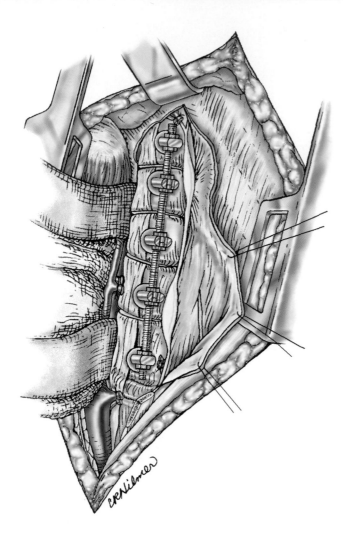

Figure 16.1 *contd*

D

Compression is applied in the corrected position, thus locking the spine in the lordotic and derotated position.

Z-Plate

The Z-Plate was designed by Zdeblick as a low profile, top-loading, dynamic device. The plate has slots at the superior end and fixed holes at the inferior end. It has a radius of curvature, so that it is more closely applied to the curvature of the vertebral body. The longer plates and the thoracic plates also have a curvature over their length to adapt to the normal kyphosis of the thoracic spine. There is both a thoracolumbar size and a thoracic size. It is recommended that the thoracic plates be used from T3 to T9. The thoracolumbar plates should be used from T9 to L4, and occasionally to L5 if the vascular anatomy permits.

The system is utilized by placing a bolt into the vertebral body above and below, as well as a screw into the vertebral body above and below. The

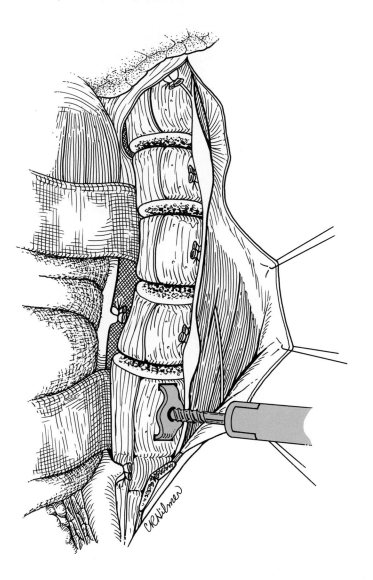

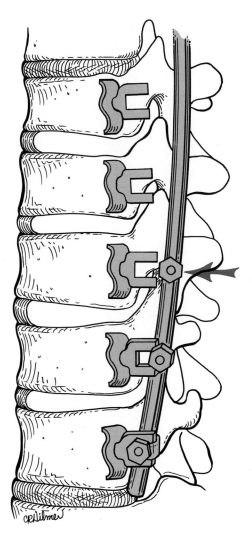

Figure 16.2

Anterior TSRH instrumentation.

A
After exposure, disc excision, and endplate preparation, the screws are placed in the posterior third of the vertebral bodies. The prongs of the staple should go into the endplate.

B
The rod is contoured for lordosis between L1 and L3 and relatively straight between T11 and L1. Eye bolts are then placed on the rod, and the rod is seated in each screw successively. The rod is seated from the caudal to the cephalad direction.

Contd

bolt–plate interface is rigid and the screw–plate interface is semi-rigid. However, this combination of a bolt and screw in each vertebra allows the system to be top-loading, as well as allowing convergence of the bolt and screw for greater pull-off strength. The bolts, once placed, can be used to provide distraction to help reduce a kyphotic deformity. The plate is then applied and the bolts are partially tightened. The slot then allows compression to be placed across the bolts, compressing the bone graft before final tightening. The screws are then placed convergent with the bolts to provide fixation into the vertebrae above and below. Finally, the nuts on the bolts are crimped, which prevents disengagement of the nuts.

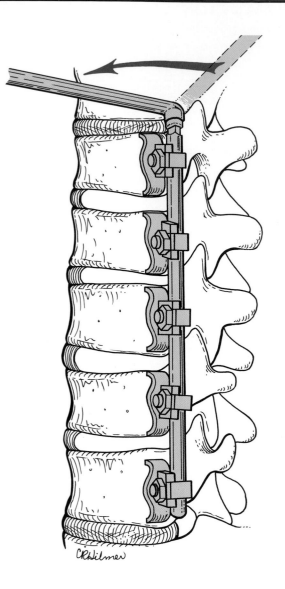

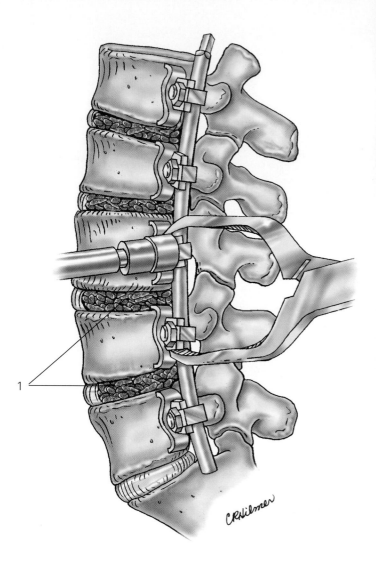

Figure 16.2 *contd*

C
The rod is rotated 90° into lordosis using the hexagonal end wrench or rod gripper.

D
The disc spaces are packed with morselized bone grafts and the instrumentation is compressed and tightened.

1 Bone graft

The thoracolumbar junction is generally approached through the bed of the 10th or 11th rib and may require partial division of the diaphragm. After exposure of the spinal segments to be instrumented, the discs above and below the area of abnormal anatomy are excised. At this time, the corpectomy is performed and canal decompression is completed. Once the corpectomy is complete, the coronal diameter of the vertebral body is measured using the anterior depth gauge. This will allow determination of the

length of the bolts and screws to be used. Measurements from preoperative computerized tomography and/or radiography can also be used to help determine the appropriate bolt and screw length. It is recommended that the screws and bolts engage the opposite cortex of the vertebral body for the most secure fixation.

Because the bolts are slightly higher profile than the screws, it is recommended that the bolts be placed posteriorly. In addition, since one can distract against

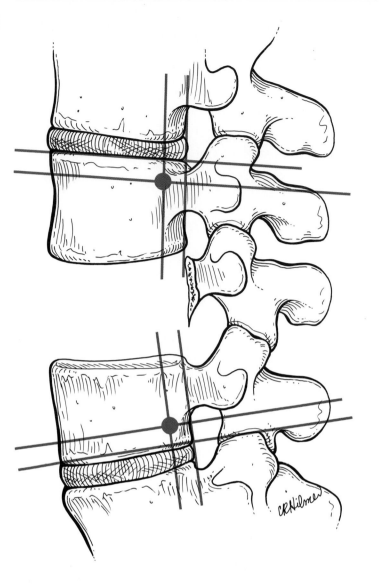

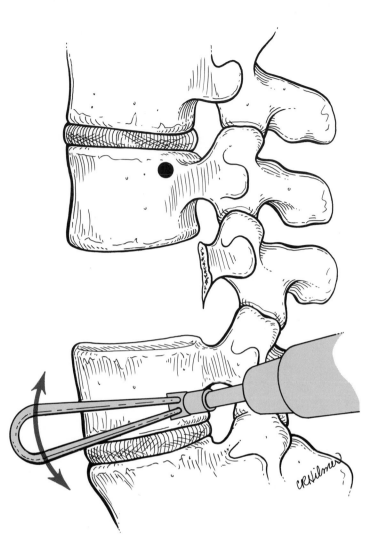

Figure 16.3

Z-Plate instrumentation.

A

The bolt starting points are determined as shown. The superior bolt is placed in the superior posterior corner of the vertebral body, and the inferior bolt placed in the inferior posterior corner of the vertebral body. These starting points are approximately 8–10 mm from the vertebral endplate and from the posterior margin of the vertebral body.

B

A starting hole is made using an awl.

Contd

these bolts, it is recommended that they be placed farther apart than the screws, i.e., the inferior bolt should be placed near the inferior endplate of the vertebral body below the fracture and the superior bolt should be placed near the superior endplate of the vertebral body above the fractured vertebra (Figure 16.3A). This will allow the relatively stronger endplate bone to support the bolts during distraction.

If no reduction is required, the appropriate plate can be used as a template to help determine the position of the starting points for the bolts. However, if reduction is required, the bolts should be placed using the hand-held guide only (Figure 16.3B). This guide will allow the bolt to be placed at an angle 10° away from the spinal canal (Figure 16.3C). The bolt should be placed parallel to the vertebral body endplate (Figure 16.3D). An awl is first used to perforate the proximal cortex and the bolt is then driven across using the bolt screwdriver. Tapping is generally not necessary in vertebral body bone. The second, or

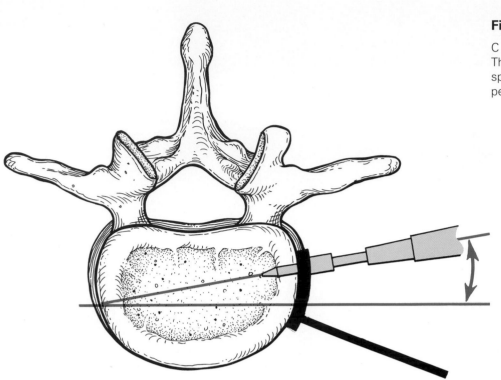

Figure 16.3 *contd*

C
The awl is angled 10° away from the spinal canal. Only the proximal cortex is perforated.

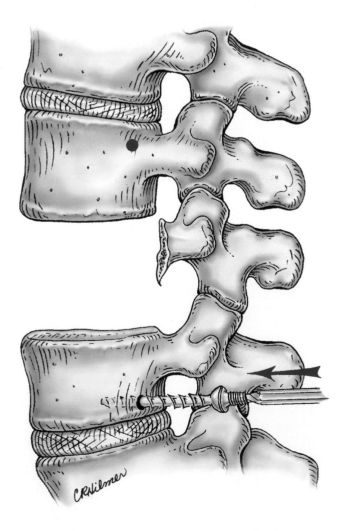

D
The 7.0 mm bolt is inserted using the screwdriver. Tapping is not necessary. Care should be taken to remain parallel to the vertebral endplate and to angle slightly away from the spinal canal.

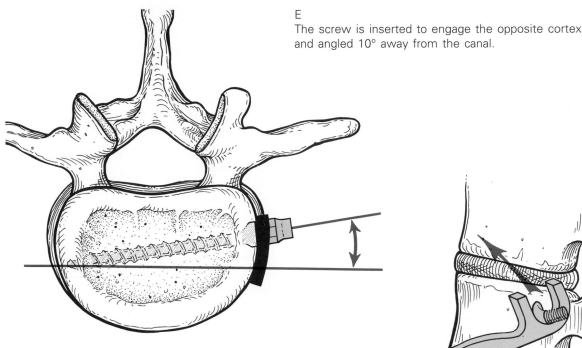

E
The screw is inserted to engage the opposite cortex and angled 10° away from the canal.

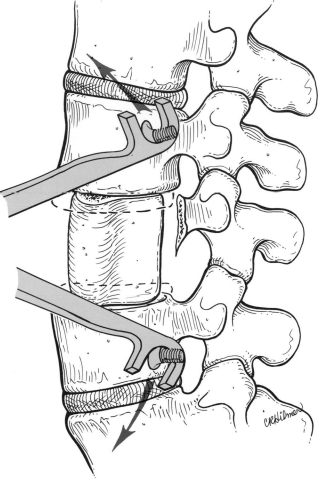

F
Once both bolts are placed, if fracture reduction is required, reduction maneuvers can be performed at this point. This includes manual pressure on the patient's back, distraction using a laminar spreader within the corpectomy defect, and distraction against the bolts using the Z-Plate distractor.

Contd

superior, bolt is then placed in a similar fashion using the hand-held starting guide and angling 10° away from the spinal canal (Figure 16.3E). Both bolts should be sunk into the vertebral body until the shoulder of the bolt is just touching the proximal cortex.

With fracture and kyphosis, reduction should be performed at this time. The reduction maneuver recommended is first to apply manual pressure over the dorsal spine at the apex of the kyphosis. A wide lamina spreader can then be placed between the vertebral endplates within the corpectomy defect to help assist in the reduction. The majority of reduction should be obtained with these two maneuvers. In cases of late correction of kyphotic deformities, the patient's blood pressure should be monitored during the corrective maneuver. Hypotension may indicate impaired vascular return to the heart, as we suspect the vena cava, now accustomed to the kyphotic spine and relatively shortened in length, is stretched and/or compressed as the spine is reduced from kyphosis to lordosis. Should hypotension be noted, the reduction maneuver should be relaxed and repeated to a lesser extent to avoid systemic vascular impairment.

The Z-Plate distractor can then be used to help hold the reduction (Figure 16.3F). This distractor is placed against the exposed threads of the vertebral body

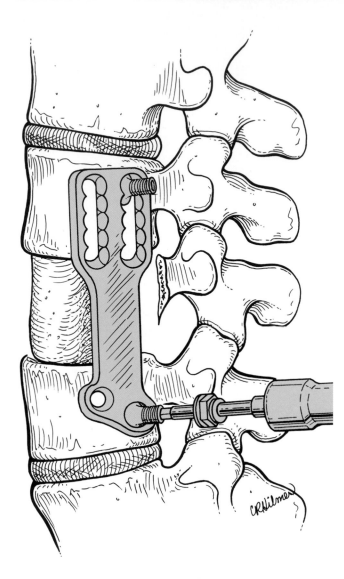

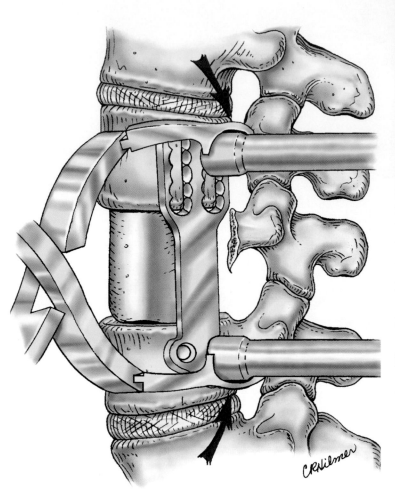

Figure 16.3 *contd*

G
The appropriate-sized Z-Plate is inserted over the bolts. The nuts are started using the nut starter shafts. The inferior nut is placed first.

H
The starter shaft is left on the inferior nut as the superior nut is seated. Prior to final tightening, compression across the bone graft can be obtained. While compression is being applied using the Z-Plate compressor, final tightening of the nuts is completed. Care should be taken to maintain the starter shafts in a parallel fashion while compression is being applied.

bolts and can also be used to provide additional distraction. Once the reduction is complete, the laminar spreader is removed from the corpectomy defect and the reduction is held with the Z-Plate distractor. One can now measure for the length of bone graft using the anterior caliper. Allograft strut grafts, such as fibula, humeral, or femoral cortical strips, or autogenous iliac crest tricortical grafts can be used according to the surgeon's preference. Once

the graft is contoured, it can be impacted in place, securing the reduced position.

One should then choose the appropriate sized Z-Plate. The slots should be positioned superiorly. To minimize impingement on the superior disc space and to allow for maximum compression, select the shortest length plate possible. Prior to placing the plate over the bolts, care should be taken in preparing a flat surface along the lateral aspect of the vertebral

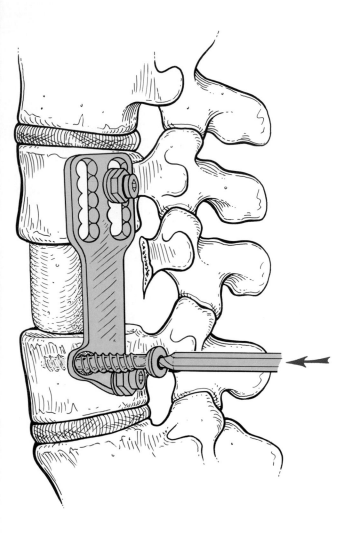

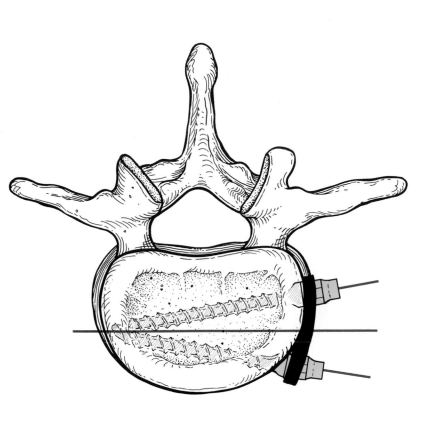

I
The two anterior 6.5 mm screws are inserted in starting points as shown.

J
The anterior screws should also engage the opposite cortex and angle slightly toward the spinal canal.

Contd

bodies. This can be done by removing the lateral prominence of the inferior endplate of the cephalad vertebral body and the superior endplate of the caudal body using a high-speed burr or rongeur. Failure to perform this step will prevent the plate from lying flush against the vertebral column and may induce a deformity in the coronal plane as the spine is reduced to the plate, and/or strip the bolts during final tightening.

Once the plate is in place and fully seated over the bolts, the spiral lock nut is implanted on to the Z-Plate nut starter shaft (Figure 16.3G). The collar of the nut is directed towards the handle. The hex end of one of the Z-Plate nut starter shafts is inserted into the recessed hex of the inferior bolt. This allows one to hold counter-torque on the handle of the shaft, preventing the bolt from being inserted further during tightening of the nut. The nut starter is then turned

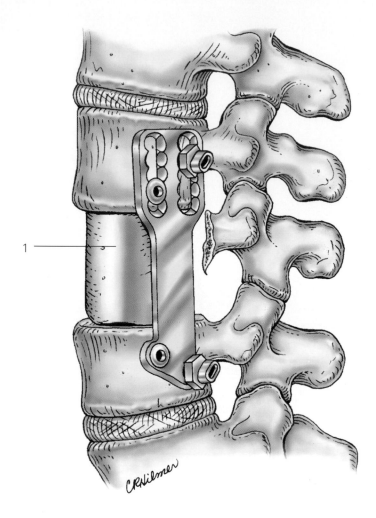

Figure 16.3 *contd*

K

The final construct shows the posterior bolts and anterior screws at different regions of the vertebral body.

1 Bone graft

until the nut drops down on to the bolt, and the spiral lock nut is partially tightened at this time. The second Z-Plate nut starter shaft is then inserted on to the superior bolt and this nut is threaded as well. The Z-Plate nut starter shafts are left in place at this time.

The Z-Plate compressor is then used to compress the bone graft prior to final nut tightening (Figure 16.3H). The surgical assistant holds the nut starter shafts in a parallel fashion while the surgeon applies the Z-Plate compressor to the base of the nut starter shaft sockets. Compression is then applied and the

nuts are fully tightened, while maintaining the parallel plane of the nut starter shafts.

Using the nut starter wrench, the inferior spiral lock nut is tightened while holding counter-torque on the shaft handle. Once the inferior nut has been tightened, the superior nut can then also be tightened, again maintaining counter-torque on the shaft handle. Compression should be maintained using the compressor during the final tightening of both nuts. The compressor can now be removed. Final tightening of the spiral lock nuts is done using the crow's foot torque wrench. Final tightening should be to a minimum of 80 inch-pounds.

The two anterior screws are now implanted (Fig. 16.3I–K). Screw placement sites are prepared using the awl. The anterior screws should be placed directly across the vertebral body perpendicular to the proximal cortex. Again, tapping is not necessary and the screws should engage the opposite cortex. In general, they will need to be 5 mm longer than the bolt implanted in the same vertebral body. When placing the screw in the slot, one should make sure that the starting guide is used with the awl to ensure that the screw head settles firmly into the base of one of the slots.

In patients with severe osteopenia, engaging the opposite cortex with the bolts and screws may not obtain sufficient purchase into the vertebral body. In this situation, fixation can be improved by either packing the screw and bolt holes with cancellous bone or injecting a small amount of thinned and cooled methylmethacrylate cement. This technique can also be used if a screw or bolt becomes stripped during insertion and an alternative insertion point cannot be utilized.

After placing the screws, a radiograph should be obtained to ensure adequate placement of all spinal hardware. The Z-Plate crimper is then used to crimp the nut collars on to the flat portion of the bolt. This will prevent postoperative disengagement of the nut from the bolt. Should the nuts ever loosen, the crimp will then prevent them from disengaging from the bolt and becoming free in the thoracic or retroperitoneal space.

Standard postoperative care should be followed. Typically, a TLSO molded brace is applied on the third postoperative day and ambulation allowed. Bracing is continued for 10 to 12 weeks or until solid fusion is noted on radiography.

University Plate

The University Plate[AM] was developed by An and McGuire as a low-profile, top loading, dynamic, and rigid plate system. This plate is similar to the Z-Plate as described above, but the plate shape is different, with more bulk and strength. Additionally, the bottom portion of plate at the bolt slot has a nest for the hexagonal bolt to link the screw rigidly to the plate once the nut is tighten on the bolt. Biomechanical rigidity of the constructs using the Kaneda rod and the University Plate was superior to the Z-Plate.

The spine is exposed one level cephalad and one level caudad to the injured segment, which is confirmed radiographically, and the segmental vessels are ligated at all three levels. The disc material and cartilaginous endplate of the cephalad and caudad level to the damaged vertebra is removed and a subtotal corpectomy and canal decompression is performed, leaving the anterior and contralateral cortices intact. A vertebral body spreader is placed inside the corpectomy site against the cephalad and caudad endplate to distract and re-establish tension in the ligamentous structures, correcting the kyphotic deformity. Distraction using vertebral screws may loosen the screws, and this technique is not recommended for the University Plate application. The graft site is then measured from endplate to endplate and an autologous tricortical iliac crest graft, other strut grafts or a cage is placed within the distracted corpectomy site. The vertebral body spreaders are removed, allowing the endplates of the cephalad and caudad vertebra to rest on the graft. Additional morselized graft is placed anteriorly to fill the void between the anterior longitudinal ligament and the strut graft. Meticulous grafting technique is a necessity, because no spinal instrumentation system will compensate for a poor, insufficient graft.

Any ridges or prominences laterally are reduced so that a flat surface is available for the plate. A drill guide template is selected to measure plate length which extends to within several millimeters of the farthest endplate of the cephalad and caudad vertebral bodies without extending into a healthy disc (Figure 16.4A). The appropriate drill guide template is then attached to the drill guide handle and placed laterally on to the vertebral bodies, spanning the graft site. The guide should be located along the posterior edge of the lateral spine to prevent extension into the anterior soft tissues and must be flush with the bone to assure correct bolt alignment. The stainless steel drill sleeves identify the posterior aspect of the guide.

The posterior drill guide positions correspond to the nests in the slot of the plate and a position is selected that will optimize bolt purchase in the vertebral body and also allow for approximately one nest of compression after the bolt is placed. The entry point for the posterior bolt should be near the endplates and posterior aspect of the vertebral body. A 3.2 mm graduated drill bit is placed through the appropriate drill guide position in either the cephalad

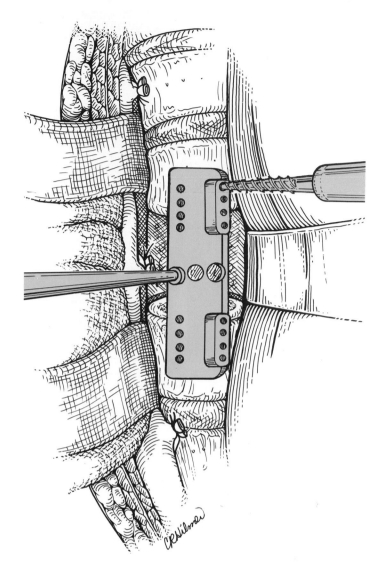

Figure 16.4

University Plate instrumentation.

A

A drill guide template is selected to measure plate length, which extends to within several millimeters of the farthest endplate of the cephalad and caudad vertebral bodies without extending into a healthy disc. The appropriate drill guide template is placed laterally on to the vertebral bodies, and the posterior drill guide positions correspond to the posterior aspect of the vertebral body. A 3.2 mm graduated drill bit is placed through the appropriate drill guide position in either the cephalad or caudad vertebra and penetrates both cortices. The drill is directed parallel to the endplate and slightly anteriorly away from the spinal canal. A pin then replaces the bit to maintain guide position while the second bolt site is prepared in a similar manner.

Contd

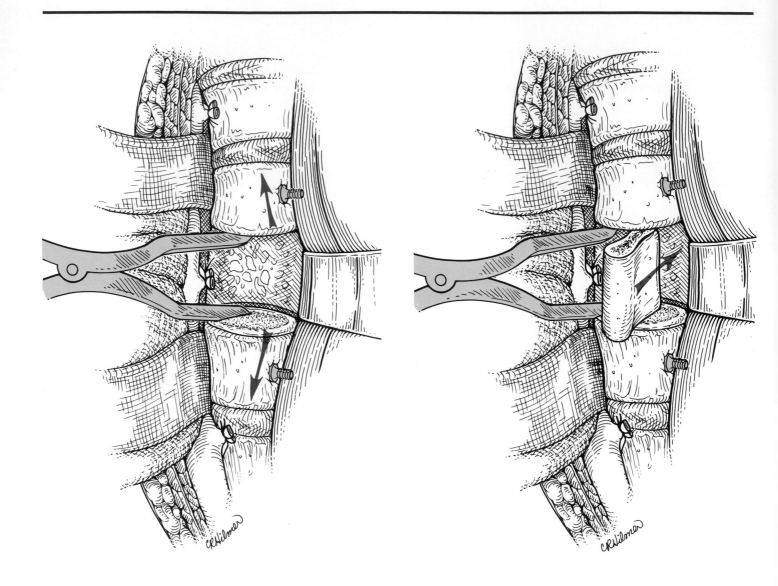

Figure 16.4 *contd*

B
After completion of the drilling, the guide is removed and the hole may be tapped and 7.0 mm bolts are inserted.

C
Following insertion of the posterior bolts, the corpectomy site is again distracted using the endplate spreader. A tricortical iliac crest strut graft or any other structural graft is placed in the corpectomy defect.

or caudad vertebra and penetrates both cortices. The drill is directed parallel to the endplate and slightly anteriorly away from the spinal canal. A pin then replaces the bit to maintain guide position while the second bolt site is prepared in a similar manner. The bolt lengths can be measured directly from the graduated drill bit.

After completion of the drilling, the guide is removed and the hole is tapped to the measured depth using the graduated tap. Tapping is not always necessary, and if tapping is done, a smaller diameter

tap than the screw diameter is recommended. The appropriate length 7.0 mm bolts are inserted (Figure 16.4B). The integral nut must sit slightly above the vertebral body and one set of parallel sides of the nut must be closely aligned along the longitudinal axis of the spine to allow the nut to engage the longitudinal slots on the bottom of the plate. Bicortical purchase is confirmed radiographically or by direct palpation.

Following insertion of the posterior bolts, the corpectomy site is again distracted using the endplate spreader. A tricortical iliac crest strut graft or any

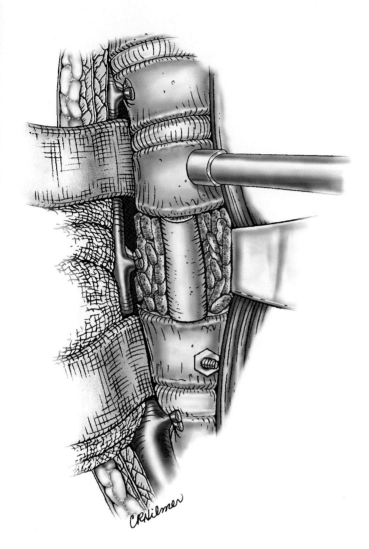

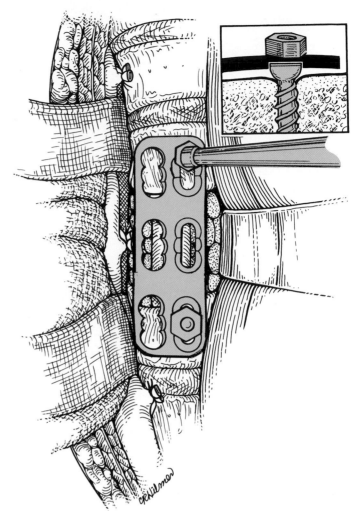

D

Additional morselized bone grafts are packed in the defects.

E

The posterior slots of the University plate are fitted over the posterior bolts and the nests exposed. The 3/8 inch (9.5 mm) tapered nuts are then placed on the exposed machine thread of each posterior bolt and spun down but not tightened securely. The plate is located in the final position relative to either the cephalad or caudal vertebral body, and the corresponding nut is tightened securely with the 3/8 inch (9.5 mm) wrench.

Contd

other structural graft is placed in the corpectomy defect. (Figure 16.4C). Additional morselized bone grafts are packed in the defects (Figure 16.4D). The posterior aspect of the plate is marked with an etched letter 'P' and is placed on the spine with the posterior nested slots fitting over the posterior bolts and the nests exposed. Correct placement of the integral nut within the slot on the undersurface of the plate is critical in preventing the bolt from advancing while tightening the tapered nut. The 3/8 inch tapered nuts are then placed on the exposed machine thread of

each posterior bolt and spun down but not tightened securely (Figure 16.4E). The plate is located in the final position relative to either the cephalad or caudal vertebral body, and the corresponding nut is tightened securely with the 3/8 inch (9.5 mm) wrench. The wrench is then placed on the remaining loose nut and the compressor is placed to anchor its tabs in the middle nested slot and around the wrench. The bolt is compressed approximately one nest and the nut is tightened to 100 inch-pounds (11.3 newton-metres) of torque (Figure 16.4F).

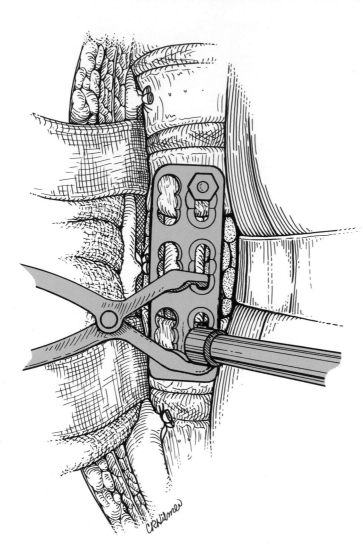
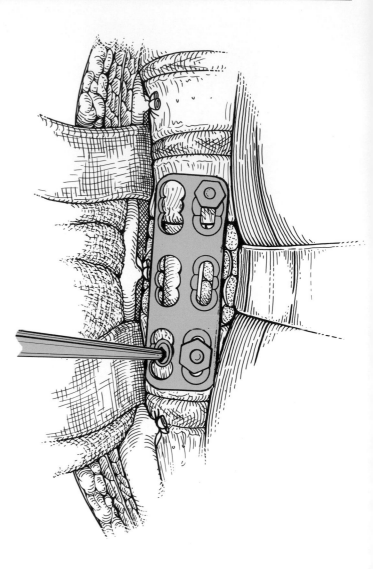

Figure 16.4 *contd*

F
The wrench is then placed on the remaining loose nut and the compressor is placed to anchor its tabs in the middle nested slot and around the wrench. The bolt is compressed approximately one nest and the nut is tightened to 100 inch-pounds of torque.

G
The anterior nest is then perforated, and the screws are inserted to engage the opposite cortex.

An anterior nest is then selected for both cephalad and caudad vertebrae to achieve maximal purchase and avoid impingement with the posterior bolt (Figures 16.4G, H). The cortex is penetrated directly beneath the selected nest with an awl and the sites are tapped bicortically and measured with a probe. Appropriate length 6.25 mm cancellous bone screws are placed with the hex head driver, and bicortical purchase is confirmed radiographically or by palpation.

Wound closure is done in a standard fashion according to the approach used and the patient is placed in a postoperative thoracolumbar spinal orthosis with activity restrictions for 3–4 months.

Kaneda system

The Kaneda system was developed by Kaneda for reconstruction of the spine following anterior decompression of thoracolumbar burst fractures and the bottom are fixed with the one-hole vertebral plate and screw. The anterior and posterior paravertebral rods are coupled with the transverse fixators. The rod of the multisegmental fixation system is flexible (the rod diameter is 4.0 mm). If the deformity is easily correctable, the rigid paravertebral rod will be applicable.

The Kaneda device can withstand both compressive and distractive forces. Either compressive or distractive forces can be applied by turning the nuts on the rods. Biomechanically, the transverse fixators are very important for elimination of rotator and flexion–extension instability.

The patient is placed in the right lateral decubitus position approaching the left portion of the spine below T9 or T10 and in the left lateral decubitus position above T9 or T10. The anterior approach utilized depends on the level of the vertebral lesion.

The thoracolumbar junction is usually approached by the extrapleural (or transpleural) and retroperitoneal route. The thoracic vertebral bodies above T9 or T10 are usually exposed by thoracotomy, and the lumbar spine by the retroperitoneal approach. Application of the Kaneda device should be on the lateral aspect of the vertebral bodies (on the right side above T9 or T10 owing to the thoracic aorta, and on the left side below T9 or T10). Placing the Kaneda vertebral plate anterolaterally increases the risk of canal penetration by the screw; therefore, the plates should be fixed on the lateral aspect of the vertebral bodies. The segmental vessels in the area of dissection are ligated and cut. The iliopsoas muscle is bluntly dissected off the spinal segments that are to be instrumented. The lateral aspect of the vertebral bodies must be well exposed for proper application of the Kaneda device implants.

The lateral aspect of the spinal column opposite the area of the exposure should be gently exposed with a finger or a long-handle nerve root retractor, and a thick sponge should be packed to protect the great vessels. The great vessels and the psoas muscle are gently retracted to expose the vertebral bodies fully. Next, the discs above and below the lesion are meticulously excised.

The vertebral body with lesion is then excised in the area. At first, the vertebra is excised with a chisel or an osteotome. Anterior spinal canal decompression is performed using instruments such as gouges, curets, rongeurs, or air-powered instruments. The spinal canal is approached through the neural foramen. The retropulsed bone or pathological lesion should be completely removed to decompress the dural sac.

Once the decompression is complete, appropriate-sized vertebral plates are tapped into place, holding the plate with the plate holder (Figure 16.5A). The plate must be positioned so that a trapezoidal configuration

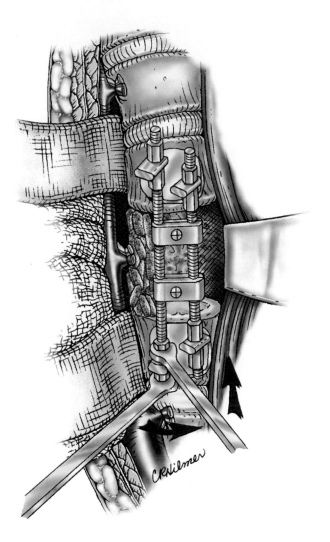

H
The final construct shows that the distal posterior bolt screw his compressed one nest of the plate, and the anterior screws are at different cephalad–caudad regions of the vertebral body.

with neurologic deficit. The Kaneda anterior spinal device consists of the vertebral plate, vertebral screw, paravertebral rod, nut, and transverse fixators. The vertebral plate has tetra-spikes, which are fixed into the lateral vertebral body. The vertebral screw is tapered and self-tapping, with a neck diameter of 6.0 mm. The diameter of the paravertebral rod is 5.5 mm. The nuts are fixed into the screw head holes on the rod from both sides. The top and bottom vertebral bodies are fixed with an ordinary plate and screws, and the vertebral bodies between the top

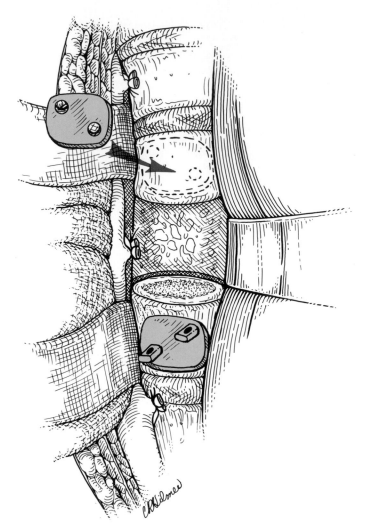

Figure 16.5

Kaneda rod instrumentation.

A
Once the decompression is complete, appropriate-sized vertebral plates are tapped into place, holding the plate with the plate holder.

B
The posterior screw is directed 10–15° anteriorly away from the spinal canal. The anterior screw must be directed transversely to the frontal plane across the vertebral body, thereby triangulating the location.

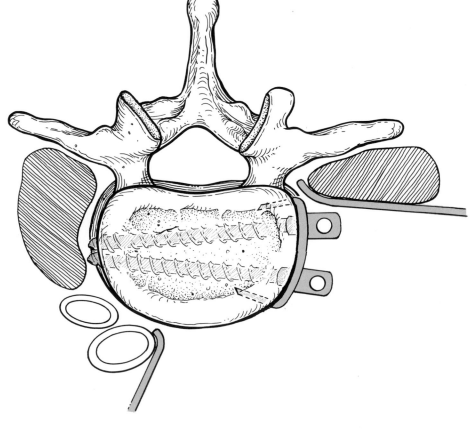

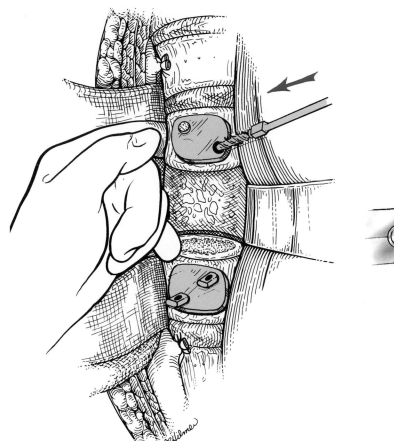

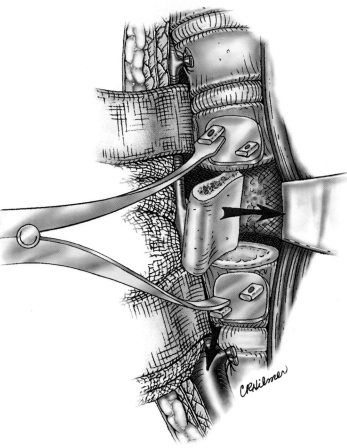

C

Direct palpation on the contralateral side must be performed to ensure penetration of the screw tip so that the penetrated screw tip does not protrude beyond the vertebral body more than 2 or 3 mm.

D

Once the screws are in place and the length is proper, correction of the kyphotic deformity is achieved by the use of the spreader between the anteriormost screwhead holes. The defect following vertebrectomy is then measured with the intervertebral scale, and an appropriate-length tricortical iliac crest bone graft is obtained to fill the defect.

Contd

of the Kaneda construct is created. This means that the anterior rod of the Kaneda device should be longer than the posterior rod.

The posterior screw is directed 10–15° anteriorly away from the spinal canal. The anterior screw must be directed transversely to the frontal plane across the vertebral body, thereby triangulating the location. The screw must be driven home so that the base of the screw head contacts the vertebral plate firmly (Figure 16.5B).

The transverse diameter of the vertebral body is measured in order to choose the most appropriate screw length, using the vertebral gauge. Direct palpation on the contralateral side must be performed to ensure penetration of the screw tip so that the penetrated screw tip does not protrude beyond the vertebral body more than 2 or 3 mm, and to guarantee that its path is straight across the vertebral body. Great care must be taken during palpation to avoid injury to the contralateral segmental vessels or the great vessels (Fig. 16.5C).

Once the screws are in place and the length is proper, correction of the kyphotic deformity is achieved by the use of the spreader between the anteriormost screwhead holes (Fig. 16.5D). If the kyphotic deformity

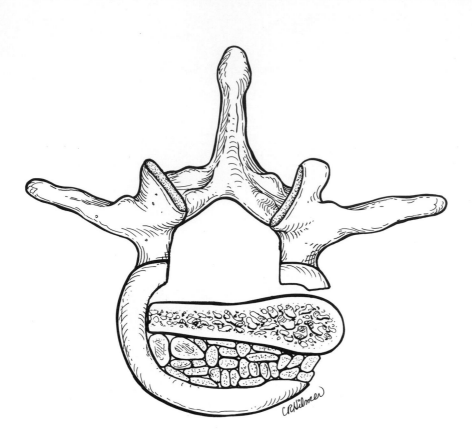

Figure 16.5 *contd*

E
Bone grafting should be done in a meticulous manner. Bone grafts consisting of the tricortical iliac crest, the rib strut taken during exposure, and the bone chips from the resected vertebral body are inserted.

F
Bone chips are packed into the defect between the anterior bony wall and the iliac crest with a bone impactor.

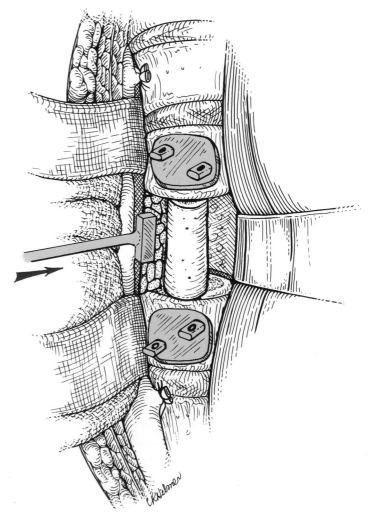

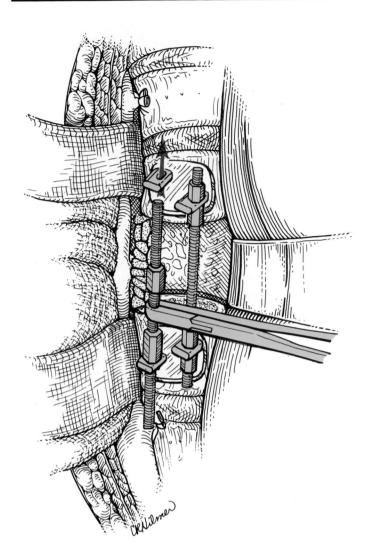

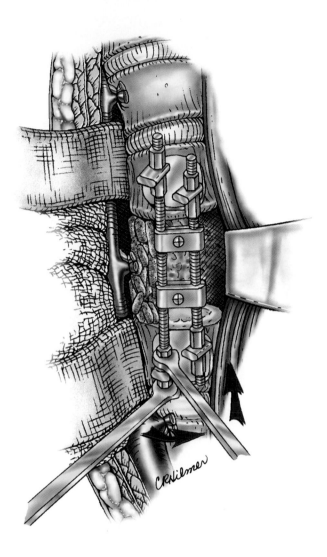

G
Appropriate-length rods that span the screw holes above and below are chosen.

H
Compression force is applied to the strut graft by tightening the nuts on the proximal and distal end of each paraspinal rod. The transverse fixators (the rod couplers) are applied to the paravertebral rods, creating a rectangular configuration.

cannot be corrected because of tension in the contractured anterior longitudinal ligament in old posttraumatic kyphosis, the ligament should be divided at the disc level using an angled curet-rongeur, which is safer than other instruments. The defect following vertebrectomy is then measured with the intervertebral scale, and an appropriate-length tricortical iliac crest bone graft is obtained to fill the defect (Figure 16.5D).

Bone grafting should be done in a meticulous manner. Bone grafts consisting of the tricortical iliac crest, the rib strut taken during exposure, and the bone chips from the resected vertebral body are inserted (Figure 16.5E). The iliac crest should be strong, wide, and long enough to share load with the implants. If the fibular strut graft is used with an iliac crest, the strut will be much stronger. The tricortical iliac crest and the rib struts are tapped into place. Bone chips are packed into the defect between the anterior bony wall and the iliac crest with a bone impactor (Figure 16.5F). Gelfoam is used over the posterior longitudinal ligament or the dura.

Appropriate-length paraspinal rods that span the screw holes above and below are chosen (Figure 16.5G). Before insertion into the holes of the screwheads, the inner nuts are placed in proper orientation on the rods. Once the distal-end nuts are added, a compression force is applied to the strut graft by tightening the nuts on the proximal and distal end of each paraspinal rod (Figure 16.5H). The importance of this maneuver cannot be overemphasized. The Kaneda device relies directly on the load transmission through the strut graft with healthy, strong tricortical iliac crest graft for secure fixation and for long-term healing. If firm compression on the graft for secure fixation and for long-term healing is not provided during instrumentation the construct will fail.

The transverse fixators (the rod couplers) are applied to the paravertebral rods, creating a rectangular configuration (Figure 16.5H). The deeper side of the transverse fixator is introduced with the holder.

Once two sets of the transverse fixators are applied firmly, the nuts must be tightened firmly to secure the rod–screwhead junctions. Overcompression may create an iatrogenic scoliosis; consequently, after tightening the nuts and the transverse fixators properly, AP radiographs should be obtained. Any lateral curvature may be corrected by adjusting the nuts. Once the instrumentation has been completed, the appropriate closing procedures should be performed step by step.

Postoperatively, the patient may ambulate with a polypropylene thoracolumbosacral orthosis (TLSO) days after surgery. Usually, a brace will be worn for 20–24 weeks.

Complications

Complications of anterior instrumentation systems can be divided into device-related and technique-related groups. Fortunately, device-related complications have been low with anterior systems. These involve fixation screw or bolt breakage, failure of the stabilizing rod, and loss of reduction with progressive kyphosis.

Technique-related complications can be avoided prior to making the surgical incision providing the patient is positioned in the true lateral position. Allowing the patient to roll posteriorly or slightly supine, without recognizing this, may risk canal penetration or injury to the contralateral thoracolumbar nerve roots during screw and bolt insertion. Allowing the patient to roll anteriorly or slightly prone may risk injury to the vascular structures on the contralateral side during the screw and bolt insertion. Both malpositions will also interfere with applying the plate flush with the spine and in correct rotation. Another avoidable technical error is selecting the improper level to approach and instrument the spine. Using the retroperitoneal approach, fixation screws

can usually be placed as high as L2. Attempting screw placement into L1 is hindered by the superior margin of the wound and may result in the screws' being placed obliquely rather than parallel to the endplates. A twelfth rib approach should be used if fixation to L1 is planned. The tenth or eleventh rib approach should be used if the lower thoracic vertebral bodies are to be instrumented. During the anterior approach to the thoracolumbar and lumbar spine, the operating table may be reflexed to facilitate exposure. This must be reversed prior to instrumentation in order to insert the bolts and screws parallel to the endplates and apply the plate flush with the spine without inducing a deformity in the coronal plane. Failure to smooth the lateral prominence of the vertebral endplates will also interfere with application of the plate and can induce a deformity in the coronal plane. Finally, all anterior instrumentation systems are designed to load-share with the bone graft interposed between the vertebral segments to be fused. Care must be taken to contour the endplates and graft to allow for a press fit and compression of the graft. Failure to accomplish this may result in a pseudarthrosis, progressive deformity, and/or hardware failure.

Conclusion

Clinical results using anterior thoracolumbar fixation systems have been quite promising. Current systems have become lower-profile, and ease of insertion has facilitated anterior instrumentation greatly. Sufficient rigidity with current systems is present and necessary to provide an excellent biomechanical environment for early anterior fusion. Postoperative maintenance of reduction has been excellent. In addition, titanium systems allow the use of postoperative MRI scans and improve the quality of CT images of the spine and neurologic elements to assess the presence of syringomyelia, tumor recurrence, and adequacy of canal decompression postoperatively. Attention to technical details will allow the surgeon to use these devices safely.

Bibliography

An HS, Lim TH, You JW et al (1985) Biomechanical evaluation of anterior throracolumbar instrumentation. *Spine*, **20**:1979–83

Bohlman HH (1985) Current concepts review. Treatment of fractures and dislocations of the thoracic and lumbar spine. *J Bone Joint Surg*, **67A**:165–9

Bohlman HH, Freehafer A, DeJak J (1975) Free anterior decompression of spinal cord injuries. *J Bone Joint Surg*, **57A**:1025

Bradford DS, McBride GG (1987) Surgical management of thoracolumbar spine fractures with incomplete neurologic deficits. *Clin Orthop*, **218**:201–16

Dunn HK (1984) Anterior stabilization of thoracolumbar injuries. *Clin Orthop*, **189**:116–24

Dwyer AF, Newton NC, Sherwood AA (1969) An anterior approach to sclerosis. *Clin Orthop*, **62**: 192–202

Flynn JC, Hoque MA (1979) Anterior fusion of the lumbar spine. End-result study with long-term follow-up. *J Bone Joint Surg*, **61A**:1143–50

Freebody D, Bendall R, Taylor RD (1971) Anterior transperitoneal lumbar fusion. *J Bone Joint Surg*, **53B** (4):617–27

Gurr KR, McAfee PC, Shih CM (1988) Biomechanical analysis of anterior and posterior instrumentation systems after corpectomy. A calf spine model. *J Bone Joint Surg*, **70A**:1182–91

Kaneda K, Abumi K, Fujiya M (1984) Burst fractures with neurologic deficits of the thoracolumbar spine. Results of anterior decompression and stabilization with anterior instrumentation. *Spine*, **9**:788–95

Kostuik JP (1983) Anterior spinal cord decompression for lesions of the thoracic and lumbar spine: techniques, new methods of internal fixation, results. *Spine*, **8**:512–31

McAfee PC, Bohlman HH, Yuan HA (1985) Anterior decompression of traumatic thoracolumbar fractures with incomplete neurological deficit using a retroperitoneal approach. *J Bone Joint Surg*, **67A**:89–104

Yuan HA, Mann KA, Found EM et al (1988) Early clinical experience with the Syracuse I-Plate: An anterior spinal fixation device. *Spine*, **13**:278–85

Zdeblick TA, Warden KE, Zou D et al (1993) Anterior spinal fixators: A biomechanical in-vitro study. *Spine*, **18**:513–17

Zielke K (1982) Ventral derotation spondylodese: Behandlungsergebnisse bei idiopathischen lumbarskoliosen. *Orthop*, **120**:320–9

17

Exposure and fixation of the sacrum and pelvis

Lee H Riley III

Introduction

Instrumentation techniques for the pelvis have already been reviewed in Chapter 14. This chapter focuses on approaches and fixation techniques for the sacroiliac joint. The sacroiliac joint can be approached either anteriorly or posteriorly. The anterior approach allows direct visualization of the sacroiliac joint during reduction, and the opportunity to denude and bone graft the joint prior to fixation. Its main disadvantage is that the L5 nerve root lies 2 cm medial to the sacroiliac joint, limiting medial exposure and placing this nerve root at risk for injury. The posterior approach allows simple, secure fixation to the sacrum using screws. Its main disadvantage is that it requires prone or lateral positioning of potentially unstable trauma patients, and no direct visualization of the sacroiliac joint. Adequate image intensification and anatomic reduction of the fracture are mandatory so that screw placement into the ala or sacral body is performed without damage to vascular and viscous structures anterior to the sacrum and the cauda equina posteriorly.

Anterior approach to the sacroiliac joint

The anterior approach allows direct access to the sacroiliac joint and inner aspect of the ala of the ilium. It is often used for fixation of sacroiliac fractures with associated iliac fractures using a single approach. Although the sacroiliac joint lies in the posterior

aspect of the pelvic ring, the oblique orientation of the joint and the posterior overhang of the posterior iliac crest makes visualization from a posterior approach next to impossible. The anterior approach allows excellent visualization of the joint and a flat surface where plates can be securely fixed.

Indications

- Sacroiliac fracture fixation
- Sacroiliac fractures with associated iliac fractures.

Procedure

The patient is positioned supine with a bump beneath the buttock. The operating room table can be further planed away from the surgeon so that the contents of the pelvis will fall away from the operative side. An incision is made over the iliac crest beginning at the level of the iliac tubercle and extending anteriorly to the anterosuperior iliac spine (Fig. 17.1A). The incision is then curved anteriorly and medially over the inguinal ligament for several centimeters.

The deep fascia is then exposed at its attachment to the iliac crest. A subperiosteal dissection of the outer lip of the anterior third of the iliac crest is then performed so that about 1 cm of the outer surface of the ilium below the crest is exposed (Fig. 17.1B). The top of the crest is predrilled for secure reattachment of the iliac crest osteotomy. An oscillating saw is then

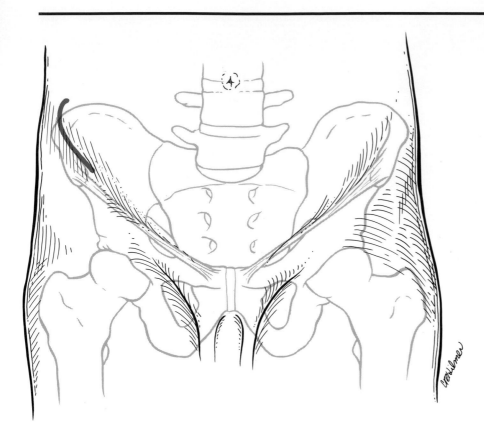

Figure 17.1

Anterior approach to the sacroiliac joint.

A

An incision is made over the iliac crest beginning at the level of the iliac tubercle, anteriorly over the anterior superior iliac spine and anteriorly and medially over the inguinal ligament.

B

Subperiosteal dissection of the outer lip of the anterior third of the iliac crest is performed prior to osteotomy.

1 Fascia over sartorius m.
2 Crest of ilium
3 Abdominal fascia
4 Drill holes
5 Gluteus medius

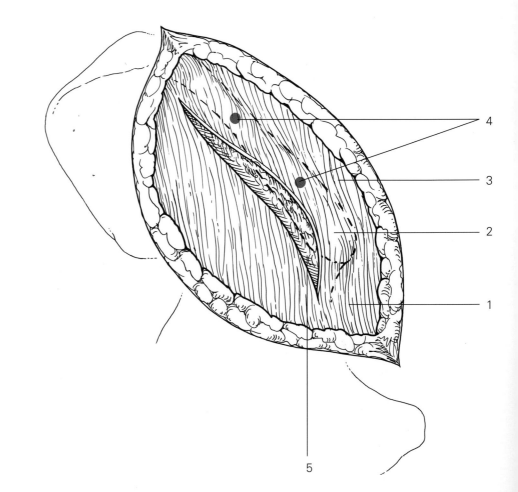

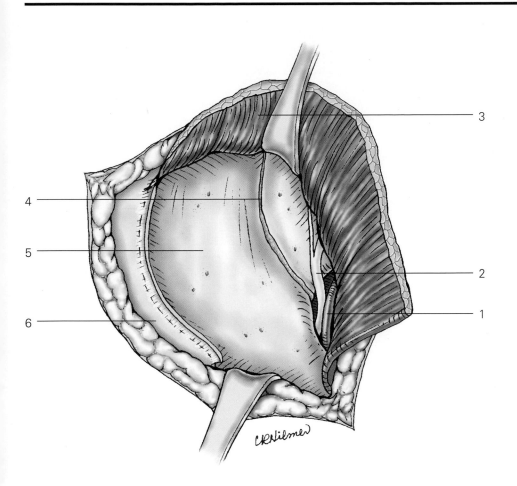

C
The dissection is carried medially to the sacroiliac joint and the lateral aspect of the sacrum.

1 Lumbar v.
2 Ventral ramus
3 Iliac m.
4 Sacroiliac joint
5 Ilium
6 Iliac crest

D
The L5 nerve root is at risk for injury, as it travels 2–3 cm medial to the sacroiliac joint.

1 Sacrospinous and sacrotuberous lig.
2 Sacrotuberous lig.
3 Sacrospinous lig.
4 Ventral sacrococcygeal lig.
5 Ant. sacroiliac lig.
6 Iliolumbar lig.
7 Ant. longitudinal lig.
8 Transverse process, L5
9 Iliac crest
10 Ant. sup. iliac spine
11 Ant. inf. iliac spine
12 Great sciatic foramen

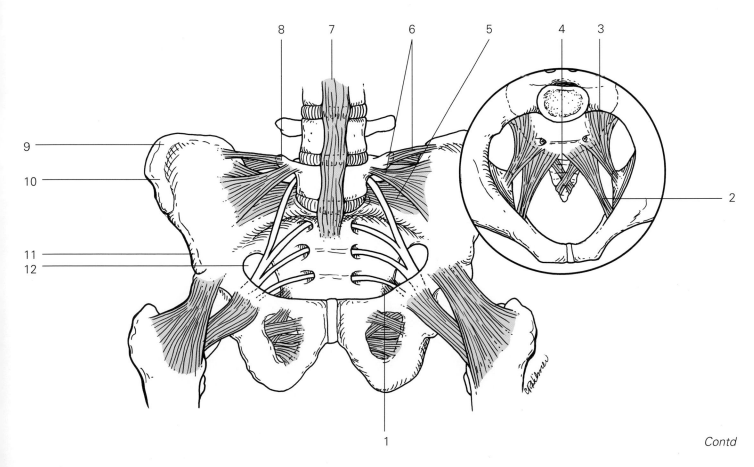

Contd

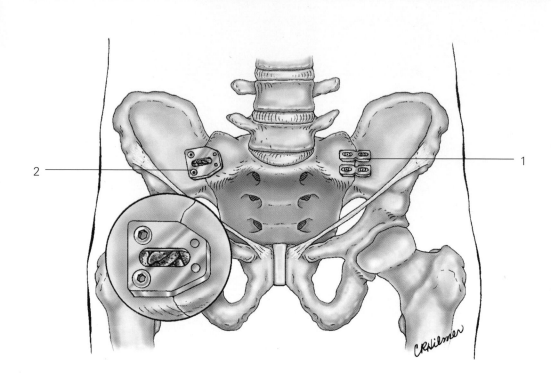

Figure 17.1 *contd*

E
Paired pelvic reconstruction
plates or specialized sacroiliac
joint plates can be used for
anterior sacral fixation. One
screw is placed in the sacral ala
parallel to the plane of the
sacroiliac joint and one or two
screws are placed in the iliac
wing.

1 Paired DCP
2 Trough with bone graft

used to perform an osteotomy of the exposed ilium
to permit detachment of the anterosuperior iliac
spine and the accompanying iliac crest. The inner
cortex of the osteotomy should be completed with an
osteotome.

A subperiosteal dissection of the inner table of the
ilium is then performed. In order to mobilize the
muscle-bone pedicle medially, fibers of the tensor
fasciae latae and sartorius muscles are divided.
Occasionally, the lateral femoral cutaneous nerve may
have to be divided to permit adequate exposure.
Nutrient vessels to the ilium will be encountered and
can be controlled with bone wax. The dissection is
then carried medially, exposing the sacroiliac joint and
the lateral aspect of the sacrum (Fig. 17.1C). The
medial dissection on to the sacrum is limited by the
L5 nerve root, which lies 2 to 3 cm medial to the
sacroiliac joint in a shallow groove. It then travels over
the anterior aspect of the sacrum before entering the
pelvis (Fig. 17.1D). The sacroiliac joint should first be
identified at the level of the sacral ala and the dissection carried down into the true pelvis to the level of
the notch. The superior gluteal artery can be damaged
if the dissection is not strictly subperiosteal.

Once the exposure has been achieved, reduction
and fixation can proceed. The sacroiliac joint on the

sacral side can be denuded to subchondral bone and
bone grafted with bone harvested from the anterior
crest. Reduction can be achieved by placing reduction
forceps on the ilial wing between the anterosuperior
and anteriorinferior iliac spines to correct posterior
translation and Schanz pins in the iliac crest to correct
rotation. Alternatively, reduction can be achieved by
placing screws in the sacral ala and the iliac wing and
using a reduction clamp to reduce the deformity. A
3.5 or 4.5 mm three or four hole reconstruction plate
or specialized sacroiliac joint plate is then contoured
and secured with one 30 or 40 mm screw placed in
the sacral ala parallel to the plane of the sacroiliac
joint and one or two screws placed in the iliac wing
(Fig. 17.1E). Reduction is then confirmed radiographically prior to closure.

Posterior approach to the sacroiliac joint

The posterior approach can be used for open reduction and internal fixation of sacroiliac joint disruptions,

open reduction and internal fixation of fractures of the ilium, sacroiliac fusions and treatment of infections of the sacroiliac joint and surrounding structures. The sacroiliac joint cannot be directly visualized with this approach without removal of the portion of the ilium overlying it. Therefore confirmation of fracture reduction is obtained radiographically and by palpation of the anterior portion of the sacroiliac joint through the greater sciatic notch.

Indications

- Sacroiliac joint disruption
- Sacroiliac joint arthritis
- Fractures of the ilium
- Infections and tumors of the sacroiliac joint and surrounding structures.

Procedure

The patient is positioned prone on a radiolucent operating room table with longitudinal bolsters or on a four-poster frame to decompress the abdomen and chest. Alternatively, the patient may be placed in the lateral decubitus position with the involved side up and the leg prepped free so that it can be manipulated to facilitate reduction. An incision is then made distal and lateral to the posterior superior iliac spine and then extended over the posterior superior iliac spine and extended along the iliac crest anteriorly and superiorly to its highest point (Fig. 17.2A). The incision is carried down to the outer border of the subcutaneous surface of the iliac crest, exposing the attachment of the gluteus maximus muscle. The origin of the gluteus maximus muscle is detached from the crest and a subperiosteal dissection of the outer wing of the ilium is then carried out (Fig. 17.2B). The inferior mobilization of the muscle will

Figure 17.2

Posterior approach to the sacroiliac joint and sacroiliac screw fixation

A
The incision is made distal and lateral to the posterior superior iliac spine and extended over the posterior superior iliac spine along the iliac crest anteriorly and superiorly to its highest point.

Contd

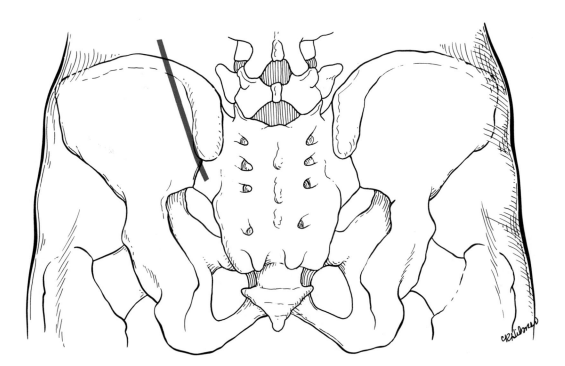

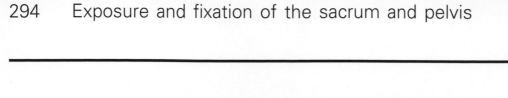

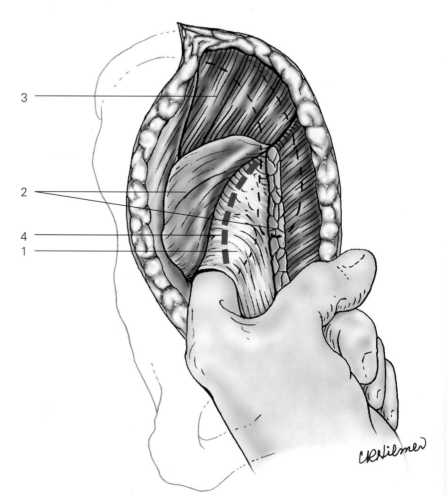

Figure 17.2 *contd*

B
The origin of the gluteus maximus muscle is detached from the iliac crest and a subperiosteal dissection of the outer wing of the ilium is performed.

1 Post. sup. iliac spine
2 Outer table of iliac wing

C
Part of the origin of the piriformis muscle may be detached from the sciatic notch to allow a finger to be inserted into the notch to palpate the anterior surface of the sacroiliac joint.

1 Greater sciatic notch
2 Gluteus maximus m.
3 Gluteus medius m.
4 Sacroiliac joint

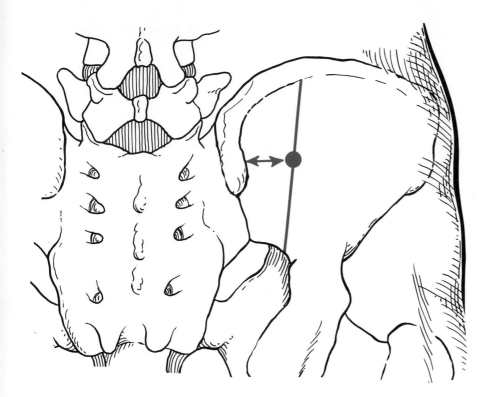

D
The starting point for screw placement is 2 cm above the greater sciatic notch and 2–3 cm lateral to the posterior superior iliac spine.

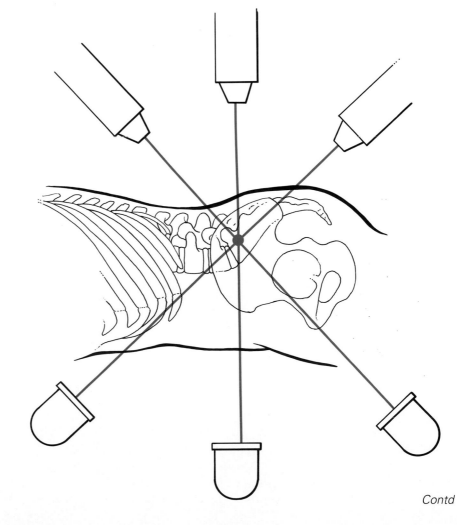

E
The anteroposterior, inlet and outlet views are used to confirm joint reduction and adequate screw placement.

Contd

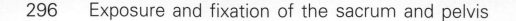

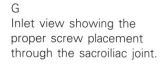

Figure 17.2 *contd*

F
Anteroposterior view showing the proper screw placement through the sacroiliac joint.

G
Inlet view showing the proper screw placement through the sacroiliac joint.

be limited by the branches of the inferior gluteal artery and the inferior gluteal nerve, which emerge from the greater sciatic notch and supply the muscle. The gluteus medius muscle is then gently elevated, the operator taking care not to disturb the superior gluteal nerve, to expose the greater sciatic notch. Part of the origin of the piriformis muscle may be detached from the sciatic notch so that a finger can be inserted into the notch to palpate the anterior surface of the sacroiliac joint (Fig. 17.2C). The sacroiliac joint can be opened with a laminar spreader and the cartilage denuded.

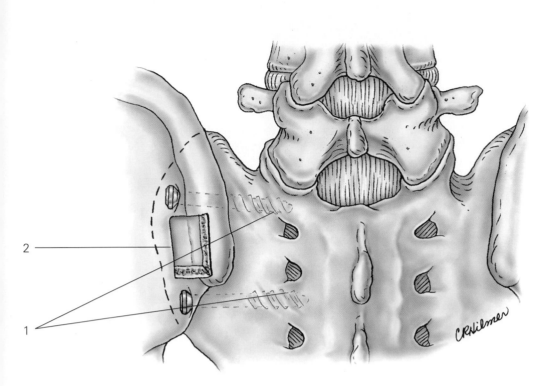

H
The window overlying the articular portion of the sacroiliac joint serves as the fusion bed for the sacroiliac fusion.

1 Fixation screws (6.5 mm cancellous)
2 Window into articular portion of sacroiliac joint

Reduction can then be determined by palpating the SI joint through the sciatic notch and superiorly along the border along the sacral ala and iliac crest. The starting point for screw placement is approximately 2 cm above the greater sciatic notch and 2–3 cm lateral to the posterosuperior iliac spine (Fig. 17.2D). Reduction and screw placement should also be confirmed radiographically using fluoroscopy or plain radiographs. Fluoroscopy has the advantage of being more time efficient. The anteroposterior, inlet and outlet views all need to be obtained to confirm screw placement (Fig. 17.2E–G). The AP and inlet views are used to confirm the anterior–posterior screw position. The outlet view is used to con screws.

Sacroiliac joint fusion can also be performed using this exposure. A window in the ilium overlying the articular portion of the sacroiliac joint is effected using an oscillating saw and osteotomes. The articular cartilage is then denuded on both sides of the joint and packed with cancellous bone. The window is then replaced and packed with cancellous bone (Fig. 17.2H). Fixation then proceeds as for a sacroiliac disruption.

Conclusions

The specific approach employed needs to be individualized for each patient. Associated injuries, the status of the soft tissues overlying the pelvis and the fracture pattern all need to be taken into consideration when deciding which approach is the most appropriate for a particular patient. This underscores the need for a careful physical examination as well as adequate radiographic imaging preoperatively so that the nature and extent of injuries is clearly understood before embarking on surgery.

Bibliography

Browner BD, Jupiter JB, Levine AM et al (eds) (1992) *Skeletal Trauma*, Vol 1. Philadelphia: WB Saunders

Matta JM, Saucedo T (1989) Internal fixation of pelvic ring fractures. *Clin Orthop*, **242**:83–97

Simpson LA, Waddell JP, Leighton RK et al (1987) Anterior approach and stabilization of the disrupted sacro-iliac joint. *J Trauma*, **27**(12):1332–9

Tile M (1995) *Fractures of the Pelvis and Acetabulum*, 2nd edn. Baltimore: Williams & Wilkins

18

Malignant tumors of the spine and sacrum

Alan M Levine
Lee H Riley III

Introduction

Malignant lesions of the spine can be divided into two groups, primary and metastatic. Metastatic lesions are forty times more common than primary malignant tumors of the spine; however, despite the lower prevalence of primary lesions, they also present both a diagnostic and a therapeutic challenge. Appropriate radiographic imaging, a carefully planned and executed biopsy that preserves the possibility of a curative resection, and an integrated treatment program involving surgical excision, adjuvant and/or neoadjuvant chemotherapy and radiation therapy are necessary for adequate treatment. This chapter reviews the surgical treatment of both metastatic and primary tumors of the spine.

Anterior resection of metastatic lesions

Removal of macroscopic disease, decompression of the spinal canal, and reconstruction of the structural defect are the basic goals of a surgical resection for metastatic lesions of the spine. Metastatic disease of the spine most commonly affects the vertebral body and in 70 per cent of patients having neurological compromise it is due to anterior compression. Therefore an anterior corpectomy and stabilization, alone or in conjunction with a posterior procedure, is most commonly performed. The spine is exposed through a standard anterior approach (Fig. 18.1A). The adjacent discs are completely removed (Fig. 18.1B). The foramen and spinal canal are then identified and

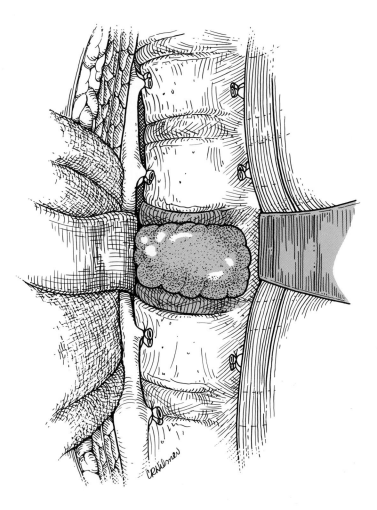

Figure 18.1

Anterior resection of metastatic lesions.

A
Exposure of the involved vertebral body.

Contd

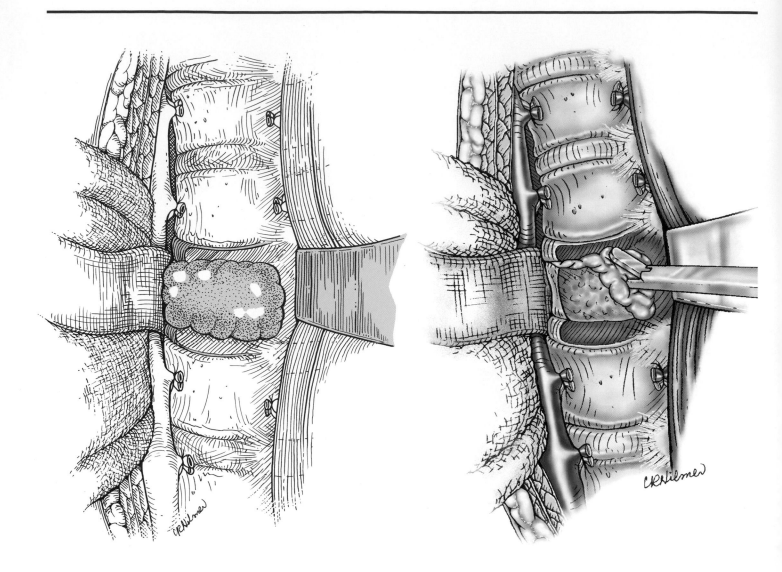

Figure 18.1 *contd*

B
The adjacent discs are removed facilitating orientation to the canal.

C
All tumor is removed and the spinal canal decompressed.

the tumor and involved bone are removed and the spinal canal decompressed (Fig. 18.1C). This may involve removal of the ligamentum flavum or partial excision of adjacent vertebral bodies in some instances. The adjacent end plates are then broached with a curved curet and a metal rod is embedded into the adjacent bodies (Fig. 18.1D). Gelfoam, alone or in combination with tongue depressors, is placed as a dam to prevent intrusion of methyl methacrylate into the spinal canal. PMMA is then mixed and allowed to thicken to a doughy consistency and carefully hand packed around the rod and into the defect, filling the void between the adjacent end plates (Fig. 181E). The PMMA is allowed to cure. A lateral radiograph is obtained to confirm the position of the implant, and the wound is closed. For additional stability a plate can be applied spanning the three levels, or if necessary a posterior procedure can be performed.

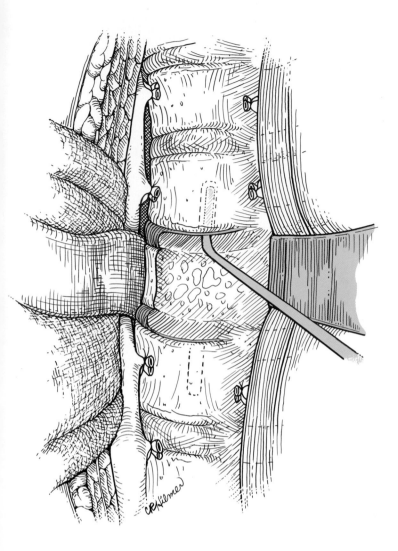

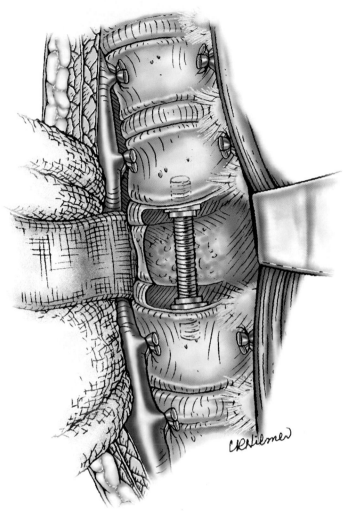

D
The adjacent endplates are breeched with a curved curet to allow insertion of the threaded rod–screw–washer construct.

E
Methyl methacrylate is packed around the construct to provide support under compression.

Anterior resection of primary cervical spine lesions

Anterior resection is performed using a vertical incision and a presternocleidomastoid approach. The skin incision should be made on the side with the most tumor involvement since the anterior approach provides less access to the opposite side. If the tumor is small, benign and localized to a single vertebral body, then the adjacent discs are removed and the tumor is excised en bloc through healthy bone using a rongeur, drill, or osteotome (Fig. 18.2A). A fine curet can be used to break through the posterior cortex and pull the specimen anteriorly. Tumors that extend laterally or into the pedicle or vertebral foramen require freeing of the transverse processes and possibly resection of the anterior border to gain access to the vertebral artery (Fig. 18.2B). The relationship of both vertebral arteries to the tumor mass must also be

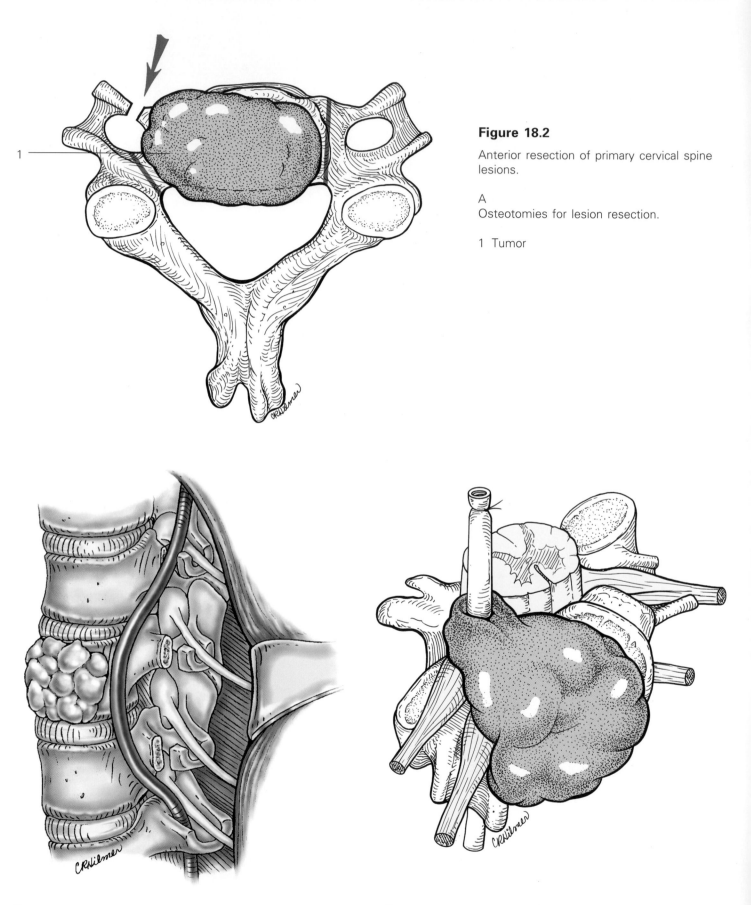

Figure 18.2

Anterior resection of primary cervical spine lesions.

A
Osteotomies for lesion resection.

1 Tumor

B
The vertebral artery should be exposed above and below the level of resection.

C
The vertebral artery should be ligated prior to removal of the tumor.

carefully considered. If one of the arteries is involved, then it needs to be either sacrificed or bypassed. The dominance of the involved vertebral artery and its importance to brain perfusion should be determined before it is sacrificed. In some cases this may involve intraoperative awake provocative testing. If the artery is to be sacrificed, then it is isolated above and below the tumor and ligated (Fig. 18.2C). If the artery is involved in the tumor but circulation on the involved side must be preserved, then it is freed from the foramen one level above and below the involved level and a bypass stent used during tumor resection. The vessel is then reconstructed as necessary. In instances where the tumor closely approximates but does not involve the vessel, the artery should be freed and protected at the involved level and the adjacent levels. The longus colli muscle can be retraced or divided transversely depending upon the size of the tumor and its invasion into the muscle. Involvement of the root, the posterior portion of the transverse process or the pedicle may mandate a posterolateral approach, which can be performed through the same incision.

Primary tumors of the thoracic spine

Several different techniques are available for the resection of primary tumors of the thoracic spine. The appropriate approach is dictated by the size and location of the tumor.

Intraosseous tumors or smaller tumors can be circumferentially resected through a posterior approach using the Roy-Camille technique. A posterior midline incision is centered over the involved vertebrae. If further exposure is necessary, then H-shaped flaps can be developed. A subperiosteal dissection of the lamina, costovertebral joints and the medial 3 cm of the ribs is performed over the segments to be resected (Fig. 18.3A). Modifications of the exposure to maintain an adequate margin will be necessary in instances of posterior tumor involvement. If no posterior element involvement is present then a laminectomy is performed at all levels. If posterior elements are involved then an en bloc resection can be done initially with transection at the level of the pedicles. The ribs are osteotomized and resected from their articulations with the vertebral bodies if they are not involved in tumor or are left with the specimen in instances where there is any doubt (Fig. 18.3B). The segmental vessels are then ligated bilaterally as close to the aorta as possible. The intercostal nerves may be cut on one side to make removal of the specimen easier and to improve anterior exposure for the subsequent anterior reconstruction. If necessary, the

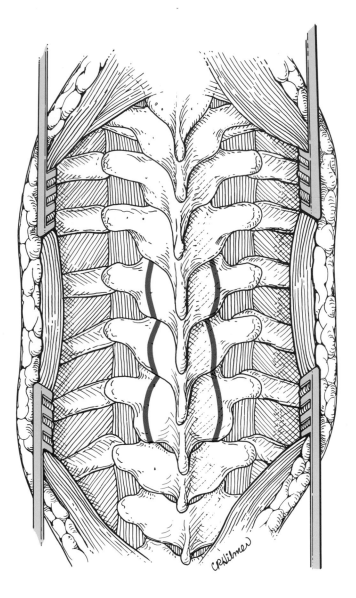

Figure 18.3

The Roy-Camille technique.

A
Posterior exposure.

Contd

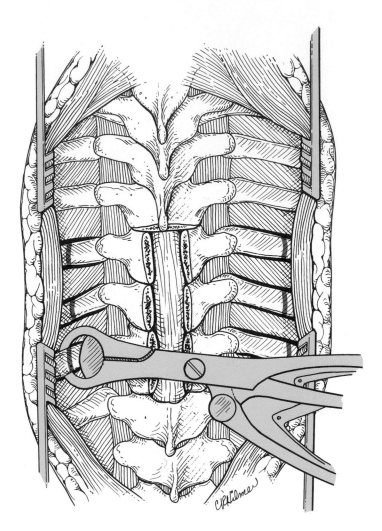

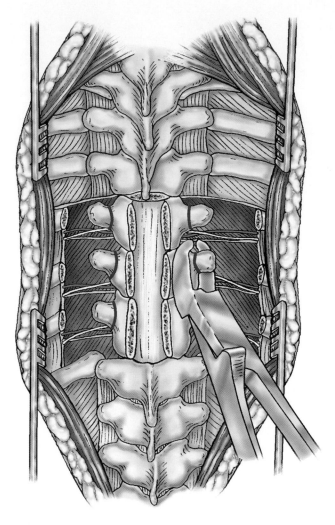

Figure 18.3 *contd*

B
Rib resection.

C
The facet joints, pars, transverse processes and uninvolved pedicles are resected to allow greater access to the anterior aspect of the vertebral body and visualization of the spinal cord.

parietal pleura can be entered. Facetectomy and removal of the pars are then performed at all levels (Fig. 18.3C). Uninvolved pedicles are resected flush with the bodies. The plane between the anterior portion of the vertebral body and the aorta is developed (Fig. 18.3D). Prior to resection, segmental fixation should be applied on one side to provide some stability. Tumor removal is facilitated if this fixation is placed on the side opposite to the side of

subsequent tumor removal. The anterior structures are then protected with malleable retractors (Fig. 18.3E). A Gigli saw is passed anterior to the vertebral bodies to allow resection adjacent to the proximal and distal end plates. The posterior longitudinal ligament is then transected under direct vision. The specimen is then rotated out. A femoral shaft allograft is then packed with cancellous bone and impacted into place. Additional anterior screw fixation can be applied if

D
The soft tissue plane is bluntly developed between the spine and the anterior structures.

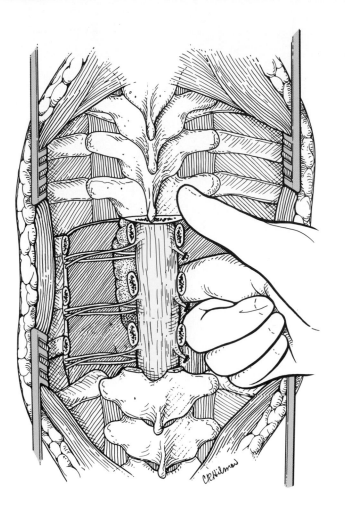

E
The anterior structures are protected with malleable retractors.

1 Aorta
2 Lung
3 Retractors
4 Azygos v.
5 Lung

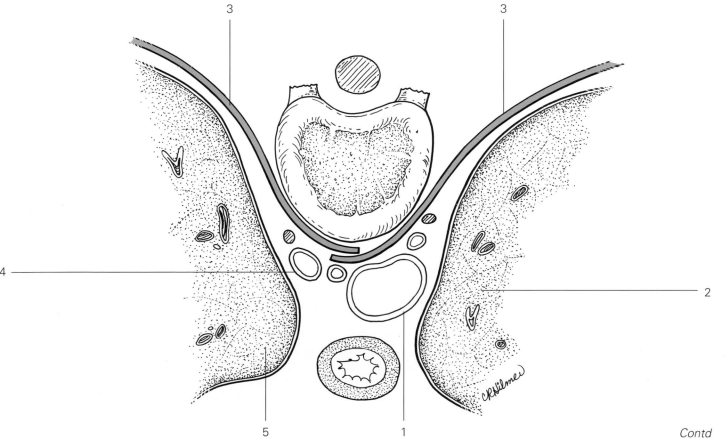

Contd

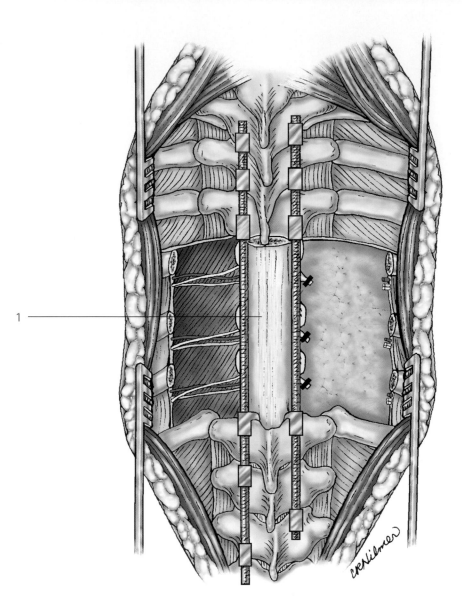

Figure 18.3 *contd*

F

Posterior reconstruction after tumor removal and anterior reconstruction.

1 Dural sac

necessary. The second posterior rod is inserted and the construct compressed for further stability. Two sets of claws proximal to the defect and one set of claws distal to the defect usually provide sufficient stability (Fig. 18.3F).

For larger lesions a posterior approach alone may not be adequate. In this instance a combined approach is needed. The posterior approach is performed first, allowing the application of stable posterior fixation. Resection of the posterior elements and dissection anteriorly from the posterior approach on the side opposite to the side of the subsequent anterior approach are necessary for complete tumor removal. This minimizes the amount of anterior dissection on the blind side during the anterior approach. A standard anterior thoracotomy approach is then performed and the lesion removed.

Resection of paraspinal sarcomas

Soft tissue sarcomas can occur in the paraspinous musculature at any level of the spinal column. They can be confined to the muscle alone or involve adjacent vertebral bodies, the chest wall, and the spinal canal in advanced stages. Usually these tumors predominantly involve one side of the spine, making a wide resection of the tumor technically feasible. Unless standard oncologic principles for resection of soft tissue sarcomas are adhered to, the local recurrence rate is very high. However, a wide resection with negative margins combined with radiation therapy can lead to a local cure. In cases where the posterior elements alone are involved the tumor is removed by transecting the pedicle and lamina, and the adjacent rib when indicated, to achieve an adequate margin (Fig. 18.4A). The pedicle is osteotomized using either a fine wire saw passed through the neuroforamen and around the pedicle or a thin curved osteotome. Involvement of the chest wall, posterior elements, and adjacent vertebral body requires an anterior and posterior approach. The anterior approach should be performed first through the first interspace above the lesion that will yield a 2–3 cm proximal margin (Fig. 18.4B). All ribs involved in the tumor are osteotomized 2–3 cm lateral to the tumor. The segmental vessels leading to the involved vertebrae as well as the normal adjacent vertebrae are ligated to allow mobilization of the aorta. The discs above and below the involved vertebrae are removed completely back to the posterior annulus. The osteotomy through the vertebral bodies is then performed (Fig. 18.4C). This is the most diffi-

Figure 18.4

Resection of paraspinal sarcomas.

A
Posterior resection with osteotomies through the rib, pedicle and opposite lamina.

1 Resection
2 Tumor

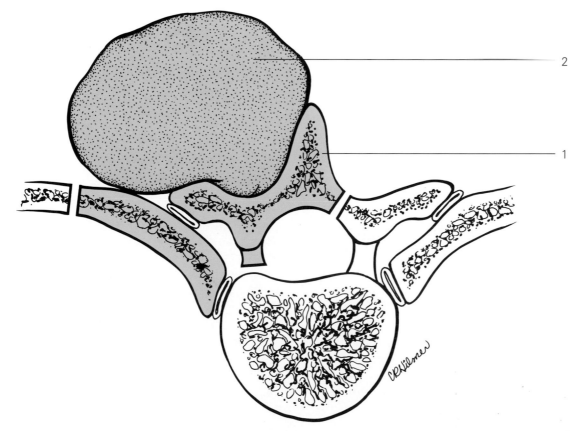

Contd

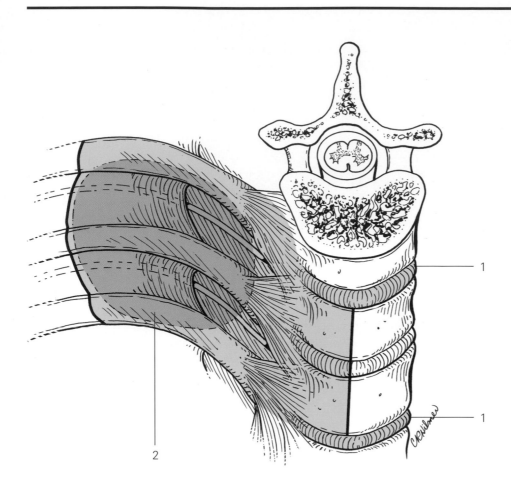

Figure 18.4 *contd*

B
A 2–3 cm tumor free margin should be maintained.

1 Discectomy
2 Tumor

C
The anterior osteotomies of the ribs and vertebral bodies are performed first.

1 Discectomy
2 Tumor

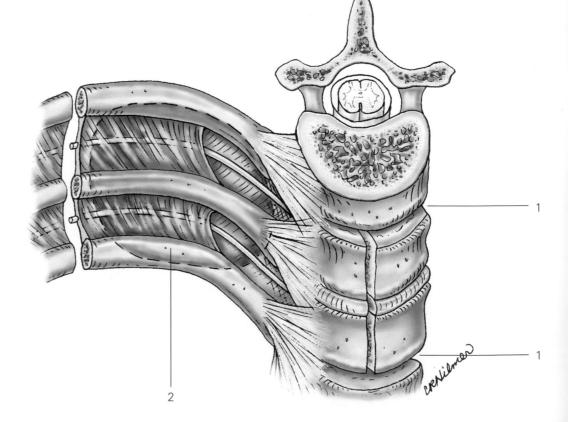

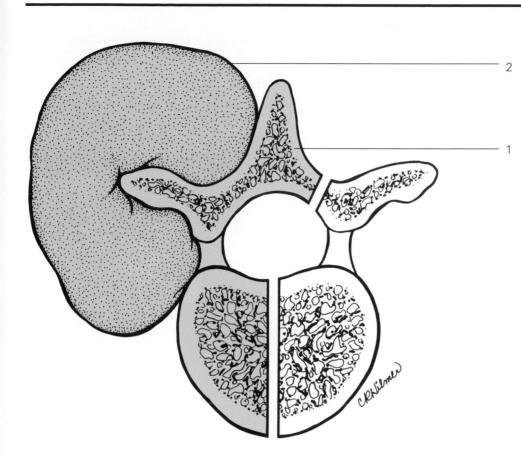

D
Cross-section demonstrating
the osteotomies of the
involved vertebral bodies.

1 Resection
2 Tumor

Contd

cult portion of the procedure because of the extensive bleeding encountered from the cancellous bone surfaces and the chance of neurologic injury during the osteotomy of the posterior cortex. Fortunately, most paraspinal lesions involve only the lateral surface of the vertebral bodies and do not extend to the central portion. A hemisection usually provides an adequate margin. The extent of tumor involvement and the dimensions of the vertebral bodies need to be determined preoperatively using CT and MRI so that the osteotomies can be appropriately planned. The vertebral osteotomy is performed using a right angled oscillating saw blade that is the exact depth of the antero-posterior dimension of the vertebral body at its midpoint (Fig. 18.4D). The posterior longitudinal ligament is preserved. The extensive bleeding encountered is controlled by placing hemostatic pads in the osteotomy site. After control of the bleeding, a chest tube is placed, the anterior approach is closed, and the patient is placed prone.

The posterior incision should include the original biopsy site. This is often off the midline, directly over the tumor mass. A vertical incision curved to include the biopsy site or H-shaped flaps is created. The laminae on the uninvolved side are then exposed and a subcutaneous flap over the tumor mass is developed. Partial laminectomies are performed above and below the levels to be resected in order to provide posterior access to the proximal and distal discectomy levels. Without violating the tumor margin, laminectomies are performed at the levels of resection (Fig. 18.4E). Because of tumor involvement, this frequently involves resection of just the opposite spinous process and a contralateral hemilaminectomy. The intercostal muscles are then divided proximal and distal to the last ribs. The intercostal neurovascular bundle is transected laterally at the level of the rib osteotomies, and the soft tissues are transected longitudinally. The parietal pleura is then incised and the chest cavity is opened through the posterior approach. The pars interarticularis and facets are removed at the terminal levels. The posterior annulus is incised using a 15 blade at the previous discectomy sites proximally and distally. This is performed from the tumor side with minimal manipulation of the neural elements. If the tumor does not have an extradural component, the roots at the

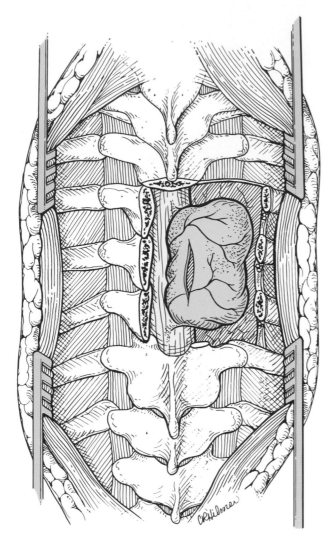 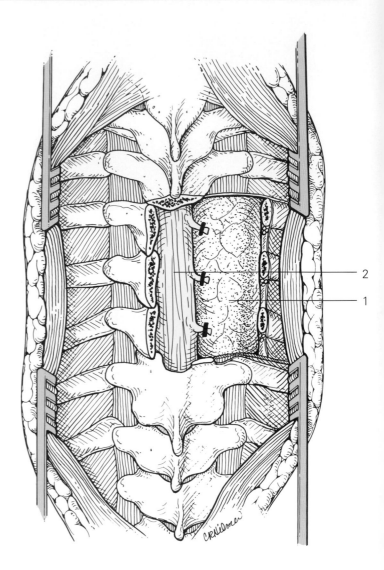

Figure 18.4 *contd*

E
Posterior laminectomies have been performed exposing the discectomy sites posteriorly and isolating the tumor mass and associated margin.

F
Surgical site prior to chest wall reconstruction.

1 Post. lung
2 Dural sac

resection levels are transected just distal to the dural sac within the spinal canal and the tumor removed (Fig. 18.4F). If an extradural component is present, then the dura is opened, the roots transected within the sac, and the anterior dura split longitudinally and left with the specimen. The posterior longitudinal ligament is then sharply transected posterior to anterior and the specimen removed. The dura is repaired using freeze dried dural allograft. The defect in the chest wall is repaired with synthetic mesh attached to the anterior edge of the vertebral bodies, proximal and distal intact ribs, and lateral rib stumps.

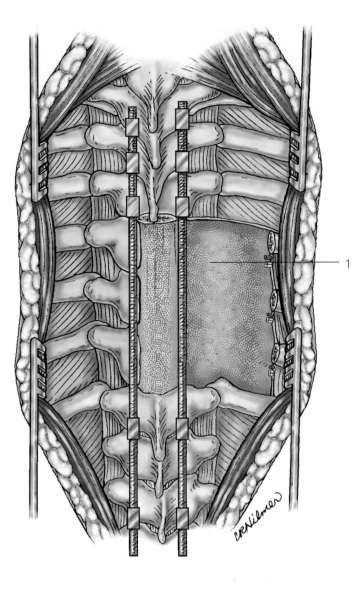

G
Surgical site following reconstruction.

1 Mesh

Posterior segmental stabilization is then performed using a multiple claw construct with two sets of direct, unilaminar claws above and one set of indirect, bilaminar claws below (Fig. 18.4G). Brachytherapy catheters can also be inserted and the incision closed over large suction drains.

Lumbar tumors

Lumbar tumors require a combined posterior and anterior approach. The posterior approach is performed first. For most malignant tumors the posterior elements are not involved. However, the tumor can extend into the pedicles. Posterior exposure extending several levels proximally and distally is performed (Fig. 18.5A). If posterior element or pedicle involvement occurs, then en bloc resection of the posterior elements is performed and the stumps of the pedicles are sealed with methyl methacrylate. Otherwise a complete laminectomy of the involved vertebra is performed as well as a partial laminectomy of the inferior aspect of the cranial lamina. The adjacent facet joints are then resected (Fig. 18.5B). If roots are involved in the tumor, they are sacrificed at the level of the dural sac after the laminectomy. If the roots are uninvolved with the tumor, the pedicle and transverse processes are resected flush with the body to allow easier removal of the specimen from the anterior approach (Fig. 18.5C). The exposed bony surfaces are then sealed with bone wax if the procedure is to be done in one stage, or with methyl methacrylate if there is to be a delay between stages. The dural sac is then mobilized and the posterior annulus of the adjacent disc is incised with a knife posteriorly as far as possible around the end plates of the adjacent bodies. This will leave the disc with the surgical specimen. Posterior stabilization is then performed. This most often involves pedicle screw fixation (Fig. 18.5D). If the tumor is predominantly anterior, corticocancellous graft can be harvested and fusion planned for the entire instrumented segment posteriorly.

Anterior resection is then performed with the patient supine. The anterior approach performed depends on the level of the lumbar spine involvement and the extraosseous soft tissue component. For tumors at the L1–L3 levels, the tumor is approached from the side of the predominant soft tissue mass through a retroperitoneal flank approach. For an L4 or L5 lesion a midline incision, transperitoneal approach and mobilization of the great vessels are performed. A retroperitoneal approach is also possible and is favored by some surgeons but makes dissection on the blind side more difficult. Intraoperative shunting followed by reanastamosis may be necessary if the vessels are involved in the tumor mass. Smaller tumors without vessel involvement can be safely resected by mobilization of the vessels. A psoas muscle margin is generally taken with any soft tissue component of the tumor. The proximal lumbar roots should be preserved when possible. The anterior and lateral portions of the adjacent discs are transected as far as possible from the involved body. The disc is then freed using an elevator from

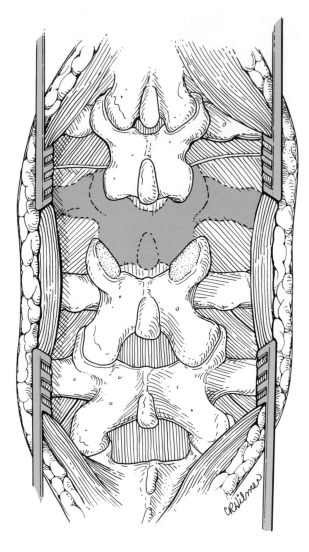 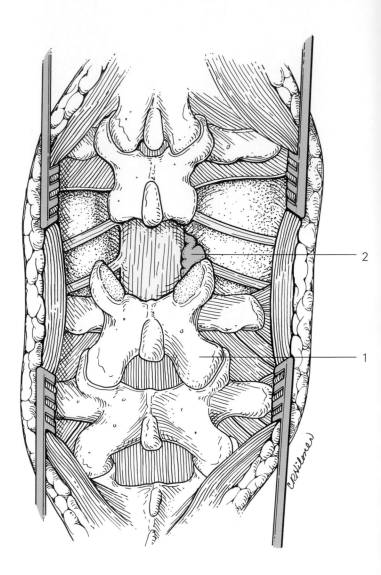

Figure 18.5

Lumbar tumors.

A
Initial exposure is performed out to the tips of the transverse processes.

B
Exposure with preservation of uninvolved nerve roots.

1 L4
2 Tumor

the adjacent end plates. A curet is passed around the posterior edge of the vertebral body and the specimen rotated free in the field. Reconstruction of the anterior defect can be performed using a femoral allograft–cancellous bone composite if the patient is not receiving adjuvant chemotherapy or radiation therapy postoperatively. If external beam radiation, or adjuvant chemotherapy is planned, then a rigid titanium cage strut with bone graft or a PMMA spacer should be used, since these constructs will bear load more effectively in the face of a prolonged time to union (Fig. 18.5E).

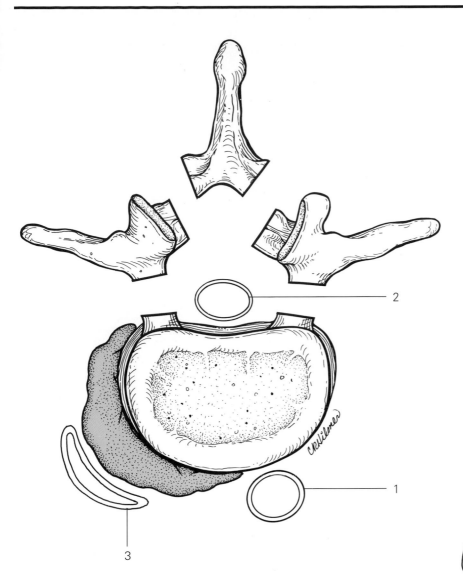

C
Cross-section demonstrating osteotomies.

1 Aorta
2 Dura
3 Inferior vena cava

D
Posterior fixation prior to anterior resection.

1 Tumor

Contd

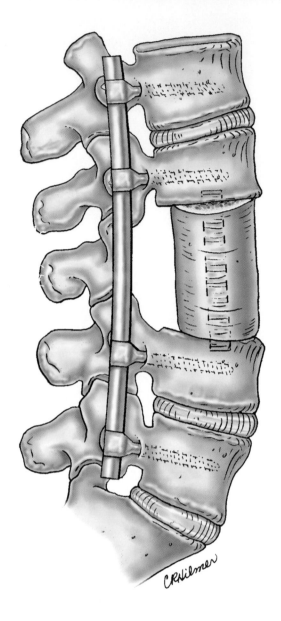

Figure 18.5 *contd*

E

Final construct.

Sacral tumors

The technique of resection of the sacrum varies with the amount of sacral involvement and the extent of soft tissue involvement. Tumors involving S3 and below can often be resected through a posterior approach alone. Involvement of either the proximal two segments or the entire sacrum need a combined approach. A posterior approach is performed for small sacral tumors distal to the S3 level not involving the rectum. The patient is given a thorough bowel preparation and is then placed in a modified knee–chest position to allow access to both the sacrum and the perineum. A purse string suture is placed around the anus. A midline incision is then used (Fig. 18.6A). This will allow total resection of the biopsy tract and distal extension to allow mobilization of the anus and rectum. Flaps superficial to the sacrospinalis muscles over the top of the iliac crest and out onto the surface of the gluteus are performed. The entire sacrum and coccyx are exposed. If the tumor has a significant posterior component, subcutaneous tissue may need to be left with the specimen. A gluteal based flap may then be rotated for coverage. If the tumor is predominantly anterior, the line of transection can be planned between the S2 and S3 dorsal foramina to include the terminal portion of the sacrospinalis musculature. Beginning at the terminal portion of the coccyx, the anus and rectum are mobilized by blunt dissection in the potential space in the presacral region. The anterior portion of the tumor can then be palpated. The dissection is further aided by mobilization of the gluteus maximus and piriformis muscles from the edge of the sacrum (Fig. 18.6 B). The sacrotuberous and sacrospinalis ligaments are transected to allow dissection of the rectum away from the tumor laterally and inferiorly. A laparotomy pad is placed between the rectum and the terminal portion of the sacrum to protect the rectum during the sacral osteotomy (Fig. 18.6C). The osteotomy can be either transverse or V-shaped; it should begin at the terminal portion of the sacroiliac joint. Transverse osteotomies are performed with a Gigli saw. V-shaped osteotomies must be performed with an osteotome (Fig. 18.6D). When the sacral canal is encountered, the distal nerve roots are divided and resected or the terminal tip of the dural sac can be ligated then transected. If the first two sacral segments are not involved, then no reconstruction is necessary. However, gluteal flaps may need to be advanced to fill in the significant dead space remaining.

Tumors involving the proximal portion of the sacrum or involving the entire sacrum require a combined anterior and posterior approach. The technique described by Stenner (Stenner and Gutenberg 1978) is the most commonly used approach. A permanent or temporary colostomy may be neces-

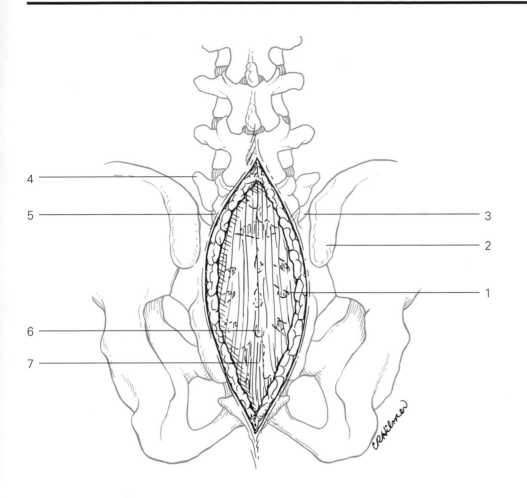

Figure 18.6

Sacral tumors.
A
The skin incision should be designed to include the biopsy tract and for excision of the tumor.

1 Dorsal sacral foramina
2 Post. sup. iliac spine
3 Sacral notch
4 Transverse process L5
5 L5–S1 facet joint
6 Median sacral notch
7 Lumbodorsal fascia

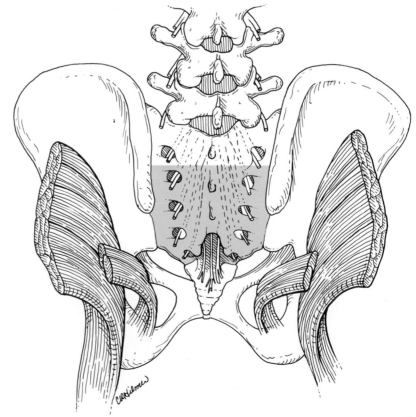

B
Posterior dissection with piriformis and gluteus maximus elevation.

Contd

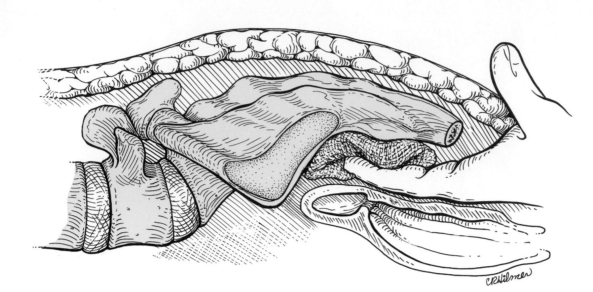

Figure 18.6 *contd*

C
A laparotomy pad can be placed to protect the rectum from perforation during the osteotomy.

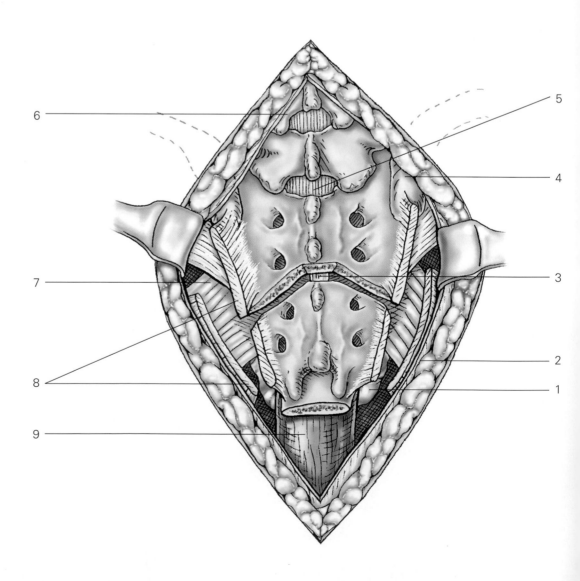

D
Osteotomy for tumor involving the distal sacrum.

1 Tumor
2 Fascia
3 Dura ligaments
4 Post. sup. iliac spine
5 L5–S1 interlaminal space
6 L4
7 Nerve roots
8 Resected sacral ligaments
9 Rectum

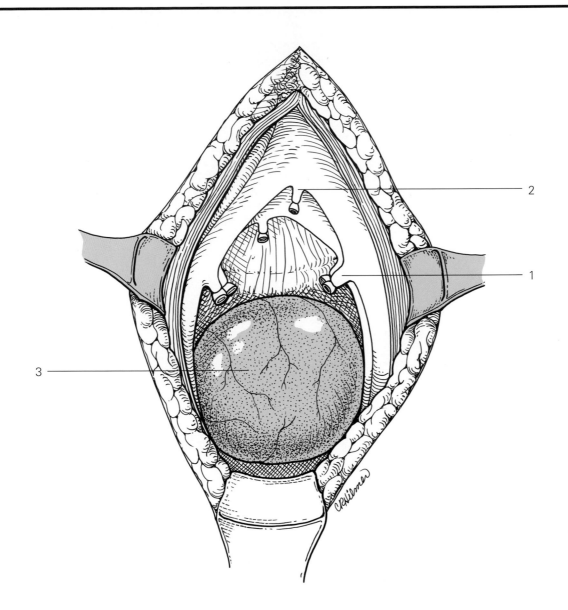

E
Anterior exposure with vessel ligation completed.

1 Int. iliac a. and v.
2 Middle sacral a. and v.
3 Tumor

Contd

sary for large tumors or tumors involving the rectum. This can be done preceding the anterior stage. The abdominal portion of the procedure is done first, with the patient in a supine position. A curvilinear or longitudinal incision can be used. An extraperitoneal or transperitoneal approach can be used for both the sacrum and the lower lumbar spine. Vessel mobilization begins at the level of the bifurcation of the aorta and vena cava. This is usually at the L4–5 disc level. Sacrifice of the internal iliac artery and vein along with the middle sacral vessels may be necessary (Fig. 18.6E). For a partial or total sacrectomy, the entire L5–S1 disc is removed with the exception of the posterior annulus. If the tumor is large, resection of the L5 body may be necessary. The L5 nerve roots are mobilized on both sides to allow exposure to the anterior portion of the sacral iliac joints. The anterior portion of the joint is divided. If segments distal to S1 or proximal to S3 are to be removed an osteotomy of the anterior cortex of the sacrum can be

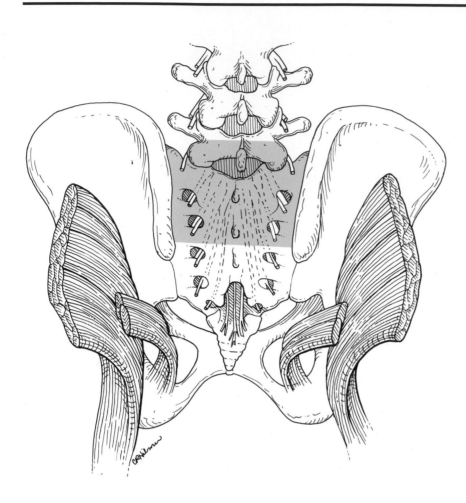

Figure 18.6 *contd*

F
Osteotomy for tumor involving the proximal sacrum.

G
Defect following osteotomy for tumor proximal to S3.

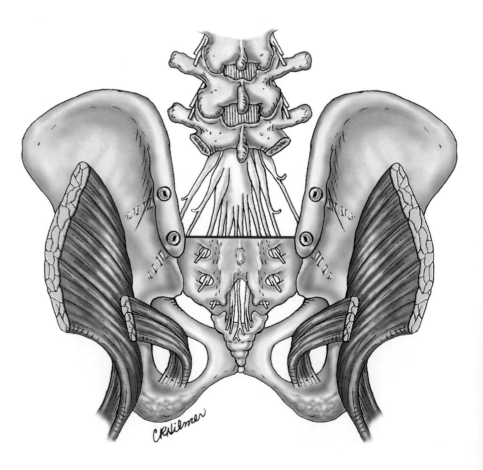

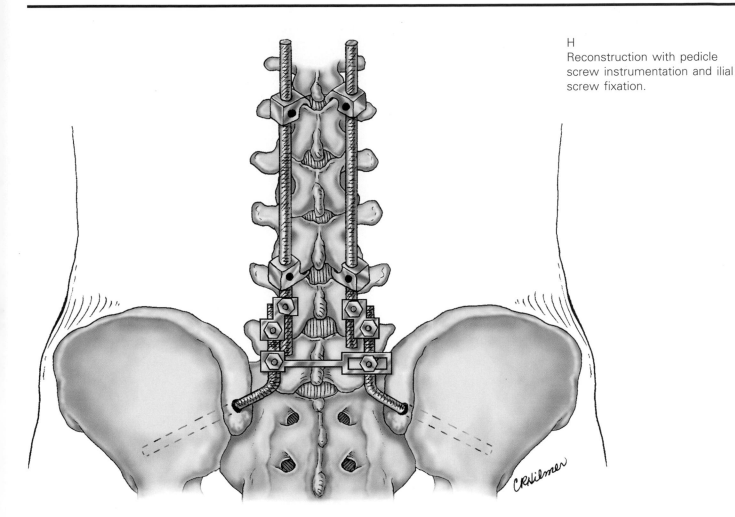

H
Reconstruction with pedicle screw instrumentation and ilial screw fixation.

performed. Before closure the sacroiliac joints are partially dissected and the proximal and distal margins of the sacral resection are established by removing the L5-S1 disc or by a sacral osteotomy. The sympathetic trunk and involved roots are divided as necessary. Several layers of laparotomy pads can be inserted between the body of the sacrum and the iliac vessels, visceral structures and lumbosacral roots before closure.

After closure of the anterior incision, the patient is placed in the prone position and a posterior midline incision is made from the base of the spinous process of L3 to the tip of the sacrum. The sacrospinalis musculature is stripped from caudal to rostral stopping at the lamina of L4 for tumors that involve the anterior portion of the sacrum. This allows exposure of the back of the sacrum and the lamina of L5. The gluteal muscles are then subperiosteally stripped from the outer side of the ilium, and the posterior iliac crest is osteotomized flush with the posterior aspect of the sacrum (Fig. 18.6F). This provides excellent exposure of the posterior aspect of the sacral iliac joint. If the entire sacrum or the upper two segments of the sacrum are to be resected, a partial L5 laminectomy is performed. The dural sac is

retracted and the posterior annulus of L5–S1 disc is completely removed. If the entire sacrum is to be removed, the dural sac is ligated and transected. If the upper segments alone are to be removed, a sacral laminectomy can be performed and a single S2 root can be sacrificed to allow space for removal of the resected sacral segment. If the S1 segment is to be preserved, a laminectomy is done in the sacral area to allow dural sac resection. The sacral joints are then divided using thin osteotomes. The ligaments of the terminal portion of the sacrum are then sectioned. The osteotomy is completed from posterior to anterior. The resected portion is then removed (Fig. 18.6G).

If the S1 segment is intact, no reconstruction is necessary. When the proximal two segments have been resected, the space can be allowed to settle and an allograft femoral shaft packed with morselized iliac crest can be inserted. Screw fixation is possible to the L5 body, but difficult to the S3 body because of the angle. This can be augmented by posterior fixation to prevent translation until healing occurs. Fixation to L5 and more cranially can be performed by using pedicle screw fixation and auxillary distal fixation into the ilium (Fig. 18.6H).

Bibliography

Bohlman HH, Sachs BH, Carter JR et al (1986) Primary neoplasms of the cervical spine. *J Bone Joint Surg*, **68A**:483

Fielding JW, Fietti VG, Hughes JEO et al (1996) Primary osteogenic sarcoma of the cervical spine. A case report. *J Bone Joint Surg*, **58A**:892

Guest C, Wong EHM, Davis A et al (1993) Paraspinal soft tissue sarcoma; classification of 14 cases. *Spine*, **18**:1292

Harrington KD (1988) Metastatic diseases of the spine. In Harrington KD (ed), *Orthopaedic Management of Metastatic Bone Disease*. St Louis: Mosby

Kaiser TE, Pritchard NJ, Unni KK (1984) Clinical pathologic studies of sacrococcygeal chordoma. *Cancer*, **54**:2574

Kibins NP, Noonan KJ, Weinstein WJN (1991) Chordoma of the lumbar spine. Surgical approach and rationale. *Contemp Orthop*, **22**:163

Levine AM (1992) Pathologic Fractures: Part I, Neoplasia. In Browner BD, Jupiter JB, Levine AM, Trafton PG (eds) *Skeletal Trauma*. Philadelphia:WB Saunders

Levine AM, Crandall DG (1997) Treatment of primary malignant tumors of the spine and sacrum. In Bridwell KH, DeWald RL (eds). *The Textbook of Spinal Surgery*. Philadelphia: Lippincott–Raven

Kawahara N, Tomita K, Baba H et al (1996) Cadaveric vascular anatomy for total en bloc spondylectomy in malignant vertebral tumors. *Spine*, **21**: 1401–7

Mankin HJ, Lang TM, Spanier S (1982) The hazards of biopsy in patients with malignant primary bone and soft tissue tumors. *J Bone Joint Surg*, **64A**:121

McCarty CS, Waugh JM, Mayo CW et al (1952) The surgical treatment of pre-sacral tumor. A combined problem. *Mayo Clin Proc*, **27**:73

Mindell ER (1981) Chordoma. *J Bone Joint Surg*, **63A**:501

Roy-Camille R, Mazel C (1991) Vertebrectomy through an enlarged posterior approach for tumor and malunion. In Bridwell K, DeWald R (eds) *Textbook of Spinal Surgery*. Philadelphia: JB Lippincott

Roy-Camille R, Saillent G, Gajna T et al (1988) Chondrosarcoma of the spine: ten cases treated surgically. *Orthop Trans*, **12**:201.

Samson IR, Springfield DS, Suit HD et al (1993) Operative treatment of sacrococcygeal chordoma. A review of 21 cases. *J Bone Joint Surg*, **75A**:1476

Shives TC, Dahlin DC, Sim FH et al (1986) Osteosarcoma of the spine. *J Bone Joint Surg*, **68A**:660

Stenner B (1978) Total spondylectomy in chondrosarcoma arising from the 7th thoracic vertebra. *J Bone Joint Surg*, **53B**:282

Stenner B (1989) Complete removal of vertebra for extirpation of tumors: a 20 year experience. *Clin Orthop*, **245**:72

Stenner B, Gutenberg B (1978) High amputation of the sacrum for extirpation of tumors: Principles and techniques. *Spine*, **3**:351

Sundaresan N, Huvos AG, Krol G et al (1989). Spinal chordoma: Results of surgical treatment. *Arch Surg*, **122**:1478

Weinstein JN, McClain RF (1987) Primary tumors of the spine. *Spine*, **12**:843

19

Osteotomies   John Kostuik

Introduction

Surgery for spinal deformity was first performed and reported by Smith-Peterson, Larson and Aufranc (1945). Since the initial description numerous techniques have been described, including modifications of the single level osteotomy with resection of the pedicles or part of the vertebral bodies in order to decrease the anterior angular height and multiple level osteotomies in the lumbar spine performed both anteriorly and posteriorly, staged or at a single sitting.

Indications

1. Flat back deformity, secondary to fusion to L5 or the sacrum in adult scoliosis
2. Flat back deformity secondary to segmental instrumentation for multiple level degenerative disease
3. Kyphosis secondary to ankylosing spondylitis
4. Frontal plane deformity in adult scoliosis.

The surgical treatment of ankylosing spondylitis

Introduction

With improvements in surgical techniques, anesthesia, internal fixation, and a better understanding of spinal biomechanics, the morbidity for surgery for ankylosing spondylitis has improved remarkably. The more typical deformity consists of a flat back as a result of loss of lumbar lordosis and an increased thoracic kyphosis. The deformities may vary in severity from mild to very severe. The head and neck tend to be thrust forward, and there may be an associated or separated flexion deformity at the cervical thoracic junction.

A severe deformity may result in considerable functional disability, including the inability to see the horizon, psychological disturbances and depression. The most common deformity occurs in the lumbar spine, followed by those of the thoracic and cervical spine respectively. The entire spine of the patient should be assessed radiographically to look for evidence of instability either at the occipital cervical, cervical, thoracic, or lumbar spine. In areas of spondylodiscitis any evidence of old fractures should be looked for. Flexion-extension radiographs of the cervical spine should be taken preoperatively to assess for any instability. The chin–brow to vertical angle should be measured with the neck in neutral position on a 3 foot standing radiograph in order to assess the patient's deformity. If there is any evidence of fracture or spondylodiscitis in the thoracic or lumbar spine, flexion-extension views should be obtained as well. The site of the primary deformity should be identified and, ideally, correction should be performed at this level. More recently, the distribution of corrective forces over multiple levels has been practiced both in the lumbar and thoracic spine.

At all times an examination of the hip joints is important, as they may be affected in ankylosing spondylitis, resulting in flexion deformities that may accentuate spinal deformity. Anesthetic problems may be significant owing to loss of chest motion, resulting in the postoperative inability to perform adequate respiratory toilet. Intubation as a result of difficulties related to the cervical spine, including cervical instability or problems with ankylosing of the temporomandibular joints, may also be encountered.

Spondyloarthropathies are often associated with ileitis or colitis that can lead to a compromised nutritional status. Significant osteopenia may compromise the use of internal fixation devices. Bone density should be determined preoperatively so that appropriate fixation and postoperative immobilization can be employed. Therefore it is important to assess pulmonary function, nutrition, and bone quality preoperatively in order to decrease morbidity.

Indications

To:
1. Correct posture
2. Relieve compression of abdominal viscera by rib margins
3. Improve diaphragmatic respiration (because of ankylosis of the costovertebral margins)
4. Broaden the operative field for upper abdominal surgery
5. Improve the patient's field of vision.

Surgical techniques

Smith-Peterson osteotomy

In the original description by Smith-Peterson of his osteotomy it was done with the patient in the prone position under general anesthesia. Adams (1952) and other surgeons preferred to perform surgery with the patients lying in the lateral decubitus position. Simmons (1972, 1977; Simmons and Duncan 1978) preferred to operate on patients with lumbar flexion deformities by performing a resection extension osteotomy under local anesthesia with sedation, and has proven this technique to be safe, reliable, and practical, although the majority of surgeons do continue to perform lumbar osteotomies under general anesthesia.

Spinal cord monitoring should be routinely used for osteotomies at any level of the spine. A nasogastric tube should be introduced, since the superior mesenteric artery may be stretched over the third part of the duodenum, with extension osteotomies resulting in gastric dilatation. The use of a radiolucent operating table facilitates the taking of intraoperative radiographs.

The chin–brow to vertical angle should be measured with the neck in neutral position on a 3 foot standing radiograph in order to assess the patient's deformity. This angle is then transposed to

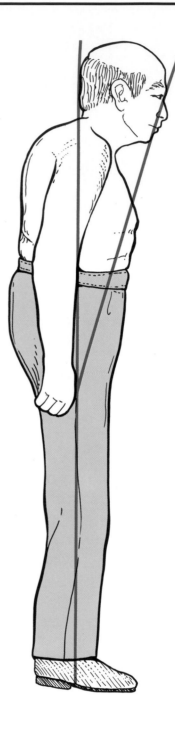

Figure 19.1

A

The chin–brow to vertical angle is measured with the neck in the neutral position, giving the angles shown.

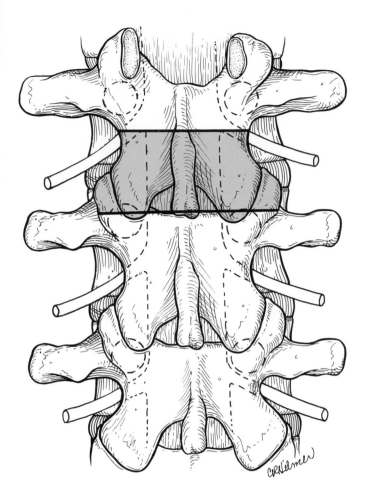

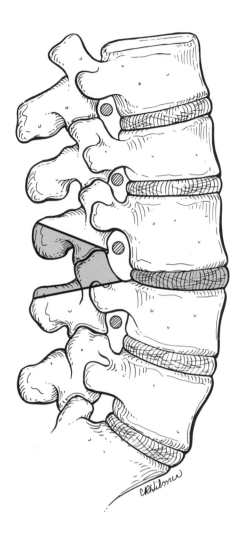

B
The chin–brow to vertical angle measurement is then transposed to the posterior margin of the L3–L4 disc space to determine the amount of bone to be resected.

C
The pars interarticularis and the inferior facet is removed along with parts of the spinous processes and lamina.

Contd

the level of the posterior longitudinal ligament of the L3–L4 disc space. The amount of bone to be resected can then be measured (Fig. 19.1 A, B). Since loss of lumbar lordosis is often associated with increased thoracic kyphosis in patients with ankylosing spondylitis, balance can only be achieved by overcorrecting the lumbar deformity in an attempt to restore the chin–brow to vertical angle to normal. Correction should be obtained so that the weightbearing line is shifted posteriorly to the osteotomy line. In this position, gravity aids in maintaining and possibly even

correcting further the deformity. This results also in increased compressive forces across the osteotomy site.

All bone removed at the site of the osteotomy should be preserved and replaced following closure of the osteotomy site for grafting purposes. Osteotomes or power burrs may be used to aid the osteotomy. The dural sac must be completely exposed bilaterally to the pedicles (Fig. 19.1 C, D). The laminae must be undercut to avoid dural impingement during extension of the spine. If the spinal canal has an

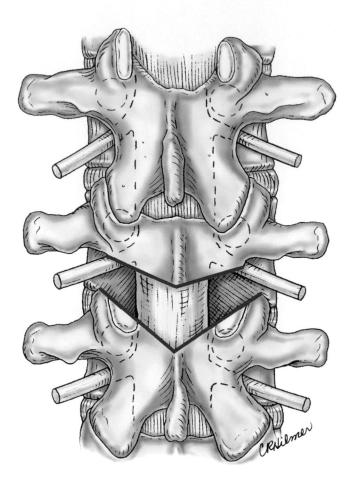

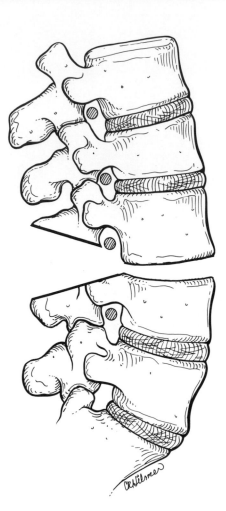

Figure 19.1 *contd*

D
A V-shaped osteotomy is performed to the level of the pedicles bilaterally. It is important to undercut the lamina to prevent dural impingement.

E
Lateral view following an osteotomy.

anterior–posterior dimension less than 20 mm, the posterior decompression must be generous, leaving an oval area open posteriorly for dural folding.

At the time of closure of the posterior osteotomy in the V-shaped wedge resection osteotomy, an anterior osteoclasis occurs (Fig. 19.1 E–G). This is possible only if the anterior disc spaces are fused. If this is performed under local anesthesia, as advocated by Simmons, short acting barbiturates are given just prior to manipulation. Osteoclasis is achieved by extension of the hips and pelvis while posterior

pressure is applied to the upper chest. Anterior pressure is applied at the level of the osteotomy by the surgeon. A distinct crack may be heard. Supplementary bone graft is not necessary posteriorly.

Manual osteoclasis may be difficult to achieve. In this case, the dura may be gently moved to one side and a thin osteotome passed anteriorly and the osteotomy performed first on one and then on the other side of the dural sac. This may not be sufficient, and then an open osteotomy must be performed anteriorly. This is more easily performed if the patient

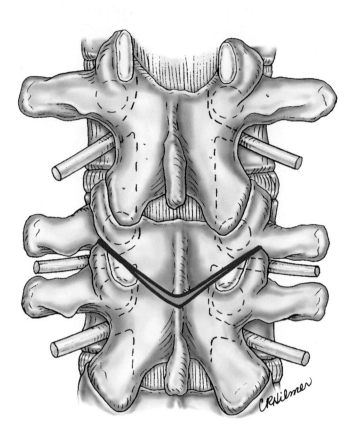

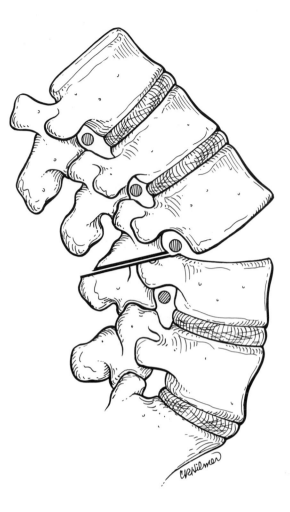

F
Anterior–posterior view following osteotomy closure. An oval area may be left open in the midline posteriorly to accommodate a dural folding if the anterior–posterior dimension preoperatively is less than 20 mm.

G
Lateral view following closure of the osteotomy.

is already in the lateral decubitus position and should be performed at the level of the posterior osteotomy. If this is done, bone graft may be placed at the open osteotomy site. If the patient is in the prone position, a supplemental posterolateral approach may be necessary, with removal of the pedicle on one side in order to weaken the anterior elements and allow for manual osteoclasis; or, at the very least, a decompression of the anterior part may be done via the pedicles.

Today either segmental instrumentation, either using four hooks, two bilaterally above and below, for a total of eight hooks, can be used; or screws are used for fixation.

Thomasen extension osteotomy

In 1985 Thomasen described a technique involving an osteotomy through the level of the vertebral body. This was felt to have less potential for stretching of the aorta, abdominal musculature and the cauda equina. The osteotomy begins with the resection of the laminae and transverse processes of L3 (Fig. 19.2A).

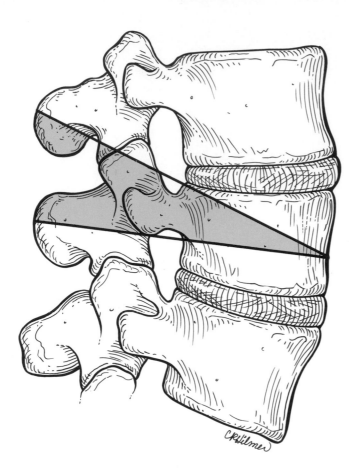 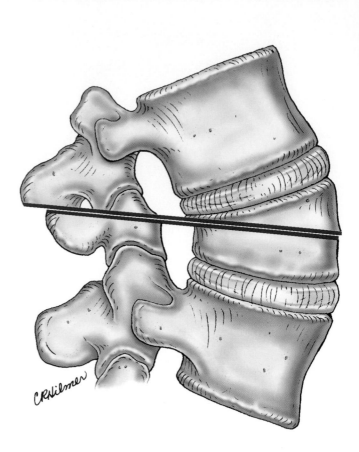

Figure 19.2

A
Osteotomy through the level of the vertebral body, as described by Thomasen (1985).

B
Osteotomy following closure.

The pedicles are subsequently removed as well as the upper part of the lamina of L3 and the articular processes of L3. The dura and spinal nerves on either side are left lying free. A narrow ronguer is introduced to remove bone in the midpoint of the vertebral body after removal of the pedicles. The side wall of the vertebral bodies and the immediate midline posterior aspect of osteo body are divided with a small osteotome. A good deal of hemorrhage may occur at this point. The patient is in the prone position and the wedge is slowly closed, followed by internal fixation (Fig. 19.2B).

Zielke technique

In 1982 Puschel and Zielke recommended multiple wedge osteotomies at three or more levels of the lumbar spine in order to reproduce lumbar lordosis. This technique is commonly used in iatrogenic flatback deformity from Harrington distraction instrumentation for scoliosis correction. Multiple partial laminectomies with extension across the pars inter-articularis following the intervertebral foramina in a V-shaped fashion are performed (Fig. 19.3). The laminae and foramen are undercut to minimize neural compres-

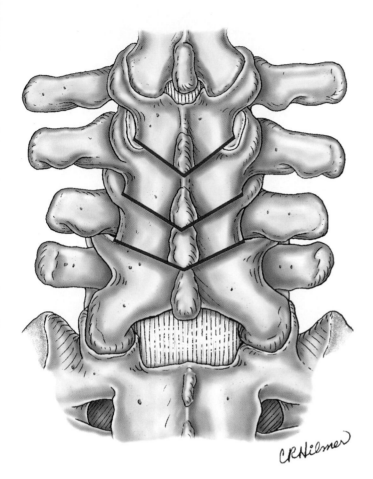

Figure 19.3

Multiple partial laminectomies with extension across the partes interarticulares should be performed in a V-shaped fashion.

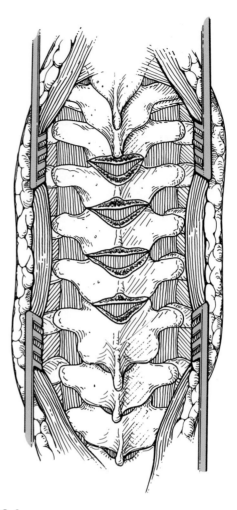

Figure 19.4

A

Multiple V-shaped resection osteotomies prior to instrumentation in the thoracic spine.

Contd

sion. Multiple level pedicle screws are used to close the osteotomy sites and restore lordosis. The use of multiple osteotomies and rigid internal fixation applied at multiple levels is a safe method of deformity reduction with minimal risk of neurological complications. The author prefers the use of multiple wedge osteotomies if the disc spaces are not fully ossified.

Thoracic osteotomy

Deformity is not usually corrected at this level because of the inherent neurological risks, although

kyphosis is always increased in the thoracic spine in ankylosing spondylitis. In the presence of an increased kyphosis of the thoracic spine associated with flattening of the lumbar spine, correction of the deformity is best achieved by performing an osteotomy in the midlumbar spine. This compensates for the thoracic kyphosis and sagittal balance can be restored. However, if the cervical and thoracic lordosis are relatively maintained and the deformity is primarily of a severe nature in the thoracic spine, then correction can be achieved in the thoracic spine through the use of multiple anterior and posterior osteotomies with

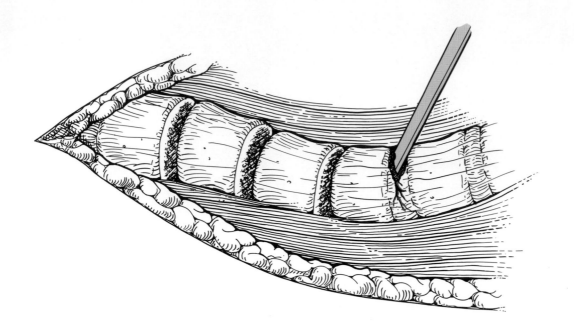

Figure 19.4 *contd*

B
An anterior approach and
anterior release may be
necessary as an initial stage.
Anterior osteotomies over
multiple levels allow
correction over a longer span
and minimize the chance of
an anterior osteotomy
propagating into the posterior
elements, resulting in
translation and spinal cord
injury.

C
Morselized bone grafts are
packed at the osteotomy
sites.

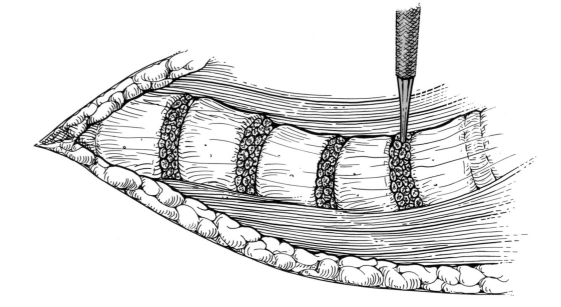

instrumentation and grafting. If there is incomplete
ossification or areas of spondylodiscitis, the correction
can be achieved first by halo dependent traction
followed by multiple posterior resection osteotomies
and instrumentation. A second stage anterior grafting
of the discitis area is then carried out using strut
grafts. If there is complete ossification anteriorly, then
osteotomies are required anteriorly. This may be
followed by a stage of halo dependent traction

followed by posterior multiple V-shaped resection
osteotomies with instrumentation (Fig. 19.4A). It may
be necessary to resect any ossified ligamentum
flavum.

The major risks of corrective osteotomies of the
thoracic spine are neurological. The contents of the
dural canal fill the bulk of the epidural space and at
this level the risk of neurological injury is high. More
recently, with improved techniques of segmental

fixation, this area has been approached more commonly. Correction is ideally achieved through multiple level osteotomies. If the disc spaces are fused anteriorly, then a first stage anterior release may be necessary (Fig. 19.4B). The anterior approach is best performed from a left thoracotomy position as described in a previous chapter. Approach through the fifth rib will allow access to T2 proximally and T12 distally. The left side is preferred, as the aorta protects the large venous structures on the righthand side from injury. Bleeding is likely to be more significant from a tear of the venous structures, which are harder to repair than possible injury to the aorta. Segmental vessels must be ligated or clipped in the midline of the vertebral bodies, and care must be taken to avoid cauterization in and around the neural foramina in order to avoid any damage to collateral circulation to the spinal cord.

Care must be taken to avoid concentration of forces at one level, as an anterior osteotomy may propagate into the posterior elements, resulting in complete fracture and possible translation with subsequent paralysis. The disc spaces should be cleansed out over as many areas as possible through a single thoracotomy approach (Fig. 19.4C). A second stage posterior procedure seven days or so later is carried out with multiple fixation, generally with the use of hooks. Segmental instrumentation is a preferable form of the fixation desired.

Eggshell procedure

This procedure can be used for rigid deformities involving one or two levels. It also allows decompression of the spinal canal through a posterior approach. This technique can be used in the thoracic, lumbar and thoracolumbar spine. The pedicle is used as a conduit to the anterior portion of the spine. The cancellous bone of the vertebral body is removed, creating an 'eggshell' of the remaining cortical bone of the vertebral body.

Once the appropriate level has been identified, the pedicle of that level is entered with progressively larger curets to create an access channel to the vertebral body for curets and pituitary rongeurs (Fig. 19.5A). The cancellous bone is then removed. If more medial access to the vertebral body is necessary, the lateral pedicle wall can be fractured to allow a more acute trajectory for instruments (Fig 19.5B).

If canal decompression is desired, as in the instance of a burst fracture with retropulsed bone, then the medial wall can be broached and retropulsed fragments can be forced anteriorly into the hollowed vertebral body. Once the desired amount of cancellous bone has been removed, the desired segmental fixation is applied. If an osteotomy is to be performed, then the lamina, pedicle and posterior wall of the

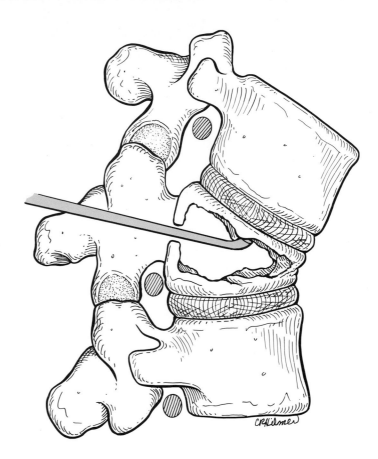

Figure 19.5

A

Transpedicular curretage is performed using curets and pituitary rongeurs.

Contd

vertebral body are removed and the lateral walls of the vertebral body are fractured or removed as necessary (Fig. 19.5C). The leading edge of the adjacent laminae may need to be removed to prevent impingement prior to deformity correction. Deformity correction is then performed using spinal monitoring (Fig. 19.5D). Segmental instrumentation is then assembled and bone grafting for fusion is performed.

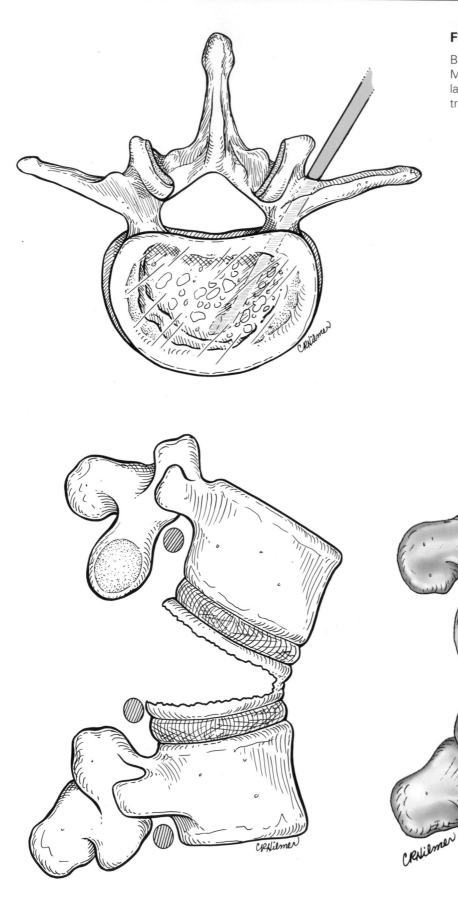

Figure 19.5 *contd*

B
Medial access can be facilitated by broaching the lateral pedicle wall to allow for a more medial trajectory for instruments.

C
Once bone resection is complete, correction should proceed after spinal instrumentation has been placed.

D
Lateral view following closure of osteotomy.

Lumbar lateral circumferential wedge osteotomy for frontal imbalance in scoliosis

Patients who are in imbalance more than 4 cm in the frontal plane may be difficult to rebalance using standard maneuvers for curve correction, particularly if the imbalance is secondary to a rigid compensatory lumbosacral curve. A similar problem exists with patients who have had a previous fusion in the lumbar or thoracolumbar spine and remained imbalanced 4 cm or more. The use of a lateral closing wedge circumferential lumbar osteotomy has been proven of value to correct such a deformity in the frontal plane.

The technique of lumbar circumferential lateral wedge osteotomy described attacks the deformity at its apex and, in those patients not previously operated upon, results in a solid fusion of the painful motion segments below their major deformity. This operation can be used to rebalance those patients who have significant pain in the major curve as well as the compensatory lumbosacral deformity where it is felt that correcting the major curve above will not suffice.

Surgical technique

Patients are operated on under general anesthetic. The apex of the deformity should lie over the break in the table to allow for reverse kidney positioning of the table to aid in closure of the osteotomy. The convexity of the curve faces upward.

A simultaneous anterior and posterior approach to the spine is taken. This is done by joining a posterior midline incision with a lateral flank incision (Fig. 19.6A). Where possible, hypertensive anesthesia is used together with infiltration with a weak solution (1:500,000) of epinephrine to control bleeding. The cell saver and spinal cord monitoring are also necessary.

After mobilization of the skin and flank musculature and subperiosteal dissection posteriorly, the transverse process at the level of the osteotomy on the convex side is removed, together usually with the more distal and proximal transverse processes. The neural foramina are then located. Anteriorly, the segmental vessels, preferably two levels proximal and two levels distal to the osteotomy site, are ligated.

The psoas muscle is then mobilized with its nerve roots. This is done by lifting the psoas off the affected vertebral bodies at the level of the osteotomy and one level distal and proximal. Broad rubber bands are passed around the psoas muscle with its contained nerve roots to help move the muscle.

The osteotomy is always performed below the conus medullaris. If there has been no previous

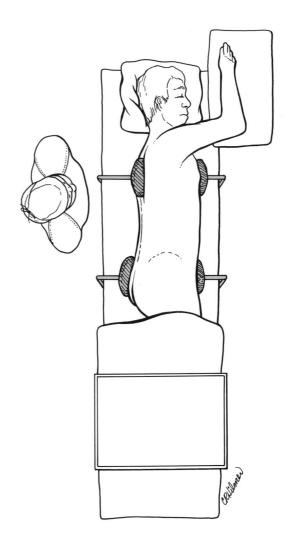

Figure 19.6

A

Patient positioning and incision.

anterior surgery, the appropriate disc at the apex of the deformity is removed. The endplate of the vertebral body interiorly is removed as well. The superior part of the vertebral body is removed on the basis of a preoperative calculation of the desired wedge to be removed.

The amount of wedge to be removed is based on calculation of pelvic obliquity, calculating the angle with the horizontal from the tops of the iliac crest and transposing that angle to the site of the proposed osteotomy in the spine (Fig. 19.6B). An intraoperative

Internal fixation is applied anteriorly in the bodies superiorly and inferiorly. If possible, pedicle screws are placed posteriorly. The osteotomy is then gradually closed by applying compression through each of the previously inserted rod–screw systems, together with flexing the operating table in reverse kidney fashion.

Following closure of the osteotomy, bone removed at the osteotomy site is applied posteriorly around the osteotomy site following pedaling of the fusion mass or laminae. Drainage tubes are placed in the retroperitoneal space and posteriorly.

Closure of the skin is preferably carried out with the use of interrupted nylon sutures, particularly at the junction of the flank wound and the posterior wound. Postoperatively, a rigid thoracolumbar spinal orthosis is used until healing occurs.

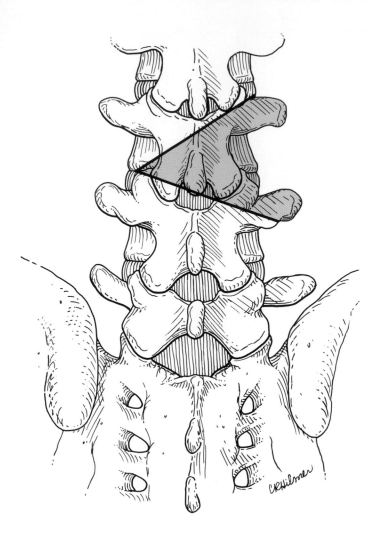

B

The amount of wedge is determined on the basis of a calculation of pelvic obliquity. This angle is transposed to the site of the proposed osteotomy, based laterally.

template or sterile goniometer is used to measure the angle.

The apex of the lateral V is based on the contralateral both anteriorly and posteriorly. If a previous anterior fusion has been done as well as a posterior fusion, then the osteotomy is carried through the site of a previous disc space. Epidural bleeding and bone bleeding is controlled by the use of thrombin-soaked sponges and large patties.

Bibliography

Adams JC (1952) Technique, dangers and safeguards in osteotomy of spine. *J Bone Joint Surg* (Br), **34**:226–32

Amamilo SC (1989) Fractures of the cervical spine in patients with ankylosing spondylitis. *Orthop Review*, **18**:339–44

Briggs H, Keats S, Schlesinger PT (1947) Wedge osteotomy of the spine with bilateral intervertebral foraminotomy: Correction of flexion deformity in five cases of ankylosing arthritis of the spine. *J Bone Joint Surg*, **29**:1075–82

Emneus H (1968) Wedge osteotomy of spine in ankylosing spondylitis. *Acta Orthop Scand*, **39**:321–6

Goel MK (1968) Vertebral osteotomy for correction of fixed flexion deformity of the spine. *J Bone Joint Surg* (Am), **50**:287–94

Graham B, Van Peteghem PK (1989) Fractures of the spine in ankylosing spondylitis. Diagnosis, treatment, and complications. *Spine*, **14**(8):803–7

Herbert JJ (1959) Vertebral osteotomy for kyphosis, especially in Marie–Strumpell Arthritis. *J Bone Joint Surg* (Am), **41**:291–302

Huaux JP, Lokietek W, Vincent A et al (1986) Place des traitements orthopédiques et chirurgicaux dans les ankyloses rachidiennes, les fractures et pseudarthroses vertébrales de la spondylarthrite ankylosante. *Acta Orthop Belg*, **52**:771–91

Jarfray D, Becker V, Eisenstein S (1992) Closing wedge osteotomy with transpedicular fixation in ankylosing spondylitis. *Clin Orthop*, **279**:122–6

LaChapelle EH (1946) Osteotomy of the lumbar spine for correction of kyphosis in a case of ankylosing spondylarthritis. *J Bone Joint Surg*, **28**:851–8

Law WA (1952) Surgical treatment of the rheumatic diseases. *J Bone Joint Surg* (Br), **34**:215–25

Law WA (1959) Lumbar spinal osteotomy. *J Bone Joint Surg* (Br), **41**:270–8

Law WA (1962) Osteotomy of the spine. *J Bone Joint Surg* (Am), **44**:1199–1206

Law WA (1969) Osteotomy of the spine. *Clin Orthop*, **66**:70–6

Lichtblau PA, Wilson PD (1956) Possible mechanism of aortic rupture in orthopaedic correction of rheumatoid spondylitis. *J Bone Joint Surg* (Am), **38**:123–7

McMaster PE (1962) Osteotomy of the spine for fixed flexion deformity. *J Bone Joint Surg* (Am), **44**:1207–16

McMaster MJ (1985) A technique for lumbar spinal osteotomy in ankylosing spondylitis. *J Bone Joint Surg* (Br), **67**:204–10

McMaster MJ, Coventry MB (1973) Spinal osteotomy in ankylosing spondylitis. Technique, complications and long-term results. *Mayo Clin Proc*, **48**:476–86

Mehdian H, Jarfray D, Eisenstein S (1992) Correction of severe cervical kyphosis in ankylosing spondylitis by traction. *Spine*, **17**(2):237–40

Pastershank SP, Resnick D (1980) Pseudoarthrosis in ankylosing spondylitis. *J Can Assoc Radiol*, **31**:234–5

Podolsky SM, Hoffman JR, Pietrafesa CA (1983) Neurologic complications following immobilization of cervical spine fracture in a patient with ankylosing spondylitis. *Ann Emerg Med*, **12**:578–80

Puschel J, Zielke K (1982) Korrekturoperation bei Bechterew-Kyphose Indikation, Technik, Ergebnisse. *Z Orthop*, **120**:338–42

Roy-Camille R, Henry P, Saillant G et al (1987) Chirurgie des grandes cyphoses vertebrales de la spondylarthrite ankylosante. *Rev Rhum*, **54**(3):261–7

Scudes VA, Calabro JJ (1963) Vertebral wedge osteotomy. Correction of rheumatoid (ankylosing) spondylitis. *JAMA*, **186**:627–31

Simmons EH (1972) The surgical correction of flexion deformity of the cervical spine in ankylosing spondylitis. *Clin Orthop*, **86**:132–43

Simmons EH (1977) Kyphotic deformity of the spine in ankylosing spondylitis. *Clin Orthop*, **128**:65–77

Simmons EH, Duncan CP (1978) Fracture of the cervical spine in ankylosing spondylitis – an analysis of its influence on severe deformity presenting for spinal osteotomy. *Clin Orthop*, **133**:277

Smith-Peterson MN, Larson CB, Aufranc OE (1945) Osteotomy of the spine for correction of flexion deformity in rheumatoid arthritis. *J Bone Joint Surg*, **27**:1–11

Styblo K, Bossers GTM, Slot GH (1985) Osteotomy for kyphosis in ankylosing spondylitis. *Acta Orthop Scand*, **56**:294–7

Surin VV (1980) Fractures of the cervical spine in patients with ankylosing spondylitis. *Acta Orthop Scand*, **51**:79–84

Thiranont N, Netrawichien P (1993) Transpedicular decancellation closed wedge vertebral osteotomy for treatment of fixed flexion deformity of spine in ankylosing spondylitis. *Spine*, **18**(16):2517–22

Thomasen E (1985) Vertebral osteotomy for correction of kyphosis in ankylosing spondylitis. *Clin Orthop*, **194**:142–6

Thorngren KG, Liedgerg E, Espelin P (1981) Fractures of the thoracic and lumbar spine in ankylosing spondylitis. *Arch Orthop Trauma Surg*, **98**:101–7

Urist MR (1958) Osteotomy of the cervical spine: Report of a case of ankylosing rheumatoid spondylitis. *J Bone Joint Surg* (Am), **40**:833–43

20

Percutaneous techniques and minimally invasive procedures

Howard S An

Introduction

Percutaneous procedures of the spine have been performed for several decades. Development of specialized needles and the availability of sophisticated imaging techniques have allowed percutaneous procedures to be performed at virtually every level of the spine. These percutaneous procedures have evolved from the biopsy technique in the diagnosis of neoplastic or infectious lesions to various therapeutic procedures. Success rates for percutaneous spine biopsy are variable depending on the technique utilized, types of lesion, the level being biopsied, and the experience of the surgeon. Percutaneous procedures are basically 'blind surgical techniques' even under imaging guidance, and therefore great caution should be taken in every step of the procedure to avoid injuries to vital structures.

Indications for biopsy

1. Presumed neoplasm in which treatment cannot be rendered without tissue diagnosis (i.e., metastatic carcinoma, primary malignant tumors, etc.)
2. Presumed discitis or osteomyelitis in which the offending organism is not known.

Techniques of biopsy

The patient should be thoroughly evaluated prior to biopsy. In addition to thorough history and physical examination, laboratory workup should include a Complete Blood Count, coagulation screen, and other appropriate tests. The radiographs, radionuclide bone scans, computerized tomography (CT) or magnetic resonance imaging should be reviewed to determine the best biopsy site. The selection of the type of needle depends on the types of lesion. For discitis or vertebral osteomyelitis, a 20 or 22 gauge needle is utilized for aspiration and tissue biopsy. For bony lesions, a 16 or 18 gauge needle is needed to perforate the outer cortex, and a larger Craig needle set may be utilized for larger samples of tissue.

Cervical spine biopsy

Biopsy of the posterior elements of the cervical spine is relatively straightforward. Either CT or fluoroscopy guided biopsy can be used for biopsy. Vertebral body lesions are more difficult and fraught with potential complications.

Vertebral body lesions of the upper three cervical vertebrae are approached most readily by the transoral approach (Fig. 20.1A). The body of C2 lies directly behind the mouth, and the C3 body lies at the level of the epiglottis. The transoral approach can reach the C1 vertebra by retracting the soft palate, and the C3 body can be approached by depressing the tongue.

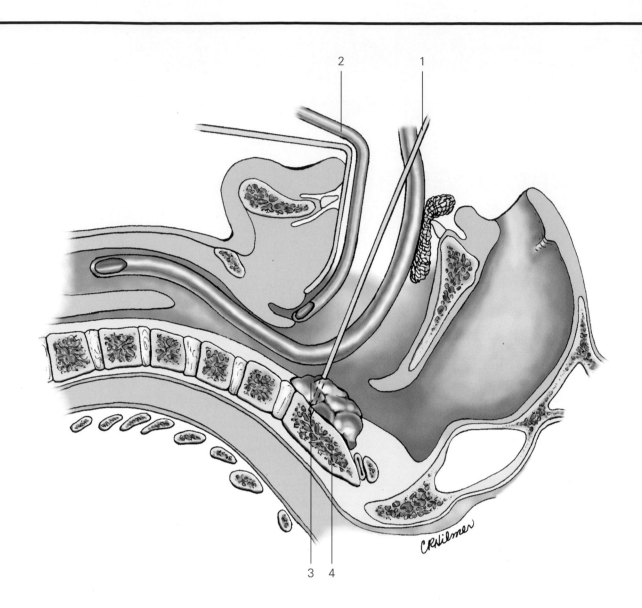

Figure 20.1

Biopsy procedures of the spine.

A
Transoral biopsy of the upper cervical spine.

1 Endotracheal tube
2 Suction
3 Abscess
4 C2

Biopsy may be carried out using an aspiration needle, as advocated by Ottolenghi and associates (1964). Complications may include an inadequate sample of tissue, vertebral artery injury, venous bleeding, pharyngeal edema, infection, dural puncture, and meningitis. All patients should be observed for pharyngeal edema and respiratory difficulty in the postoperative period. Antibiotics should cover the organisms in the oral flora in the perioperative period.

Percutaneous biopsy of the lower cervical vertebrae may be approached posterior or anterior to the sternocleidomastoid muscle (Fig. 20.1B). Prebiopsy imaging studies should determine which route is more likely to be successful and safer. For the lateral approach, the needle is inserted posterior to the sternocleidomastoid muscle and enters the vertebral body from the lateral aspect. The needle should not extend too far, to avoid injury to the esophagus. Alternatively, the needle may be inserted anterior to the sternocleidomastoid

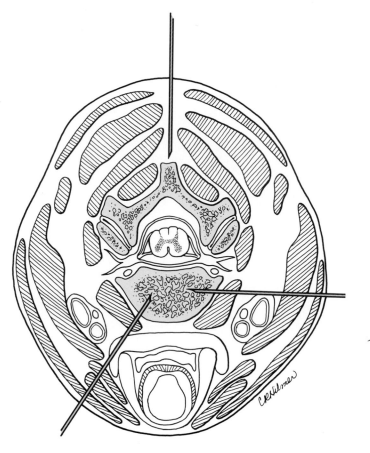

B
Lesions in the spinous process or lamina may be approached posteriorly. Lesions in the vertebral body can be approached laterally posterior to the carotid content or anterolaterally anterior to the carotid content.

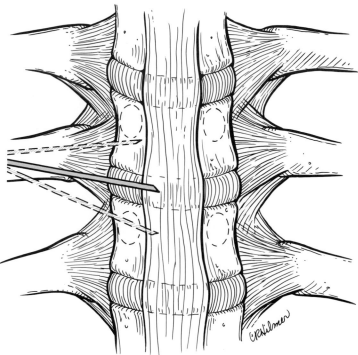

C
The thoracic spine is approached posterolaterally, and the biopsy needle may be directed to enter the disc or vertebral body above or below.

Contd

muscle. The sternocleidomastoid muscle and carotid contents are retracted laterally, and the needle is introduced to the anterolateral aspect of the vertebral body. The possible complications include injuries to the carotid contents, recurrent laryngeal nerves, thyroid vessels, esophagus, nerve root, and spinal cord. Because of these risks of percutaneous biopsy of the cervical spine, the use of CT-guided biopsy or open biopsy is preferred in the majority of cases.

Thoracic spine biopsy

Percutaneous biopsy of the thoracic spine may be done under fluoroscopy, but the CT-guided technique is preferred. The needle should be inserted about 4 cm from the midline. The angle of insertion is 35° and angled slightly cephalad or caudad depending on the

location of the lesion (Fig. 20.1C). Alternatively, transpedicular thoracic biopsy may be performed. The entry point is more medial and the angle of insertion is less than in the posterolateral technique. Great caution should be taken to avoid medial penetration of the pedicle. Penetration of the pedicle laterally is less dangerous, but may cause significant bleeding if segmental vessels are injured. A small-bore aspiration needle is preferred over the larger Craig needle in the thoracic spine. The most common complication of thoracic spine biopsy is pneumothorax. The use of CT-guided biopsy has reduced the incidence of this complication.

Lumbar spine biopsy

The larger lumbar vertebrae lend themselves to percutaneous procedures. Percutaneous biopsies of the

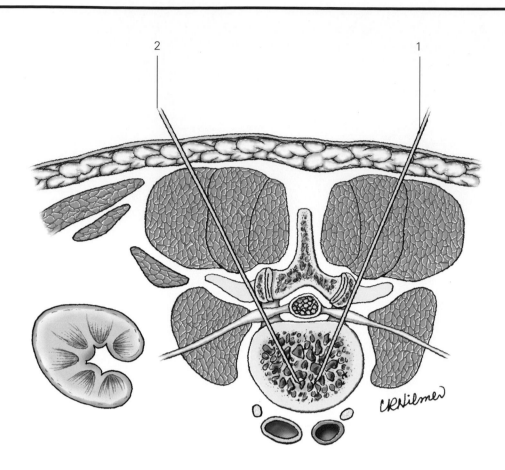

Figure 20.1 *contd*

D

The vertebral body of the lumbar spine can be approached
posterolaterally or through the pedicle as shown.

1 Transpedicular
2 Posterolateral

vertebral body or intervertebral disc may be
performed under fluoroscopy or CT. Percutaneous
transpedicular procedures of the lumbar spine are
safer than those of the thoracic spine.

For the percutaneous biopsy procedure, the patient
is placed in the prone position. The entry position is
about 6–7 cm from the midline and the direction of
the needle is approximately 45° for the posterolateral
approach (Fig. 20.1D). The transpedicular approach
enters more medially and is directed more vertically
(Fig. 20.1D). After local anesthesia, a long 22 gauge
needle is guided fluoroscopically to the vertebral
body. If the patient should report radicular pain or
sensations during insertion of the needle, it must be
redirected to avoid injury to the nerve root. After
confirming the correct placement of the needle on
both AP and lateral planes, the trocar of the Craig
needle is advanced in the same path. When the
position of the trocar is satisfactory, the cannula is
advanced over the trocar and held firmly against the
vertebral body. The trocar is removed, and the inner
trephine needle is advanced for biopsy.

Percutaneous lumbar discectomy

In recent years, significant advances have been made
in minimally invasive surgery, particularly in percutaneous lumbar discectomy procedures. There are
numerous techniques available, and results vary
depending on different series. The success of lumbar
disc surgery is mainly dependent on patient selection.
The indications for the percutaneous procedures
should be the same as for the open procedure. The
surgical patient should have persistent radiculopathy
with tension signs or neurologic deficits, a positive
neuroimaging study that correlates clinically, and have
failed an appropriate course of conservative treatment
for at least 6 weeks. It should be realized that the
percutaneous procedures have less predictable clinical results, and extruded or sequestered herniated
discs are not amenable to percutaneous procedures
unless the technique involves endoscopic visualization of the extruded fragment.

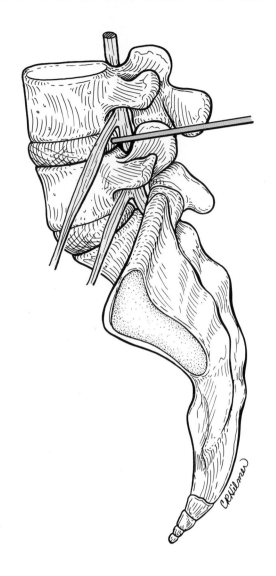

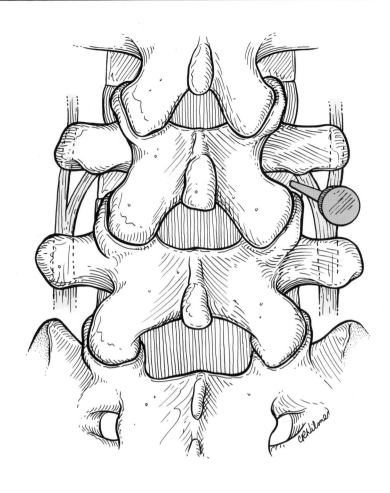

Figure 20.2

Percutaneous techniques involving the lower lumbar discs.

A
The triangular working zone is bordered by the thecal sac medially, the exiting root laterally, and the endplate inferiorly.

B
The AP view shows the needle position just lateral to the superior facet and medial to the exiting nerve root.

Contd

The most common surgical technique used is the posterolateral approach to the triangular working zone (Fig. 20.2A,B). This zone is the site of surgical access used in discography, automated nucleotomy, and arthroscopic or endoscopic discectomy. It is anatomically described as a right triangle over the dorsolateral aspect of the intervertebral disc whose hypotenuse is formed by the spinal nerve, with its base (width) defined by the horizontal superior border of the next inferior vertebral body. The height of the triangle, which runs parallel to the axis of the

vertebral column, is formed by the structure dorsal to the intervertebral foramen, and its superior angle is formed by the axilla of the exiting nerve. The exiting nerve is consistently at 40°, and the dimensions of this triangular working zone are 18.9 mm in width, 12.5 mm in height, and 23 mm for the hypotenuse (Fig. 20.2A,B). The size of needle and cannula should not exceed these dimensions.

The patient is positioned prone or in lateral decubitus. The entry point is 8–11 cm from the midline. The needle is advanced to the annulus fibrosus under

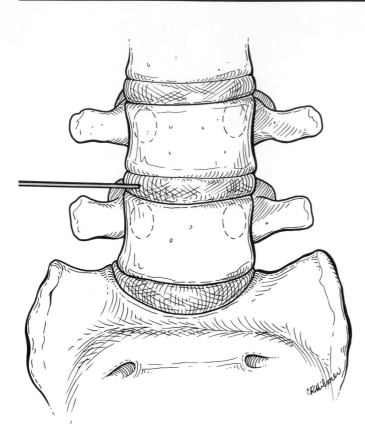

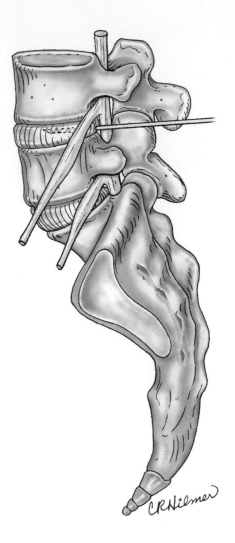

Figure 20.2 *contd*

C
The anteroposterior view shows that the needle has penetrated to the annulus fibrosus and advanced to a level corresponding to the middle of the pedicle.

D
Following radiographic confirmation in both anteroposterior and lateral planes, the needle is advanced to the middle of the intervertebral disc.

fluoroscopic control. The tip of the needle should be seen at the midpedicular line in the anteroposterior view (Fig. 20.2C), and the tip should be in line with the posterior border of the adjacent vertebral bodies. Following radiographic confirmation in both antero-posterior and lateral planes, the needle is advanced to the middle of the intervertebral disc (Fig. 20.2D). For the discectomy procedure, the needle has the stylet, which can be interchanged with a guide wire for obturator and cannula insertions. Uniportal or bipor-tal techniques are reported along with various endoscopic systems (Fig. 20.2E).

The entry into the L5–S1 disc is more difficult because the iliac crest is too high and the angle between the posterior rim of the iliac bone and the lumbar vertebral column is too acute. Furthermore, in males the iliac crest tends to be positioned more medially, making access to the L5–S1 level more difficult. The angle of trajectory should be about 10–12 cm from the midline at the level of L4–5 disc and directed medially and caudad toward the L5–S1 disc (Fig. 20.2F,G). The approach to the L5–S1 disc may be aided by a curved needle (Fig. 20.2H).

The posterolateral approach may be used to perform arthroscopic or percutaneous fusion. The interverte-

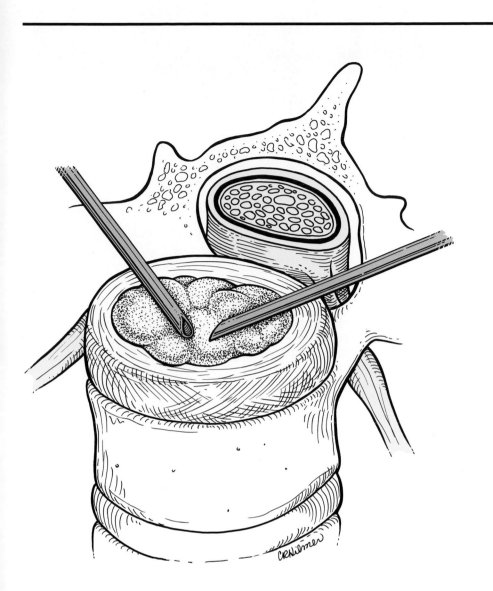

E
For the discectomy procedure, the needle has the stylet, which can be interchanged with a guide wire for obturator and cannula insertions. Biportal technique is illustrated.

F
The entry into the L5–S1 disc is more difficult because of the high riding iliac crest. The angle of trajectory should be about 10–12 cm from the midline at the level of the L4–5 disc and directed medially and caudad toward the L5–S1 disc.

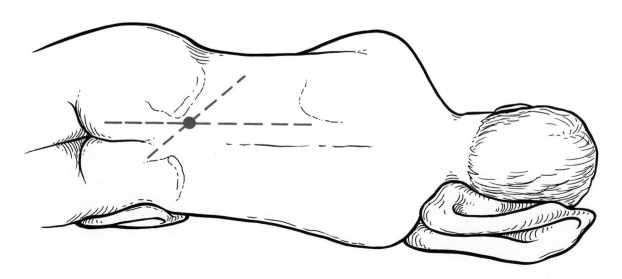

Contd

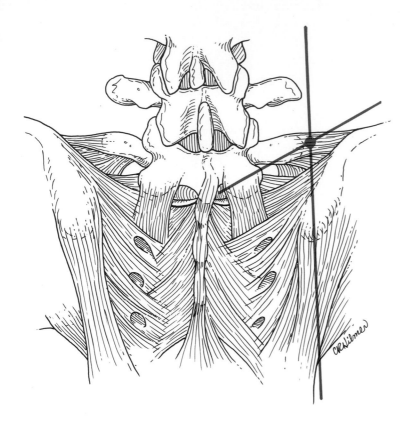

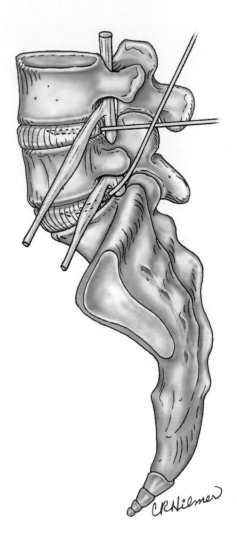

Figure 20.2 *contd*

G
The L5–S1 disc is approached by angulating the needle distally.

H
Approach to the L5–S1 disc may be aided by a curved needle.

bral foramen may be approached using the endoscopic technique. The trocar is directed more horizontally toward the epidural space from the foramen. This approach may allow for removal of extruded disc fragments, but the nerve root is more likely to be injured and epidural bleeding may be problematic.

improve shoulder girdle function early as compared to formal thoracotomy procedures. These video thoracoscopic surgery techniques have been applied to treat multiple diseases of the thoracic spine such as disc herniation, vertebral abscesses, tumors, fractures and spinal deformities.

Thoracoscopic spinal procedures

Thoracoscopic diagnostic procedures have been utilized for over eighty years, and in recent years, more complex therapeutic procedures have been performed by the thoracic surgeon. Thoracoscopic procedures can reduce postoperative pain, minimize respiratory difficulties, shorten hospital stays, and

Indications

1. Disc herniation
2. Vertebral abscess
3. Spinal tumors
4. Spinal fractures
5. Spinal deformities.

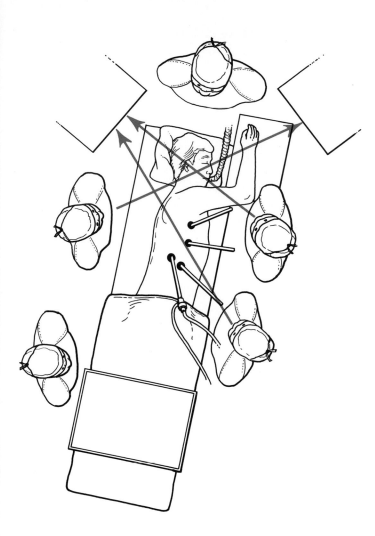

Figure 20.3

Thoracoscopic procedures.

A
Operating room setup for the thoracoscopic spinal
procedures. The surgeon and the assistant should view
separate monitors.

B
The thoracoscope is usually placed in the midaxillary line over
the sixth intercostal space. Working ports are then placed in
the posterior axillary line and higher in the midaxillary line. A
fan retractor may be placed through a separate portal to
retract the lung. The ports can be interchanged for
thoracoscope or instruments as necessary.

Contd

Surgical techniques

General anesthesia with a double lumen intubation is
recommended. The patient is placed in a lateral
position, and the ipsilateral lung is collapsed. The table
is also flexed to widen the intercostal spaces. The
entire chest should be prepped to allow conversion to
an open thoracotomy should the need arise during the
procedure. The surgeon and the assistant should view
separate monitors (Fig. 20.3A). Typically a 1 cm
incision is made in the midaxillary line over the sixth
intercostal space (Fig. 20.3B). The skin and the intercostal muscles are spread using a hemostat. Blunt
dissection with a finger creates an opening into the
pleural space. Any pleural adhesions should be released
prior to insertion of the trocar. A 1 cm trocar is placed

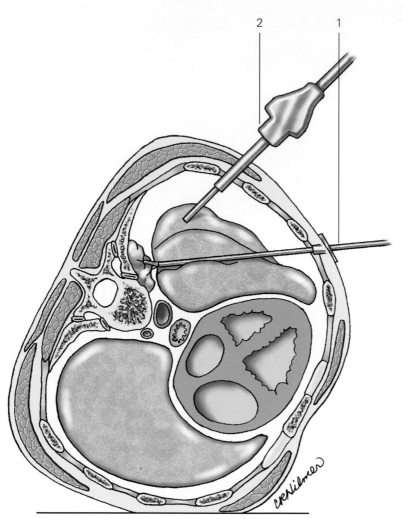

Figure 20.3 *contd*

C
Gravity, by the Trendelenburg or reverse Trendelenburg position, or tilting the table forward, can also enhance retraction of the lung.

1 Instrument
2 Camera

D
The upper thoracic region and lower thoracic region can be approached thoracoscopically by placing the portals at higher levels.

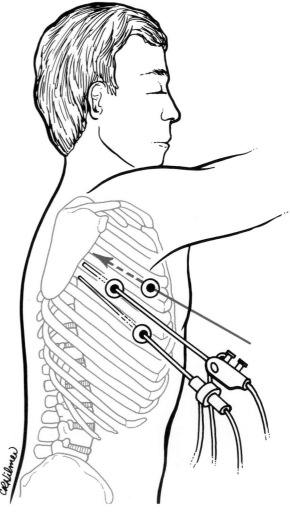

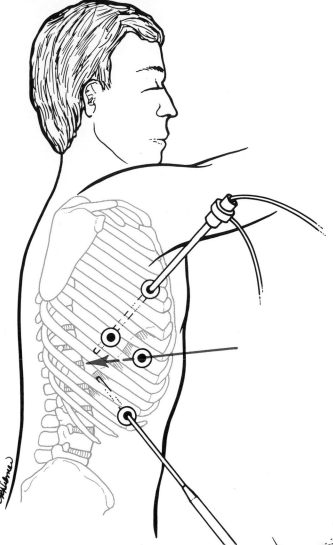

E

The lower thoracic region is more difficult to approach owing to the presence of the diaphragm, but it is possible to expose the lower thoracic region through lower portals and partially detaching the diaphragm.

F

The anatomy of thoracoscopic exposure includes ribs, segmental vessels, sympathetic chain, vertebral body, intervertebral discs and great vessels.

1 Intervertebral disc
2 Sympathetic chain
3 Rib
4 Vertebral body
5 Segmental vessels

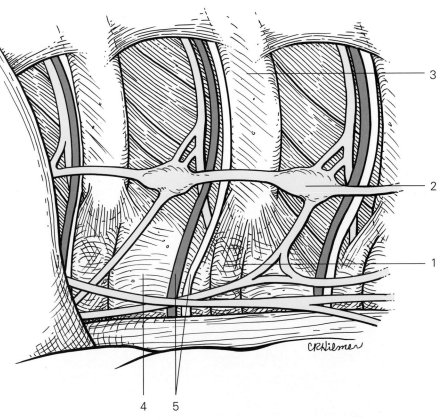

Contd

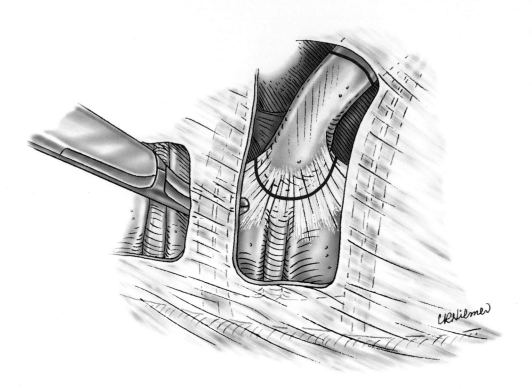

Figure 20.3 *contd*

G
Following division of the pleura, the segmental vessels are mobilized, clipped and ligated.

H
For the purpose of thoracic discectomy and spinal cord decompression, the rib head is removed. An endoscopic power burr may be used to cut the rib head.

1 Costovertebral articulation

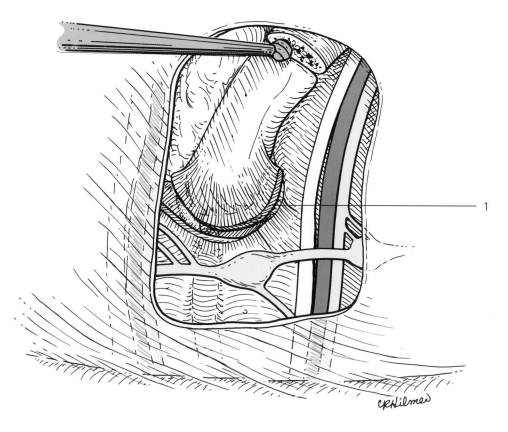

1

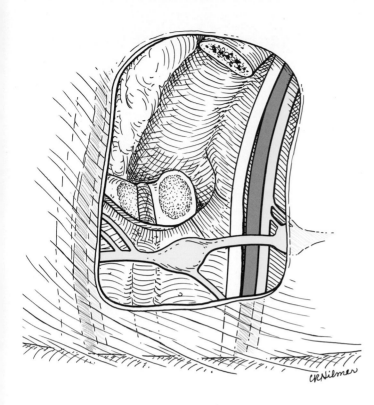

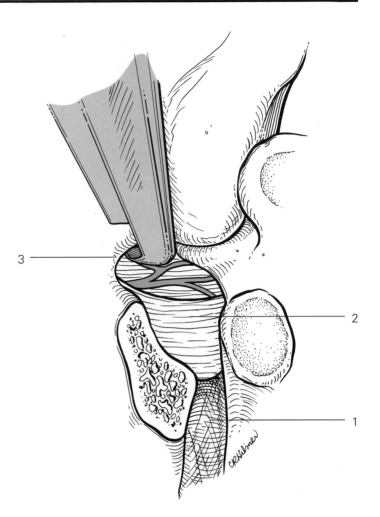

I

A 3 cm piece of the rib is removed by dividing the costovertebral and costotransverse ligaments and cutting the rib.

J

The superior portion of the pedicle is then removed to expose the lateral aspect of the thecal sac.

1 Disc
2 Dura
3 Pedicle

Contd

through the intercostal opening for insertion of the thoracoscope into the chest cavity. Placement of the initial trocar is variable, depending on the level of the thoracic spine to be accessed. A 1 cm rigid 30° angled scope is placed, and exploratory thoracoscopy is then performed. In those patients in whom complete resorptive atelectasis and lung collapse does not occur, temporary CO_2 insufflation can expedite and enhance collapse for better visualization. Gravity with the position Trendelenburg or reverse Trendelenburg or tilting the table forward can also enhance retraction of the lung (Fig. 20.3C). Working ports are then placed in the posterior axillary line and higher in the anterior axillary line. A fan retractor may be placed through a separate portal to retract the lung. The upper thoracic region and lower thoracic region can be approached thoracoscopically by placing the portals at appropriate levels (Fig. 20.3D,E).

Once the thoracic spine is visualized through the parietal pleura, the correct level is ascertained by counting the ribs as well as through a radiograph with a laparoscopic needle placed into the disc space. The pleura is divided over the spine to be exposed (Fig. 20.3F). Thoracoscopic electrocautery is used to divide the pleura. The segmental vessels are mobilized, clipped, and ligated (Fig. 20.3G). For spinal cord decom-

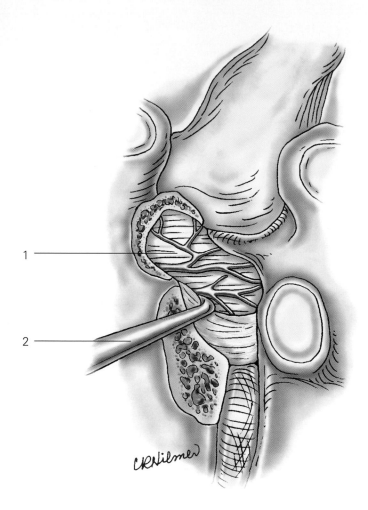

Figure 20.3 *contd*

K
Discectomy is completed by removing the herniated disc away from the thecal sac.

1 Dura
2 Angled curet

pression in thoracic herniated disc cases, rib osteotomy is first performed (Fig. 20.3H). A 3 cm piece of the rib is removed by dividing the costovertebral and costotransverse ligaments and cutting the rib (Fig 20.3I). The superior portion of the pedicle is then removed to expose the lateral aspect of the thecal sac (Fig. 20.3J). Discectomy is completed by removing the herniated disc away from the thecal sac (Fig. 20.3K). In addition to discectomy, other procedures such as corpectomy, fusion, and even instrumentation may be performed through this thoracoscopic approach.

Laparoscopic procedures of the lumbar spine

Laparoscopic procedures are common in general surgery, but laparoscopic lumbar spinal surgery is relatively new. The lower lumbar discs may be excised and fused through the laparoscopic technique, and it may be advantageous in preventing the posterior muscular dissection and fibrosis associated with posterior fusion procedures. The upper lumbar spine may also be approached with an expandable balloon that dilates the potential retroperitoneal space. The technique of laparoscopic spinal surgery is exacting, and complications may be devastating. Furthermore, the long-term results of laparoscopic spinal procedures are not available, and strict indications for these procedures should be followed.

Indications

1. Disc herniation or degenerative disc disease
2. Intervertebral discitis.

Surgical techniques

The patient is supine in a 20–30° Trendelenburg position on the radiolucent table with a C-arm fluoroscope ready (Fig. 20.4A,B). Lumbar lordosis should be maintained, and draping is done widely. Necessary equipment includes CO_2 insufflation, a 30° endoscope, laparoscopic trocars with adapters. The first portal is typically placed at the umbilicus (Fig. 20.4C). The incision is made with direct visualization, and CO_2 insufflation to 15 mmHg is maintained. The 30° scope is safely entered. Working portals are lateral to the epigastric vessel. The left trocar is used to mobilize the sigmoid colon from right to left, and two right-sided trocars are inserted in such a way as to avoid instrument crowding (Fig. 20.4D).

The dissection proceeds with monopolar endoshears to incise the peritoneum along reflection (Fig. 20.4E). The sigmoid colon mesentery is approached from the right side, and incised longitudinally. The ureters are identified and protected. Blunt spreading technique is used to expose the aortic bifurcation. The middle sacral artery is mobilized and ligated with hemoclips and divided (Fig. 20.4F). The bifurcation of the inferior vena cava and inferior hypogastric sympathetic plexus must be protected to avoid retrograde ejaculation in males. Monopolar coagulation must be

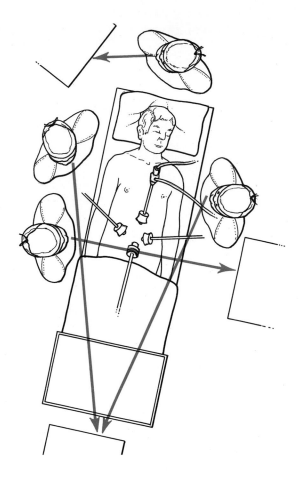

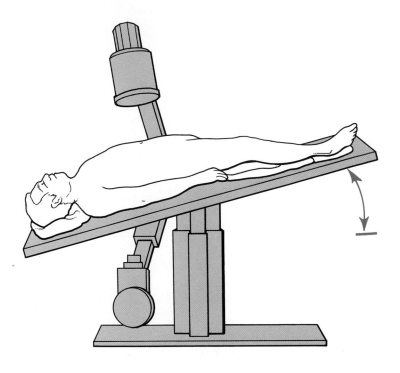

B
The operating room table should be in the Trendelenburg position to mobilize the bowel contents from the lower lumbar region.

Figure 20.4

Laparoscopic procedures of the lumbar spine.

A
Operating room setup for the laparoscopic procedures of the lumbar spine.

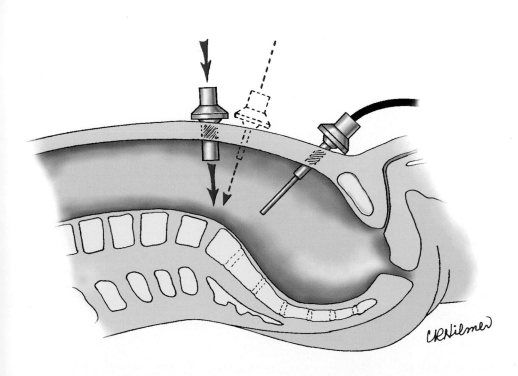

C
The initial portal is placed in the umbilicus. The incision is made with direct visualization, and CO_2 insufflation to 15 mmHg is maintained. The 30° scope is safely entered. The suprapubic portal is over the L5–S1 disc space.

Contd

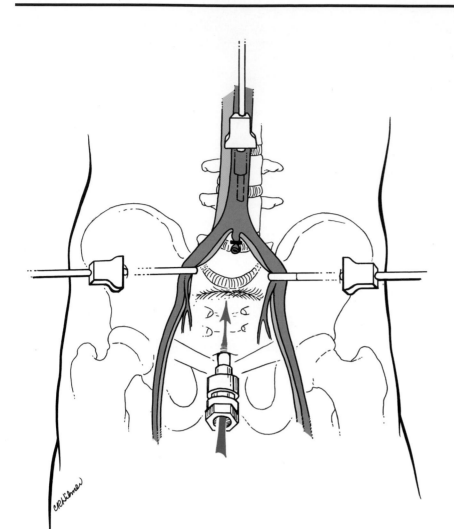

Figure 20.4 *contd*

D

Working portals are lateral to the epigastric vessel. The left trocar is used to mobilize the sigmoid colon from right to left and two right-sided trocars are inserted in such a way as to avoid instrument crowding.

E

The dissection proceeds with monopolar endoshears to incise the peritoneum along reflection. The sigmoid colon mesentery is approached from the right side, and incised longitudinally. The ureters are identified and protected. Blunt spreading technique is used to expose the aortic bifurcation.

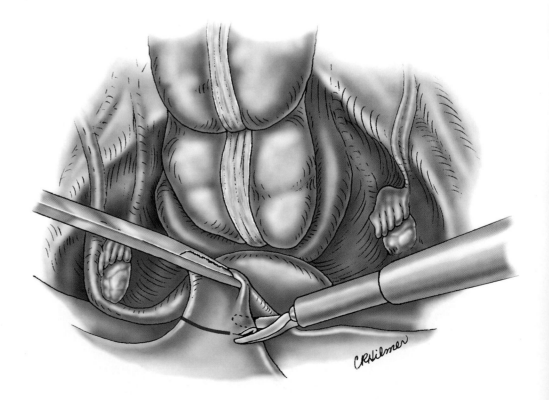

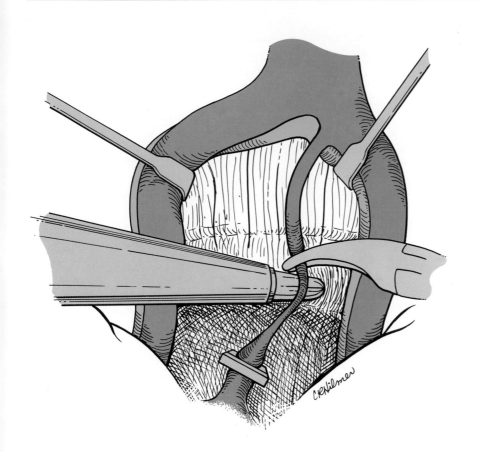

F
The middle sacral artery is mobilized and ligated with hemoclips and divided.

G
Retraction of vessels will expose the L5–S1 disc.

1 Left iliac a. and v.
2 Anterior longitudinal ligament
3 Right iliac a. and v.
4 Middle sacral a.

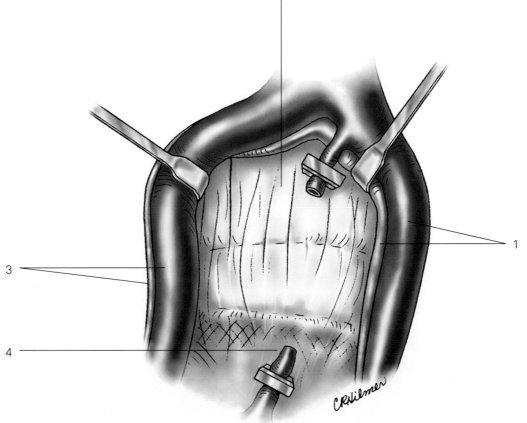

Contd

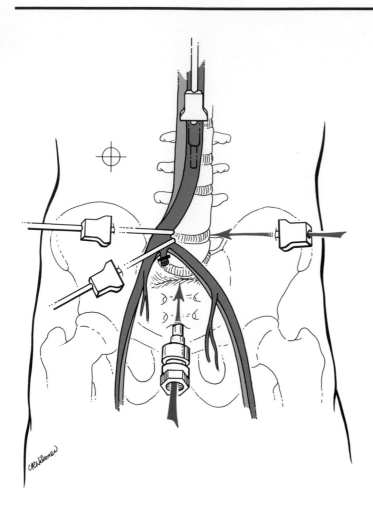

divided for mobilization of the great vessels. Fluoroscopic discectomy and instrumentation can be performed in the disc spaces with the aid of the fluoroscope. At the completion of the procedure, the surgical field should be thoroughly inspected for bleeding as the CO_2 insufflation is reduced to 10 mmHG. The posterior peritoneum is closed with a running laparoscopic suture. The portals are examined for any bleeding, and closed with sutures.

Complications associated with thoracoscopic and laparoscopic procedures include great vessel injuries, trocar site bleeding, injuries to the visceral structures, and spine related problems including epidural bleeding, dural tear, spinal cord injury, inadequate discectomy, and poor fusion constructs. Postoperatively, hypotensive episodes, ileus, hemorrhage, and construct failure may occur.

In summary, the percutaneous and minimally invasive procedures of the spine are significant advances in the field of spine surgery. The morbidity of surgery, the duration of hospitalization, and the outcome may be significantly different in minimally invasive techniques when compared with traditional techniques. However, the most important factors for the successful outcome of surgery are proper patient selection, meticulous techniques, and prevention of complications, whichever procedure is performed.

Figure 20.4 *contd*

H
The access to the L4–5 disc is more difficult, but the left common iliac artery and vein can be mobilized from left to right. The iliolumbar vein on the left must be identified, ligated and divided for mobilization of the great vessels.

avoided in this area. Retraction of the right iliac vein and left iliac artery exposes the L5–S1 disc (Fig. 20.4G). The suprapubic portal is directed to the L5–S1 disc space. The access to the L4–5 disc is more difficult, but the left common iliac artery and vein can be mobilized from left to right (Fig. 20.4H). The iliolumbar vein on the left must be identified, ligated and

Bibiography

Cloward RB (1958) Cervical discography: technique, indications, and use in the diagnosis of ruptured intervertebral discs. *Am J Neurosurg,* **79**:563–74

Craig FS (1956) Vertebral body biopsy. *J Bone Joint Surg,* **38A**:93–102

Mirkovic SR, Schwartz DG (1995) Anatomic consideration in lumbar posterolateral procedures. *Spine,* **20**:1965–71

Ottolenghi CE, Schajowicz F, DeSchant FA (1964) Aspiration biopsy of the cervical spine. *J Bone Joint Surg,* **46A**:715–33

Regan JJ, Mack MJ, Picetti GD (1995) A technical report on video-assisted thoracoscopy in thoracic spinal surgery. *Spine,* **20**:831–7

Schaffer JL, Kambin P (1991) Percutaneous posterolateral lumbar discectomy and decompression with a 6.9 mm cannula: Analysis of operative failures and complications. *J Bone Joint Surg,* **73A**:822–31

Zucherman JF, Zdeblick TA, Bailey SA et al (1995) Instrumented laparascopic spinal fusion: Preliminary results. *Spine,* **20**:2029–35

21

Intradural lesions

Don M Long

Introduction

Intradural techniques focus upon the exposed nervous system. Every spinal surgeon should recognize when such an operation is indicated and understand the general principles applied during the procedure. However, the tissue manipulation required once the dura is exposed is strikingly different from the techniques that are valid for extradural procedures. Neural tissue not protected by cerebrospinal fluid (CSF), and dura is more vulnerable to injury from manipulation and herniation. Therefore, only those trained and experienced in manipulation of nervous tissue should attempt intradural surgery.

Tumor removal constitutes the majority of intradural procedures in the spine. Tumors of the spinal column are traditionally divided into extradural, intradural–extramedullary, and intramedullary categories on the basis of their anatomical location (Brotchi et al 1992; Masaryk 1991; McCormick and Stein 1990). Extradural tumors are virtually always metastatic in origin and become intradural very rarely. Their management was discussed in detail in Chapter 18 and that discussion will not be repeated here. However, the management of intradural tumors will be discussed. Additionally, correction of congenital abnormalities and intradural excision of disc herniations will be reviewed.

Tumors of the spinal cord and spinal nerves

Intradural–extramedullary tumors

Schwannomas, meningiomas, or myxopapillary ependymomas of the filum terminale constitute the majority of the intradural–extramedullary tumors seen. Rarely a dermoid or hemangioblastoma may be encountered, particularly in the region of the cauda equina.

Schwannomas

Schwannomas characteristically occur on the posterior roots and thus are located in the posterolateral quadrant. They are best diagnosed by MRI, and are rarely mistaken for any other tumor. They are most common in the thoracic region, and then occur most often in the cervical area; and the number in the lumbar area are nearly equivalent to those occurring in the cervical segments. They are usually single except in neurofibromatosis. Tumors may grow to very large size before significant symptoms develop.

The operation is carried out under general anesthesia in the prone position. The techniques for cervical and thoracic tumor removal are virtually identical. Some modifications of the technique are required in the lumbar spine. A major extraspinal component may require more lateral exposure.

Localization of the lesion is paramount. In the cervical region this is generally not difficult to do. In the thoracic region radiography may be necessary for accurate localization. A full laminectomy is preferred because it is safer when spinal cord retraction is required. Removal by hemilaminectomy tends to be the exception. Bone should be removed until the upper and lower margins of the tumor are clearly visible. When there is no contraindication, one full level above and below the lesion should be removed. The laminectomy should be wide enough that the lateral margin of the tumor in the spinal canal can be reached. The extraforaminal extent of the tumor must be determined preoperatively and reassessed intraoperatively. It is usually possible to follow the tumor out through the neural foramen and remove the extraforaminal expansion by simply expanding the

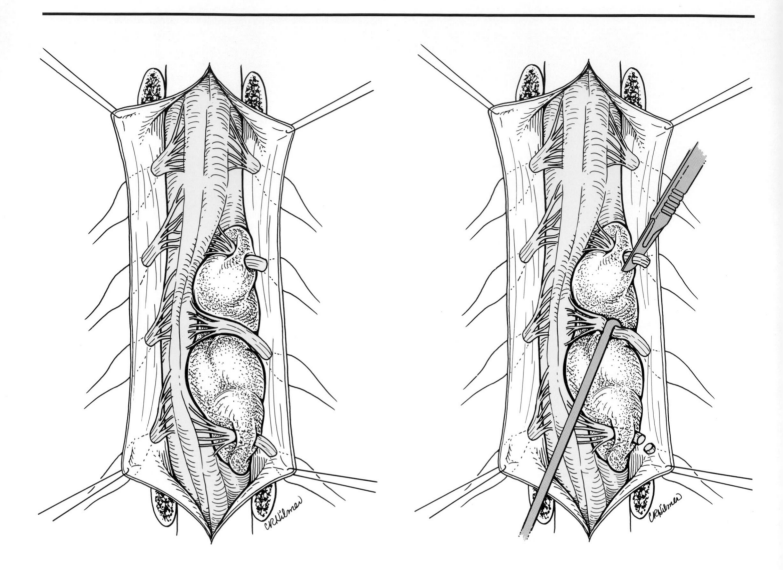

Figure 21.1

A
The tumor is widely exposed so that the margins of the tumor are easily visible.

B
The tumor must be freed from the nerve roots and all nerve roots not entering the tumor mass should be preserved.

muscular retraction laterally. In these cases an ample skin incision facilitates lateral retraction. The intradural removal is performed first so that the cord is no longer compressed during removal of the remainder of the extraspinal tumor. When it is substantial, a second stage operation may be necessary.

Immaculate extradural hemostasis is required. The gutters should be packed with hemostatic agents until there is no blood at all. At this point the operating microscope is brought into the field and the remainder of the operation is carried out under appropriate magnification.

The dura should be opened in the midline from above downward, with due attention to the displacement of the spinal cord. It is extremely important to open the dura leaving the arachnoid intact, so that CSF is not lost and to prevent cord herniation or injury with the knife blade. The dural margins should be tied back to bone or retracted by sutures weighted with clamps. This will provide good hemostasis and expose the tumor widely. Then the arachnoid is opened on the lateral side of the tumor from the top to the bottom of the incision. This will usually allow good visualization of the spinal cord and the superior

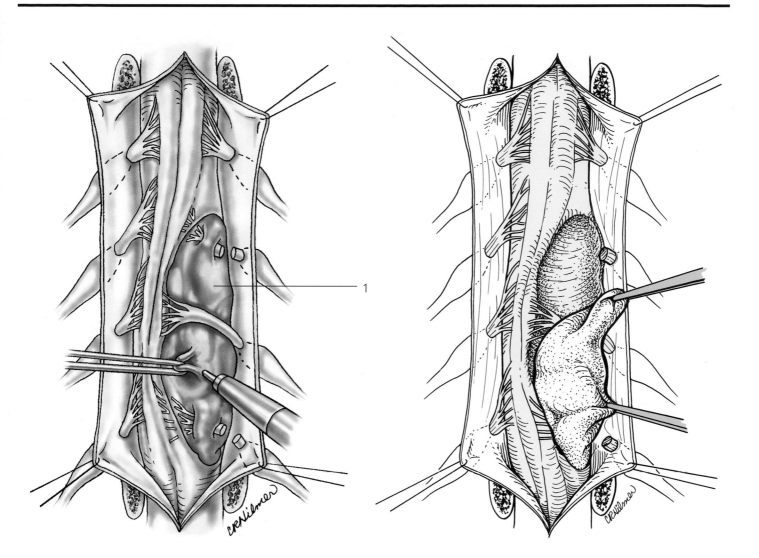

C
Intracapsular removal should be performed before
manipulation of the cord.

1 Tumor

D
Capsular removal is performed with as little manipulation of
the cord as possible. Sharp dissection and coagulation
should be employed.

Contd

and inferior margins of the tumor (Fig. 21.1A). The
adhesions of the lateral margin of the spinal cord to
tumor should be freed by sharp dissection. If coagulation is used, it should always be on the tumor side,
not near the cord. The relationships of nerve roots to
the tumor are then defined. All nerve roots not entering the tumor mass should be dissected free. Those
that obviously enter the tumor may be cut at this
point (Fig. 21.1B). It is easy to be initially misled into
thinking that a dissectable root is entering the tumor,
so time should be taken to identify and separate all
uninvolved nerve roots. In the thoracic region or the

upper cervical region, where loss of a single posterior
root is unimportant, it may be reasonable simply to
cut them all at this point. However, in the brachial
plexus or at the thoracolumbar junction all possible
roots must be preserved.

Intracapsular removal should be performed before
manipulation in order to minimize cord trauma (Fig.
21.1C). The tumor should be entered near its lateral
dural attachment and removed by ultrasonic dissection, suction, laser, or forceps. When the bulk of the
tumor is removed, the capsule can be slowly mobilized
and dissected free from spinal cord (Fig. 21.1D).

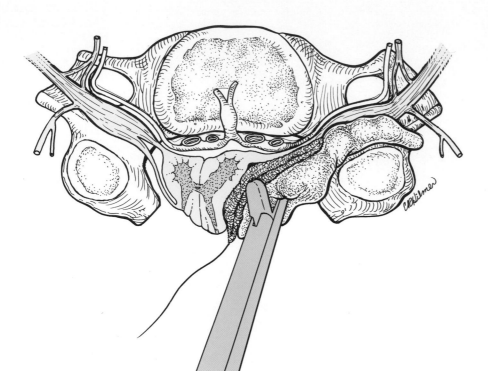

Figure 21.1 *contd*

E
The spinal cord can be protected with cottonoids when removing the extraforaminal component of the tumor.

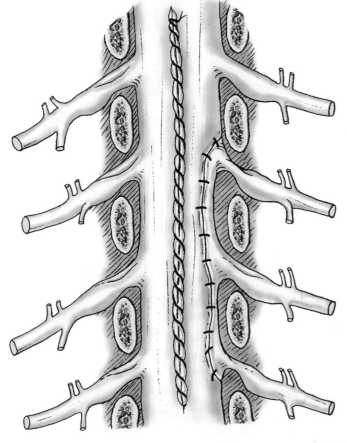

F
Watertight closure employing local fascial graft or allograft needs to be performed so that a pseudomeningocele is avoided.

Crossing blood vessels should be coagulated near the tumor and cut. Coagulation and sharp dissection is preferable to blunt dissection, which may injure the cord. These maneuvers will allow the tumor to be gradually extracted from the spinal cord and mobilized from medial to lateral, leading to spinal cord decompression.

The capsule is then removed. A cuff will remain exiting from the dura. In areas where the anterior roots are important, they should be examined and freed from tumor. The tumor can then be mobilized from the margins of the dura and followed out into the extraforaminal space. Cottonoids can be used to protect the spinal cord so that it is not injured by any movement of the instruments directed to the extraforaminal component of the tumor. The tumor is followed out into the space through the foramen and the capsule gradually mobilized (Fig. 21.1E). It is usually possible to free the capsule completely, coagulate it distally, and cut the residual capsule, with total removal of the tumor. In the cervical spine the vertebral artery is likely to be adherent anteriorly to a sizable tumor mass. The nerve roots should not be injured during the dissection. If the vertebral artery does bleed, it is best controlled by packing. Venous bleeding around the tumor may be substantial as the tumor is debulked, and should be packed off as the dissection continues.

If it is impossible to remove all the extraforaminal tumor distally, the procedure should be terminated at this point and a second stage anterior removal performed. This is rarely necessary.

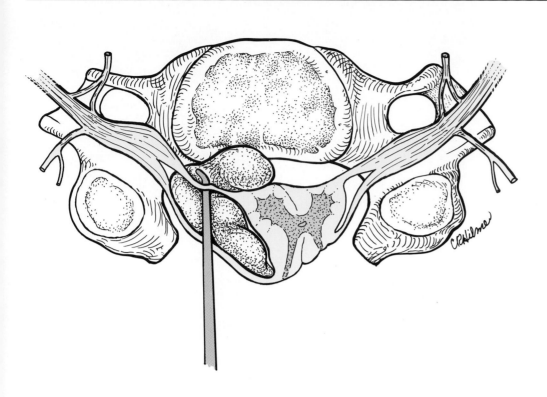

Figure 21.2

A
Great care should be taken to resect nerve roots free of the tumor mass.

1 Tumor

Contd

When tumor removal is complete, it is important to reconstitute the dura. The midline incision is easily closed. It is always the large dural defect left by removal of the tumor that is a problem. A local fascial graft or allograft is sutured circumferentially in a watertight fashion using fine sutures (Fig. 21.1F). Pseudomeningocele is an irritating complication that may prolong hospitalization.

If it was necessary to divide an important motor or sensory root, every effort should be made to reapproximate them. If it is not possible to reapproximate the ends, the greater occipital nerve or, better, the sural nerve previously prepared for this purpose can be used to graft an important anterior cervical root. In the lumbar region there is nearly always enough redundant root to gain first intention approximation. The recovery of function for this rare eventuality has been uniformly good.

The wound is then closed in anatomical layers as after any spinal operation. If a watertight closure has been obtained, there is no reason to restrict postoperative mobility.

Intradural meningiomas

Meningiomas are commonly found in the anterolateral quadrant of the canal. They typically displace the cord posteriorly and laterally. Occasionally one may be found directly in front of the cord. It is important to recognize this situation on the preoperative MRI so that an intramedullary tumor is not mistakenly diagnosed.

The operation for meningioma is identical to that for schwannoma or neurofibroma until the tumor is actually exposed. The meningioma will not have the same smooth capsule and cannot be dissected free as easily from surrounding structures. Once the meningioma is exposed above and below, the spinal cord should be dissected free from the meningioma throughout the length of the tumor. Nerve roots ought to be separated as well. The nerve roots will all be salvageable, so great care should be taken dissecting them free from the tumor mass (Fig. 21.2A). An intracapsular removal allows the tumor to be gradually dissected free and brought from medial to lateral. The ultrasonic dissector is the most effective way to remove the tumor and, if there is adequate exposure, will allow the meningioma to be removed with great precision without risk of injury to the spinal cord (Fig. 21.2B). Occasionally one of these tumors is calcified and virtually rock hard. Such tumors usually have to be cut and removed piecemeal.

After the tumor mass is removed, there will be residual involvement of the dura. There are two ways to manage this problem. One is simply to excise the dura and replace the removed dura with a patch. Total excision has less risk of recurrence, but exposes the spinal cord to increased risk. Alternatively a laser can be used to vaporize all residual tumor back to normal dura (Fig. 21.2C). The laser offers the advantage of allowing

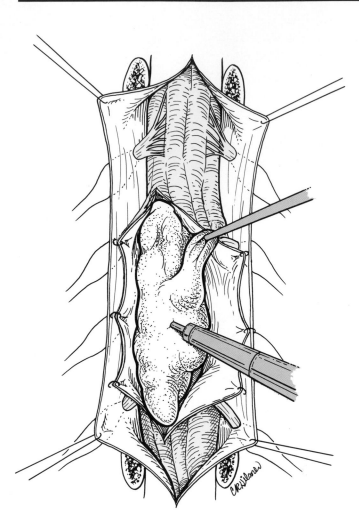 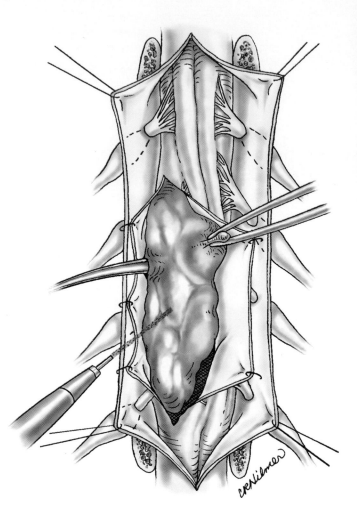

Figure 21.2 *contd*

B
Removal of the meningioma is facilitated by using an ultrasonic dissector.

C
Laser vaporization of residual tumor on the dura offers the advantage of allowing simultaneous vaporization of tumor and coagulation of the extradural veins.

simultaneous vaporization of all involved dura and coagulation of the extradural veins. The laser has an excellent capacity for vaporization of tumor, but there remains an increased risk of recurrence. The author has not had a recurrence with this technique. The closure is identical to that employed for other spinal operations.

Schwannomas of the cauda equina

The procedure for removal of tumors of the cauda equina is somewhat different from that used for tumors at the cord level. The roots of the cauda must be separated from the tumor, to which they are frequently adherent. This should be done without entering the capsule of the tumor (Fig. 21.3A). A small cataract knife can be used, unless the roots come off easily with blunt dissection. When all the uninvolved roots are clearly free from the tumor, it should be possible to identify those roots that actually enter and exit the tumor. Some of these tumors will be true neurofibromas. It is frequently more difficult to isolate the roots that are actually involved in the tumor down to one or a few filaments in neurofibromas as compared with schwannomas.

Following dissection, the distal roots are stimulated to determine what muscles are involved. Important

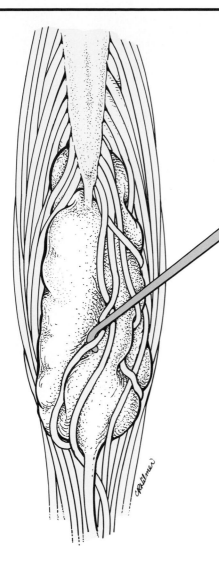

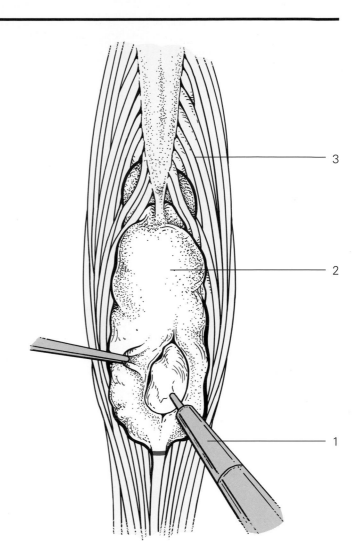

Figure 21.3

A

The cauda equina should be separated from the tumor without entering the capsule.

B

If the tumor is large, intracapsular removal after tumor isolation may be necessary. The tumor and capsule should be entirely removed.

1 Debulking the tumor
2 Tumor
3 Cauda

Contd

motor roots are resutured if their division has been necessary.

When the tumor is large, intracapsular removal may be necessary (Fig. 21.3B). The tumor is debulked with ultrasonic suction or bipolar forceps until the residual tumor capsule can be mobilized out of the field.

If the tumor is relatively small and can be easily brought out of the intraspinal space, it can be removed in its entirety. The root above is cut without coagulation or clamping if it is to be reapproximated. If not, it can be clamped and cut. The same is true distally. Fine suture tags should be placed on both ends of the roots if they will be reapproximated (Fig.

21.3C). Approximation of important root is usually possible with one or two fine sutures. There is frequently enough redundant root to bring the two ends together without difficulty. However, occasionally grafting may be required. The dura should be closed in a watertight fashion and the wound repaired like any other spinal wound.

Myxopapillary ependymoma of the filum terminale

These tumors are exposed in exactly the same way as was described for schwannoma. The dura is opened in the midline and at least one segment above and

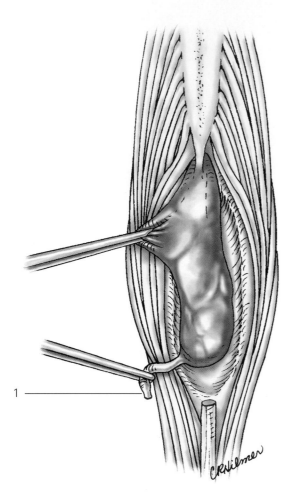

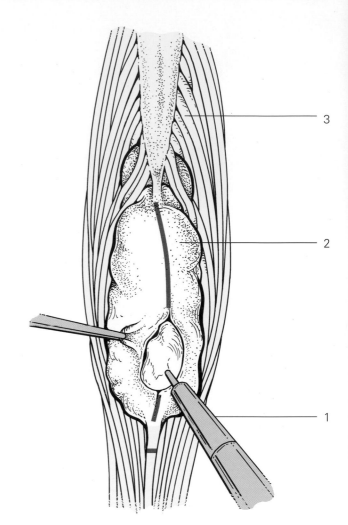

Figure 21.3 *contd*

C
Nerve roots should be repaired with fine suture tags if possible.

1 Cut end of nerve root

Figure 21.4

Dermoid tumors can be removed piecemeal using an ultrasonic dissector after careful dissection of the nerve roots.

1 Debulking the tumor
2 Tumor
3 Cauda roots

below the tumor should be exposed. Then the nerves must be dissected from the tumor. With these tumors it is extremely important not to spill cells into the subarachnoid space, for implantation may occur and multiple intraspinal metastases may result. Therefore the subarachnoid space should be packed with soft cottonoids before beginning tumor removal. Using high magnification all nerve roots and vessels are dissected from the capsule. This will allow identification of the filum, which can be coagulated and cut above and below the tumor. Small tumors are then lifted out of their bed and all nerve roots are dissected

free. Larger tumors may have to be entered and debulked. These tumors are very soft, and the Cavitron will remove them quickly. The capsule should not be entered to avoid injury to the nerve roots.

Once the tumor removal is complete, copious irrigation should be used to make certain that any cells that have seeded the area are washed out. Only then should the cottonoid dams which have protected the rest of the subarachnoid space be removed and the whole field be irrigated again. The dura is then closed in a watertight fashion and the wound closed in the usual fashion in anatomical layers.

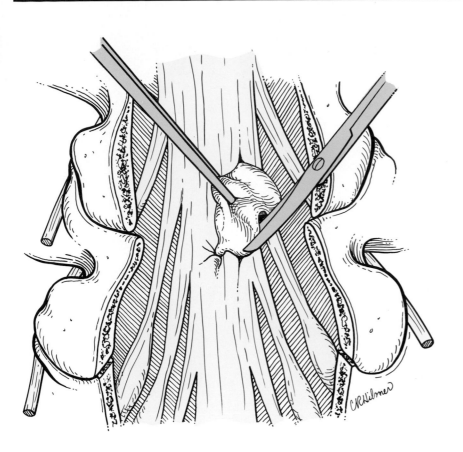

Figure 21.5

It is important to mark the extent the cyst and excise all the cyst wall and associated arachnoid.

Unusual intradural–extramedullary tumors

Occasionally unusual tumors such as dermoids, epidermoids, or lipomas are encountered. Dermoids and epidermoids contain noxious materials which must be kept from the subarachnoid space. Otherwise they require no special techniques. The key is to dissect all nerve roots free. When small, they do not represent a serious problem. Unfortunately, some of them are enormous, and may fill the entire spinal canal from the conus well down into the sacrum. Removal of the cholesterol material that constitutes the bulk of the tumor is not difficult. These tumors should be removed piecemeal after opening the dura to be certain that all the noxious material is out (Fig. 21.4). Copious irrigation is required after they are removed. Adherence of the capsule to dura and the nerves may be undefinable and inextricable. High magnification and a great deal of patience must be used to try carefully to separate the capsular material with adherent arachnoid from nerve roots. This may be an impossible job. It is particularly difficult in patients who have failed previous attempts at surgery. These are unusual tumors, and should not be approached by anyone who is not thoroughly skilled

in their removal and willing to spend the time required in the tedious dissections. Even so, it may not be possible to cure these tumors.

With large epidermoid tumors the dura can be left open so that the tumor can grow into an expanded extradural space without recompressing nerve roots. This technique has resulted in long-term palliation and makes reoperation for evacuation of accumulated cholesterol crystals substantially easier.

Arachnoid cysts

Arachnoid cysts are functionally intradural–extramedullary tumors. The cyst should not be entered while opening the dura, or it may be very difficult to determine its margins and remove it totally. These cysts are usually elliptical masses clearly separable from the remainder of the subarachnoid space. Some can be dissected free in their entirety, virtually like a tumor and removed. Most will be opened before this, and then the cyst disappears. For that reason it is very important to recognize its extent beforehand, mark it above and below, and then excise all the cyst wall and associated arachnoid until the mass is gone (Fig. 21.5). If any part of the cyst is left behind, it increases the

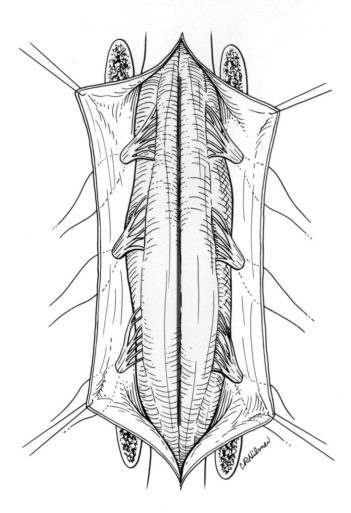

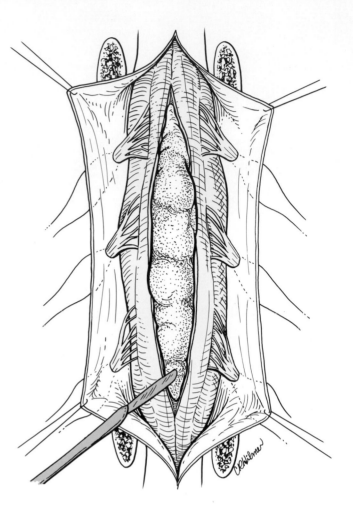

Figure 21.6

A
After ultrasound localization of the tumor, the dura should be opened in the midline well above and below its cranial and caudal extent.

B
The cord should be opened in the midline, beginning in a place where it is most abnormal and the cyst closest to the surface.

risk of recurrent loculation. In spite of extensive removal of abnormal arachnoid, there is a tendency for reloculation of spinal fluid in the area. Therefore, it is important to be certain that spinal fluid flow is reconstituted in an unimpeded fashion above and below, posteriorly and anteriorly around the dentate ligament. Most arachnoid cysts occur in the posterior region, where they are of easy access. Cutting the dentate ligament and opening the arachnoid anteriorly decreases the risk that loculation can recur.

Intramedullary tumors

Astrocytomas and ependymomas each make up nearly 50% of intramedullary neoplasms. These tumors can

be identified with great accuracy now with MRI. Cystic components are seen. The extent and nature of the tumor can usually be determined with great accuracy using MRI.

The surgery should be planned to be two full segments above and two below whenever possible. One segment above and below is a necessity. The operation is carried out under general anesthesia with the patient in the prone position. A midline incision is used and a laminectomy is performed.

Ultrasound may be utilized to locate the tumor with accuracy once the laminectomy is complete. The dura is then opened from above down in the midline. Immaculate hemostasis is required, so that there is no bleeding to distract the surgeon and obscure the field during the operation (Fig. 21.6A).

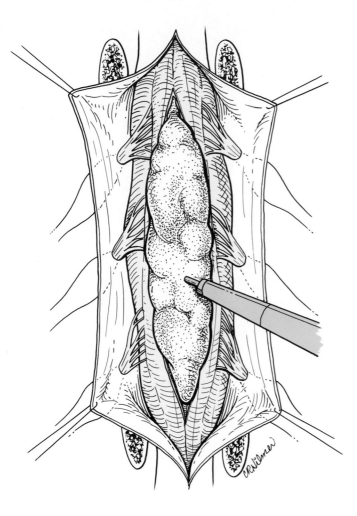

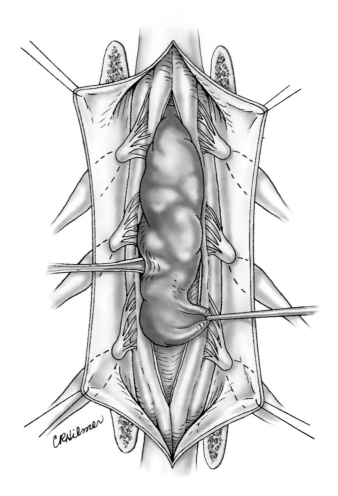

C
High grade astrocytomas can be debulked by using an ultrasonic dissector.

D
Every effort should be made to remove an ependymoma in its entirety, since they can be cured by surgery.

From this point forward the operating microscope is used at high magnification. Ultrasound is useful to verify the area of the cord which is increased in size, particularly if there is an associated cyst.

The cord is then opened in the midline. Fine 6–0, or 7–0 retention pial sutures are used to keep the cord open so that it is not traumatized by retraction. Beginning in a convenient place, where the cord is most abnormal and where it appears the tumor is closest to the surface, a midline myelotomy is performed using a fine arachnoid knife and careful midline dissection (Fig. 21.6B). Micro-dissecting knives (Rosen) are good tools in the avascular plane. The tumor is then biopsied. Astrocytomas are rarely encapsulated, usually infiltrative, and usually difficult to differentiate from spinal cord. They may have a pseudoencapsulated appearance, and can then be removed. Ependymomas, by contrast, are well encapsulated and usually separate relatively easily from the surrounding cord. Since ependymomas can be cured by surgery and astrocytomas probably cannot, it is extremely important to determine which one is present. Other masses such as sarcoid or acute inflammatory processes generally do not need to be removed, but the biopsy will verify their nature. Oddities such as schwannoma can be removed, as can hemangioblastoma.

Laminoplasty is preferable to laminectomy in children. If laminectomy is used, posterior fusion should follow in the cervical region in children. Fusion is not usually required in adults. Remember that both children and adults must be followed postoperatively for the development of a swan neck deformity.

Management of high grade astrocytoma

If the tumor is a high grade astrocytoma, then the prognosis is virtually hopeless since no cure has yet been reported. However, to preserve function as long as possible, it is usually feasible to remove the bulk of the tumor. They tend to be soft, separable from the remainder of the cord, and removed by suction or ultrasonic dissection (Fig. 21.6C).

Another technique used is to carry out this removal in two stages. The first stage is a midline myelotomy to the extremities of the tumor. The wound is then closed, leaving the dura open. The surgeon then returns seven to ten days later and removes the bulk of the tumor, which has become exophytic through the long myelotomy. This will often palliate the neurological deficit. However, these tumors tend to spread rapidly, and death from intracranial extension is the rule. Radiation therapy is employed postoperatively, but is uncertain in its effect.

Radical cordectomy going well above the tumor has been described, but the author's limited experience with this technique in four patients has been disappointing. Three of the four died of intracranial tumor in less than one year.

Management of low grade astrocytoma

Most low grade tumors are not separable from the cord. The myelotomy should be large enough to explore the tumor and determine if it has a pseudo-encapsulated appearance. If it does, it may be possible to separate tumor from cord, using precise microsurgical techniques, and remove a substantial part of the mass. Cure is not probable. However, the patient may be palliated by removal of a portion of a compressive mass. Attempting to remove tumor is terminated when separation from surrounding tissue becomes too difficult.

All of this removal is carried out using spinal evoked sensory potentials and motor stimulation. Substantial degradation of the responses may lead to cessation of the surgery.

If an excellent decompression has been obtained, it may be possible to close the dura primarily. However, it is more likely that a dural patch will be required. Dorsal fascia, fascia lata, or a dural substitute may be employed, and should be circumferentially sutured to the defect precisely. In order to provide maximum decompression the dural retention sutures can be left in place and the patch sutured into the expanded dural pouch. Once this is accomplished, the wound is closed in anatomical layers.

Intramedullary ependymoma

Ependymomas can be cured surgically, and therefore radical surgery is warranted. Once the dura is opened and the nature of the tumor has been identified, its extent should be determined with accuracy using direct observation and ultrasound. The myelotomy should extend from top to bottom and a little beyond obvious tumor, because there tend to be small tails of tumor going up and down the central canal. Again, pial retention sutures are used. The dissection of the overlying cord from capsule can usually be done bluntly or with Micro-knives. Blood vessels are coagulated on the tumor side as they are encountered, and cut. Sharp dissection is generally used to reduce the risk of trauma to the cord. Evoked potential and motor stimulation monitoring are used throughout and the technique is modified if changes in wave forms or responsivity occur. The tumor mass is gradually isolated from top to bottom and then laterally (Fig. 21.6D). It may be necessary to open into the tumor and reduce its bulk if the mass is a particularly large one. The cystic cavities that commonly are associated with these tumors usually occur at the extremities, and we need not be concerned with them during the dissection of the main tumor mass. Remember, these tumors can spread in the subarachnoid space, so, if the capsule is entered, it is important to create dams above and below to prevent tumor spread. The tumors are dissected free circumferentially. Blood vessels typically enter in the midline anteriorly, and should be coagulated as the tumor is removed. The small extensions that go superiorly and interiorly should be followed so that no tumor is left. If there is a substantial syrinx cavity, the wall should be biopsied to be certain that it is not tumor. Usually there is no tumor in the wall of the cavity, but occasionally the cavity will have actually occurred within the capsule of the tumor, and it is important to know this so that no tumor is left behind.

When the tumor is completely removed, hemostasis should be obtained without coagulating in the tumor bed. Do not resuture the cord, because that may lead to postoperative syrinx formation. The dura is reconstituted in the midline, and grafting is virtually never required.

Radiotherapy is commonly used for tumors in which removal is incomplete. The use of radiotherapy probably compounds the issue of bone deformity, because it interferes with appropriate bone growth and maturation. It may also interfere with fusion healing.

Extensive laminectomies in children may lead to a serious postoperative deformity. The surgeon has the option of carrying out the exposure and closure by means of laminoplasty or postoperative fusion using a lateral technique.

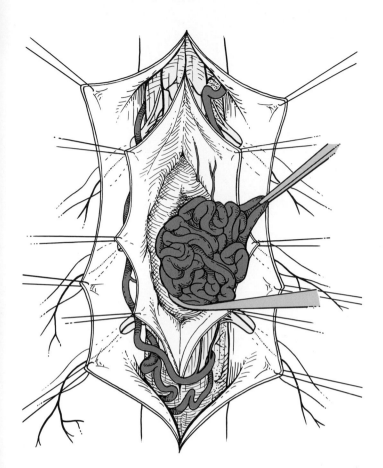

Figure 21.7

A
Hemangiomas should be dissected circumferentially without entering the capsule. The blood vessels should be coagulated as they are encountered.

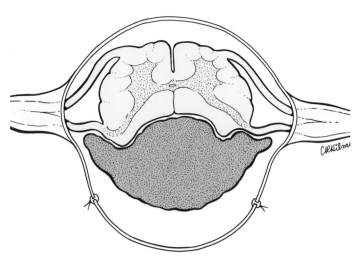

B
Decompression and untethering of the spinal cord exophytic lipomatous mass and dural grafting are all that is required for the treatment of intramedullary lipomas.

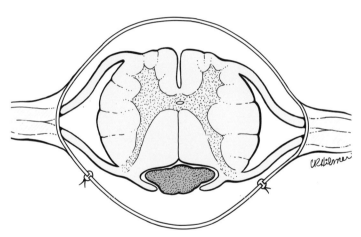

C
Elimination of the compression and tethering of the spinal cord by removal of the exophytic mass and a dural graft.

Hemangioma, lipoma, and other unusual intramedullary tumors

Hemangiomas are handled almost exactly like ependymomas. The tumor should be dissected circumferentially without entering the capsule. Feeding blood vessels should be coagulated and cut as encountered (Fig. 21.7A). Cure is probable. An occasional ependymoma may be so vascular that it appears to be a hemangioblastoma or hemangioma.

Lipomas tend to be intramedullary, with exophytic masses outside the cord (Fig. 21.7B). Once their nature is identified and they are decompressed, they do not need to be removed. Elimination of the compression, tethering of the spinal cord by removal of the exophytic mass, and a dural graft are all that is required (Fig. 21.7C).

Occasionally other rare tumors can be encountered. Intramedullary schwannomas are removed in exactly the same way that an ependymoma is approached. Intramedullary meningioma has now been reported. Because of the rarity of this tumor, no surgical rules have been established; but it is probable that such a tumor would be treated in the way described for ependymoma.

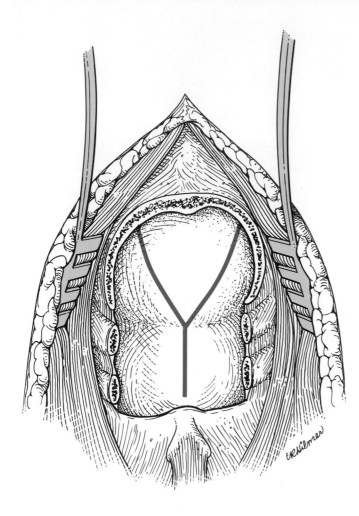

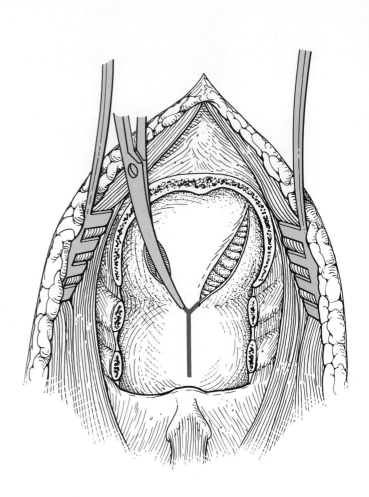

Figure 21.8

A
Laminectomy, removing the base of the occiput followed by C1 and C2.

B
Y-shaped opening of the dura.

Congenital anomalies of the spine

There are four congenital anomalies that routinely require intradural exploration: the Chiari malformation and attendant syringomyelia; diastematomyelia; the various forms of arteriovenous malformations; and the tethered cord syndrome.

Surgery for the Chiari malformation

These operations are carried out under general anesthesia with the patient in the prone position and the head in skeletal fixation. A skin incision is made from the inion to the spine of C3 or C4, depending upon the extent of the tonsillar herniation through the foramen magnum. Bones are exposed by typical subperiosteal dissection until the occipital bones are exposed from mastoid process to mastoid process. The arch of C1 is exposed to just medial to the vertebral arteries, and the spine and laminae of C2 are completely exposed to the zygapophyseal joints. In the rare case in which the tonsils are really herniated far into the cervical cord, exposure to one level below the lowest tonsil will be required.

A laminectomy is then performed, removing the occipital bone first, then C1, and finally C2 (Fig. 21.8A). This sequence is usually required because the

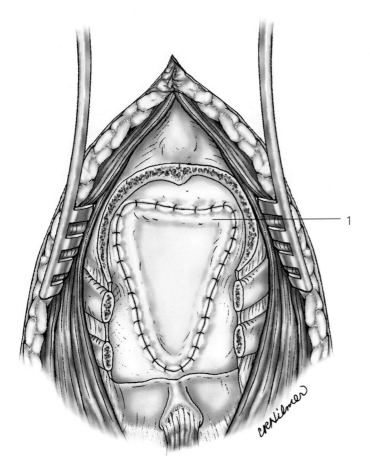

C
Fascial graft occupying the dural opening.

1 Dural patch

There is considerable disagreement among surgeons about the extent of the decompression necessary. Some believe that all the potential dural adhesions in the area should be sectioned surgically, and others do nothing to them. Some advocate exploration of the posterior fossa and even placement of a small pledget of muscle in the obex to try to prevent CSF from entering the central canal. Others omit this step. Some believe that a compressive tonsil should be removed. Others indicate this is never necessary. The only rule to follow is that the cervicomedullary junction must be decompressed, and it is important to do whatever is required for this.

Once this decompression is satisfactory, and it is clear that there is free communication from posterior fossa subarachnoid space into the same space in the cervical spine, closure can follow. A graft of fascia lata, cervical fascia, or dural substitute is formed as a triangle to fit the Y-shaped opening. It is then sutured circumferentially in a watertight fashion (Fig. 21.8C). A pseudomeningocele is very prone to develop if a watertight closure is not obtained. Bony stabilization is usually not necessary, so the remainder of the closure is what would be typical for any cervical spine operation.

Syringomyelia

Management of the syrinx is a matter of considerable debate. The majority opinion seems to be to do nothing directly when an associated symptomatic Chiari malformation has been appropriately decompressed. The supposition is that restoration of normal CSF dynamics around the foramen magnum will cause collapse of the syrinx. The weight of opinion favors this approach now, but definitive data to support this opinion are still lacking.

Other options are to open the syrinx and create a cyst subarachnoid shunt or to open the syrinx and create a shunt into another body cavity, usually the pleura.

Other syringomyelic cysts do not communicate with the fourth ventricle or are not associated with a Chiari malformation, and may require direct treatment. Furthermore, small tumors are sometimes associated with large cysts, and it is very important to be certain of the nature of the cyst before deciding that a shunt alone is adequate.

When opening the cyst and shunting is required, the operation is performed as if for tumor removal, but in a much more limited way. Fortunately, MRI with gadolinium enhancement will now identify most tumors, so extensive decompressive laminectomy for exploration is not required. The author prefers to enter the cyst in the least critical area, where the cyst is easily accessible. A one level laminectomy or even hemilaminectomy is all that is required. The dura is

arch of C1 may be under the rim of the foramen magnum and very difficult to reach. The author prefers to remove the foramen magnum with high speed drills and rongeurs. The arch of C1 and C2 can usually be removed by rongeurs alone.

Once hemostasis is adequate, the dura is opened in a Y-shaped fashion, beginning in the midline just above C3, with the arms of the Y emanating from the foramen magnum upwards (Fig. 21.8B). Dural venous anomalies are extremely common, and venous bleeding may be brisk here. It may be necessary to coagulate the edges thoroughly, or even to apply clips, to obtain adequate hemostasis. This will usually give adequate decompression.

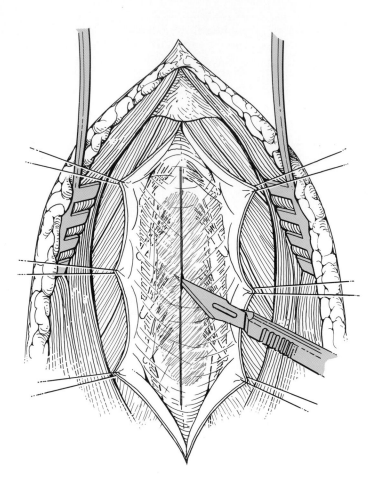 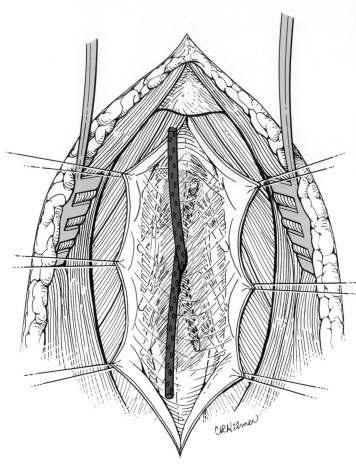

Figure 21.9

A

Once the cyst is identified, a small incision through the midline raphe is made into it.

B

Shunts are placed inside the cyst inferiorly and superiorly and brought out through the same midline incision.

then opened in the midline, and the presence of the cyst is verified. A small incision into the cord through the midline raphe is made and the cyst is entered (Fig. 21.9A). The cyst should not be allowed to empty, or it may be hard to get the shunts in place. Myelotomy can be above the dentate ligament, through the thinning which routinely occurs there.

A variety of shunts are possible. Commercially available lumbar shunt or T-tubes cut to size without a valve and with multiple holes both inside the cyst and in the subarachnoid space are commonly used. One is placed inferiorly in the cyst and one superiorly, bringing them out through the same midline incision (Fig. 21.9B). They should be sutured in position with a fine

suture attached to the pia or the arachnoid. The ends must be well into the subarachnoid space if they are to function. It does no good to place them in the extra-arachnoid subdural space, where they will not flow for long. The dura is then closed in the midline and the wound closed in the usual fashion. If shunting to the pleura or the peritoneum is required, the technique has only to be slightly modified. The same cystostomy is done, but a single shunt tube is used, and it is placed so that the greater part of it is in the dependent portion of the cyst. The catheter is then brought out and tunneled to the appropriate pleural or peritoneal space, and the remainder of the shunt is completed.

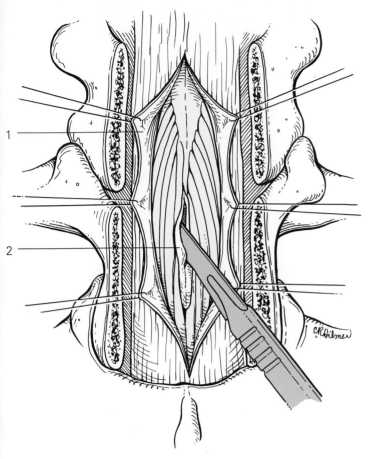

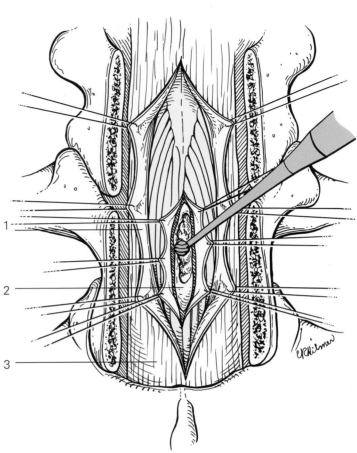

Figure 21.10

A
Bony spicule is exposed.

1 Posterior dura
2 Anterior dura over spicule

B
Bony spicule removed.

1 Anterior dura
2 Spicule
3 Posterior dura

Contd

Diastematomyelia

This unusual anomaly consists of a spike of bone or band of heavy fibrous tissue which divides the dura, usually connecting vertebral body with laminae in the midline. The anomalies that can occur with it are many. There may be a temporary split in an otherwise normal cord, or there may be true diplomyelia, with separate divided cords and dural tubes below. MRI and CT now identify the nature of the anomaly with great accuracy.

The operation is carried out under general anesthesia, with the patient in the prone position. These anomalies occur almost exclusively in the thoracic region. A subperiosteal dissection of muscles from spine and laminae is carried out and the location of the anomaly is identified by radiography. A laminectomy to expose the dural tube one segment above and below the anomaly is required. The procedure is then tailored to the specific anomaly present. The typical abnormality is completely extradural, with an intact dural tube surrounding it on both sides. In this case the operating microscope is used for the remainder of the operation. A high speed drill is used to remove the bony spicule by drilling it right down to the base. Once it is gone nothing further is required if that is the only abnormality. Occasionally, the abnormality is truly intradural, and then the dura must be opened

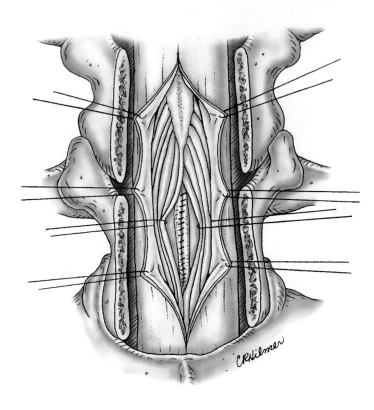

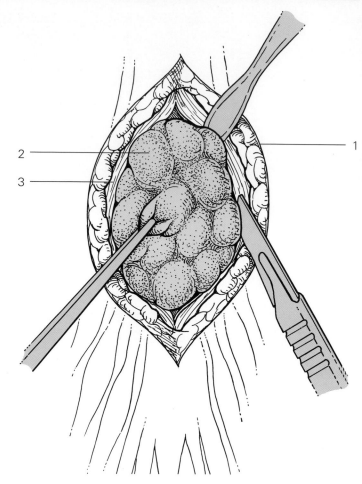

Figure 21.10 *contd*

C

Anterior dura as well as posterior dura is closed in a watertight fashion.

Figure 21.11

A

Extradural lipoma being removed.

1 Midline incision
2 Lipoma
3 Dura

above, on both sides of, and below the anomaly, so that it is completely exposed (Fig. 21.10A). It is then removed with high speed drill, laser, or fine rongeurs, depending upon its nature (Fig. 21.10B). Occasionally a fibrous band can just be cut anteriorly and posteriorly and removed.

Once the offending mass is removed, the dura should be reconstituted in a watertight fashion (Fig. 21.10C). When the mass has been purely extradural, nothing is required except anatomical closure of the wound.

Tethered cord syndrome

These operations are carried out under general anesthesia with the patient in prone position on an appropriate spinal frame or support. A midline

incision is made which will expose the area to be repaired. A subperiosteal dissection of muscles from spines and laminae is then carried out; care must be taken not to enter the dura or injure nerve root through a bony anomaly. Posterior decompression is required. Occasionally one of these patients will be unstable enough to require fusion, but this is usually determined from the analysis of the bony anomaly prior to surgery.

If there is a subcutaneous lipoma, it should be removed. These anomalies often have tracks that go down to the dura. These should be followed and all extradural abnormal tissue removed (Fig. 21.11A). Do not compromise later skin closure by excessive tissue removal.

Then the dura is opened above the area of abnormality and followed down until the tract can be circumscribed. Sometimes the roots are quite adherent posteriorly, and this must be taken into consideration in opening the dura (Fig. 21.11B).

Once the dura is opened a number of associated anomalies can be found. When the abnormality is a thickened, shortened filum terminale, the filum should be stimulated to be sure it is not a nerve root, and then divided. The filum is then coagulated and a centimeter or so is removed to prevent any possibility of readherence. When there is an associated intradural lipoma, the mass must be removed if it is compressive or tethering (Fig. 21.11C). Then the nerve roots have to be dissected, at least partially, using exact microtechniques until the mass of tissue is adequately removed to untether the cord. The mass has to be detached circumferentially so that no further tethering can occur. The filum is then identified and cut. Sometimes the lipoma and the filum are all the same mass, and then cutting the filum above and removing all possible lipoma is all that is required. There is no reason to try to remove the lipoma totally, because it will not grow, and the goal of the operation is untethering. Sometimes the lipoma and cord are fused; radical removal is not necessary, since untethering is accomplished.

Then the dura needs to be closed in a watertight fashion and, if a patch is required, this should be harvested or a dural substitute should be used. A generous patch reduces the risk of scar retethering the cord. Watertight closure is important. Then the wound is reconstituted in anatomical layers.

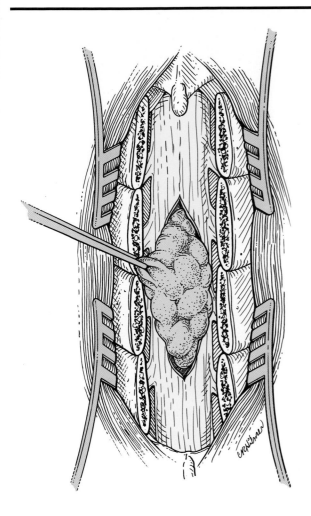

B
Opening of the dura.

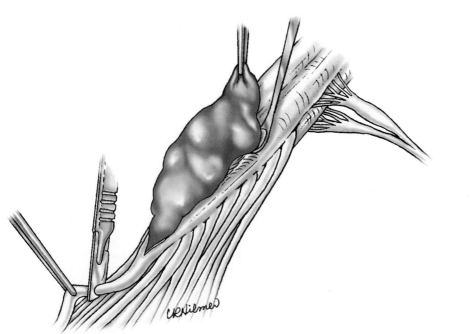

C
Removal of intradural lipoma.

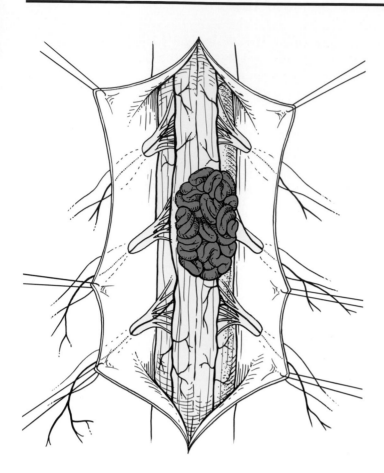

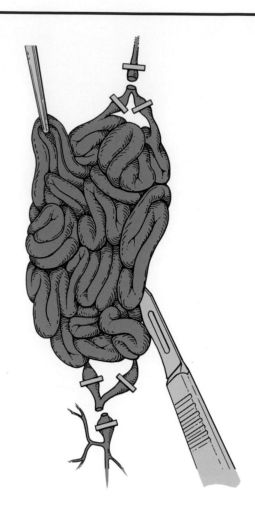

Figure 21.12

A
Isolation and ligation of feeding vessels and fistula.

B
Removal of AVM connection.

Dural arteriovenous fistulae and true arteriovenous malformations

The arteriovenous malformations (AVMs) involving the spinal cord are of three basic kinds. There is an intramedullary type with multiple feeding arteries and veins which is generally inextricable from the spinal cord and can only rarely be treated successfully. There is another related form of arteriovenous malformation which is largely extramedullary, though often compressing and invading the spinal cord, in which total removal is possible. There is the dural fistula, which occurs at the root entry zone and is associated with symptoms secondary to increased venous pressure in the spinal cord. These can virtually always be obliterated by simple blockade of the fistula.

Dural arteriovenous fistula

The abnormalities usually occur at a single level identified by myelography. Most commonly these are treated by a curative endovascular technique.

When embolization is not curative, it is possible to obliterate them directly. Careful localization is required to be certain that the exposure is at the proper level. Usually exposing only the segment to be removed is all that is required. A laminectomy is done at the level to be exposed with enough bony removal above and below to be certain that the whole fistula is reached. It is usually possible to find the feeding vessels intradurally and ligate them, thus eliminating the increased venous pressure in the cord. The fistula itself should be coagulated (Fig. 21.12A). If there is any

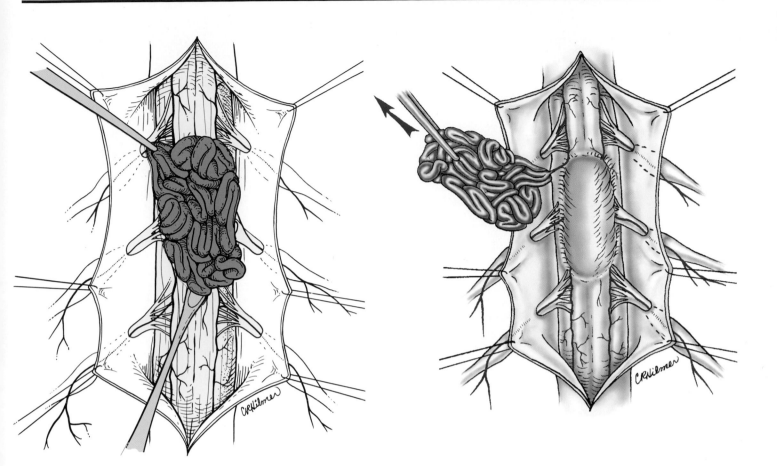

C
Extramedullary AVM with ligation of residual feeder vessels.

D
Removal of mass.

question, the whole dura of the root exit area can be excised, and then it is certain that the fistula is gone (Fig. 21.12B). Thoracic roots can be sacrificed with impunity when the vascular anatomy is known and it is certain that in so doing the cord is not devascularized. Such radical removal is not possible in lumbar or cervical areas. The wound is then closed in anatomical layers after posterior dural closure.

The extramedullary arteriovenous malformation

Occasionally one of these large arteriovenous malformations is virtually outside the cord and markedly compressing it. These are treated like any extramedullary intradural tumor, except that their extreme vascularity and high flow mandate control of the feeding vessels. Usually some or all of these feeders will have been embolized preoperatively. Then its dissection from the cord becomes straightforward. A laminectomy exposure of at least one segment above and below the mass is performed. The dura is opened in the midline and the mass exposed. Using high magnification and careful microdissection, all residual feeding vessels are identified, ligated, and cut (Fig. 21.12C). Then the mass is dissected free from underlying cord using fine micro bipolar coagulation and sharp dissection. The separation must be precise, but is usually not difficult, and the mass can be removed in its entirety (Fig. 21.12D). This is curative. The dura is then closed and anatomical reconstruction of the wound is required.

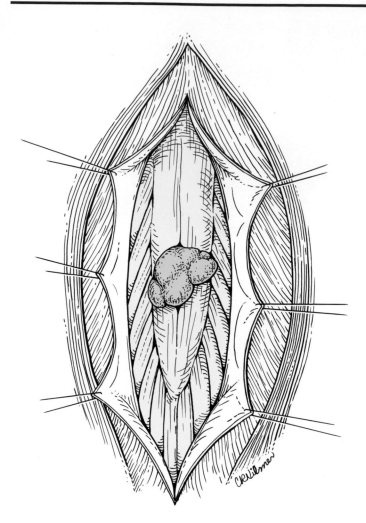

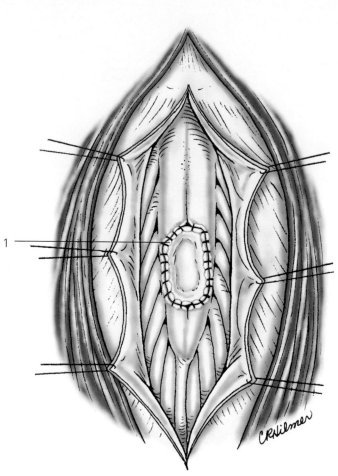

Figure 21.13

A
Intradural lumbar disc being freed from surrounding nerve roots.

B
Dural closure with anterior patch for anterior dural defect.

1 Disk fragment

The intramedullary arteriovenous malformation

Operations on intramedullary malformations are rarely performed. They frequently can be at least partially devascularized by embolization of feeding vessels. In an occasional patient with progressive neurological deficit they cannot be treated in any way other than excision, and then a rare favorable mass may be excised directly. However, for the most part it is not possible to cure these lesions surgically, except at great risk. Occasionally it may be required to expose one and actually ligate feeding vessels that cannot be embolized appropriately. The operation is no different from that described for the dural fistula.

Intradural lumbar disc herniation

A rare lumbar disc herniates intradurally. This is most common in patients who have undergone one previous operation. The traditional discectomy approach must be modified to allow transdural removal.

A complete laminectomy is performed to allow exposure of the mass. The dura is opened either in the midline or to either side, depending on the location of the mass. It is well not to try to do this operation through a small incision. The roots are intimately adherent to the disc mass, and room to manipulate the nerve roots and free them using microtechniques is often necessary.

Once the dura is opened, the disc is usually immediately seen. Using a microscope each individual nerve root is freed from the disc, which is gradually teased out of the subarachnoid space (Fig. 21.13A). If it has been within the dura for a while, the adherence of the mass is likely to be substantial.

Once the disc fragment is out the hole in the ligament in the adherent dura is usually easily seen. An experienced intradural surgeon can remove the remainder of the degenerated disc through this approach. However, for most others it is better to go back to the extradural space and remove any residual degenerated disc in the usual way. There is a great propensity for more disc herniation to occur through this hole, so it is important to remove as much degenerated disc material as possible, even if it requires a bilateral incision of the ligament.

If the anterior defect in the dura is substantial, a small piece of fat can be harvested and slid into the interspace to occlude the hole (Fig. 21.13B). Then the dura is closed posteriorly and the wound reconstituted in anatomical layers.

Unusual approaches to intradural tumors

Most intradural tumors are approached by the direct posterior route. Occasionally an unusual approach is required. These are most commonly necessary at the cervicomedullary junction. Intramedullary meningiomas and schwannomas located directly in front of the cervicomedullary junction may be difficult to expose by a direct posterior approach. In this case a far lateral approach with unilateral removal of the C1–2 and C1–occipital articulations may be required.

Even more unusual is the direct anterior transoral approach to such a lesion. The descriptions of these unusual operations are included elsewhere.

The transoral operation provides excellent access to the cervicomedullary junction, and only requires removal of the arch of C1, the odontoid and occasionally the lower third of the clivus. The issue is obtaining a watertight closure. It may be very difficult or impossible to close the dura. Packing with fat and meticulous closure of the oropharynx coupled with spinal drainage will usually prevent CSF leak, but infection remains a serious issue.

What to do when the dura is inadvertently opened

An unexpected laceration of the dura during extradural surgery is not uncommon. The loss of spinal fluid may reduce tamponade and lead to excessive extradural bleeding, but usually the dural tear does not reduce the quality of the outcome of surgery. To be certain this is the case, it is necessary to understand how such tears can be treated. The typical abnormality is just a small pinhole with a patch of arachnoid through it. A single fine suture (4-0 or smaller) suffices to close the defect. If the laceration is larger, it may require several stitches to close. The important thing is to remove bone until the entire laceration can be visualized and then close the margins of the dural tear carefully with fine sutures. Be certain no nerve roots are adherent around the laceration, so that the nerve roots are not incorporated into the closure. Nerve roots tend to pouch through the defect, and may have to be held in place with small cottonoid pledgets. A watertight closure should be obtained. Sometimes the laceration is in a place that simply cannot be sutured well. This is particularly true with reoperations or when the laceration is around the nerve root. Posteriorly placed lacerations or defects can be closed by sewing a small graft of fascia or a small pledget of muscle or fat over the hole. Sometimes, when the laceration is on the root sheath, it might really compromise the root to try to close the dural defect. Then packing with fat or muscle is an acceptable alternative. Closing or packing should be adequate to allow the anesthesiologist to increase intrathoracic pressure dramatically without evidence of CSF leak.

When the CSF space has been entered, it is important to reconstitute CSF volume by the injection of saline to recreate the tamponade in the epidural space. Special care must be taken to close the wound solidly, so that a pseudomeningocele or cutaneous leak cannot occur.

Conclusions

Most spinal surgery is extradural only. The procedures that require intradural exploration are fewer in number. It is important to understand that the techniques utilized for intradural surgery are very different from those required when the operation is extradural only. Intradural procedures should be carried out by those who have been trained to handle nervous tissue and are familiar with both the anatomy and the function of intradural surgery. Therefore the spine surgery team needs a member skilled in intradural surgery as an integral part of its function.

Bibliography

Anson JA, Spetzler RF (1992) Interventional neuroradiology for spinal pathology [Review]. *Clin Neurosurg*, **39**:388–417

Brotchi J, Noterman J, Baleriaux D (1992) Surgery of intramedullary spinal cord tumours. *Acta Neurochir (Wien)*, **116**(2–4):176–8

Chapman PH, Davis KR (1993) Surgical treatment of spinal lipomas in childhood. *Pediatr Neurosurg*, **19**(5):267–75

Crockard HA, Sen CN (1991) The transoral approach for the management of intradural lesions at the craniovertebral junction: review of 7 cases. *Neurosurgery*, **28**(1):88–97, discussion 97–8

Dernevik L, Larsson S (1990) Management of dumbbell tumours. Reports of seven cases. *Scand J Thorac Cardiovasc Surg*, **24**(1):47–51

Dorizzi A, Crivelli G, Marra et al (1992) Associated cervical schwannoma and dorsal meningioma. Case report and review of the literature [Review]. *J Neurosurg Sci*, **36**(3):173–6

Epstein FJ, Farmer JP (1990) Pediatric spinal cord tumor surgery [Review]. *Neurosurg Clin N Am*, **1**(3):569–90

Friedman DP, Tartaglino LM, Flanders AE (1992) Intradural schwannomas of the spine: MR findings with emphasis on contrast-enhancement characteristics. *Am J Roentgenol*, **158**(6):1347–50

Gundry CR, Heithoff KB (1994) Imaging evaluation of patients with spinal deformity [Review]. *Orthop Clin North Am*, **25**(2):247–64

Isu T, Chono Y, Iwasaki Y et al (1992) Scoliosis associated with syringomyelia presenting in children. *Child's Nerv Syst*, **8**(2):97–100

Kanzer MD, Parisi JE (1990) Case for diagnosis. Myxopapillary ependymoma. *Military Medicine*, **155**(2):87, 90

Li MH, Holtas S (1991) MR imaging of spinal intramedullary tumors. *Acta Radiol*, **32**(6):505–13

Linn RM, Ford LT (1994) Adult diastematomyelia. *Spine*, **19**(7):852–4

Lunardi P, Licastro G, Missori P et al (1993) Management of intramedullary tumours in children. *Acta Neurochir (Wien)*, **120**(1–2):59–65

McCormick PC, Post KD, Stein BM (1990) Intradural extramedullary tumors in adults [Review]. *Neurosurg Clin N Am*, **1**(3):591–608

McCormick PC, Stein BM (1990) Miscellaneous intradural pathology [Review]. *Neurosurg Clin N Am*, **1**(3):687–99

Masaryk TJ (1991) Neoplastic disease of the spine [Review]. *Radiol Clin North Am*, **29**(4):829–45

Milhorat TH, Johnson WD, Miller JI et al (1992) Surgical treatment of syringomyelia based on magnetic resonance imaging criteria. *Neurosurgery*, **31**(2):231–44, discussion 244–5

Ozer AF, Ozek MM, Pamir MN et al (1994) Intradural rupture of cervical vertebral disc [Review]. *Spine*, **19**(7):843–5

Pagni CA, Canavero S, Giordana MT et al (1992) Spinal intramedullary subependymomas: case report and review of the literature [Review]. *Neurosurgery*, **30**(1):115–17

Pulst SM, Riccardi VM, Fain P et al (1991) Familial spinal neurofibromatosis: clinical and DNA linkage analysis. *Neurology*, **41**(12):1923–7

Rabb CH, McComb JG, Raffel C et al (1992) Spinal arachnoid cysts in the pediatric age group: an association with neural tube defects. *J Neurosurg*, **77**(3):369–72

Sanguinetti C, Specchia N, Gigante A et al (1993) Clinical and pathological aspects of solitary spinal neurofibroma. *J Bone Joint Surg* (Br), **75**(1):141–7

Sen CN, Sekhar LN (1990) An extreme lateral approach to intradural lesions of the cervical spine and foramen magnum. *Neurosurgery*, **27**(2):197–204

Seppala MT, Haltia MJ (1993) Spinal malignant nerve-sheath tumor or cellular schwannoma? A striking difference in prognosis. *J Neurosurg*, **79**(4):528–32

Steck JC, Dietze DD, Fessler RG (1994) Posterolateral approach to intradural extramedullary thoracic tumors. *J Neurosurg*, **81**(2):202–5

Stiller CA, Bunch KJ (1992) Brain and spinal tumours in children aged under two years: incidence and survival in Britain, 1971–85. *Br J Cancer Suppl*, **18**:S50–3

Tatter SB, Borges LF, Louis DN (1994) Central neurocytomas of the cervical spinal cord. Report of two cases. *J Neurosurg*, **81**(2):288–93

Ulmer JL, Elster AD, Ginsberg LE et al (1993) Klippel–Feil syndrome: CT and MR of acquired and congenital abnormalities of cervical spine and cord. *J Comput Assist Tomogr*, **17**(2):215–24

van Velthoven V, Jost M, Siekmann R et al (1993) Surgical strategies and results in syringomyelia. *Acta Neurochir (Wien)*, **123**(3–4):199–201

Venkataramana NK, Kolluri VR, Narayana Swamy KS et al (1990) Exophytic gliomas of the spinal cord. *Acta Neurochir (Wien)*, **107**(1–2):44–6

Index